Hypopigmentation

Hypopigmentation

Edited by

Electra Nicolaidou, MD, PhD
Associate Professor of Dermatology and Venereology
1st Department of Dermatology and Venereology
National and Kapodistrian University of Athens

"Andreas Sygros" Hospital for Skin and Venereal Diseases
Athens, Greece

Clio Dessinioti, MD, MSc, PhD
Clinical Fellow
1st Department of Dermatology and Venereology
National and Kapodistrian University of Athens

"Andreas Sygros" Hospital for Skin and Venereal Diseases
Athens, Greece

Andreas D. Katsambas, MD, PhD
Emeritus Professor of Dermatology and Venereology
National and Kapodistrian University of Athens

Head
Dermatology Clinic
Hygeia Hospital
Athens, Greece

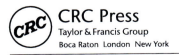

CRC Press is an imprint of the
Taylor & Francis Group, an **informa** business

CRC Press
Taylor & Francis Group
6000 Broken Sound Parkway NW, Suite 300
Boca Raton, FL 33487-2742

© 2020 by Taylor & Francis Group, LLC
CRC Press is an imprint of Taylor & Francis Group, an Informa business

No claim to original U.S. Government works

Printed on acid-free paper

International Standard Book Number-13: 978-1-138-50523-0 (Hardback)

This book contains information obtained from authentic and highly regarded sources. While all reasonable efforts have been made to publish reliable data and information, neither the author[s] nor the publisher can accept any legal responsibility or liability for any errors or omissions that may be made. The publishers wish to make clear that any views or opinions expressed in this book by individual editors, authors or contributors are personal to them and do not necessarily reflect the views/opinions of the publishers. The information or guidance contained in this book is intended for use by medical, scientific or health-care professionals and is provided strictly as a supplement to the medical or other professional's own judgement, their knowledge of the patient's medical history, relevant manufacturer's instructions and the appropriate best practice guidelines. Because of the rapid advances in medical science, any information or advice on dosages, procedures or diagnoses should be independently verified. The reader is strongly urged to consult the relevant national drug formulary and the drug companies' and device or material manufacturers' printed instructions, and their websites, before administering or utilizing any of the drugs, devices or materials mentioned in this book. This book does not indicate whether a particular treatment is appropriate or suitable for a particular individual. Ultimately it is the sole responsibility of the medical professional to make his or her own professional judgements, so as to advise and treat patients appropriately. The authors and publishers have also attempted to trace the copyright holders of all material reproduced in this publication and apologize to copyright holders if permission to publish in this form has not been obtained. If any copyright material has not been acknowledged please write and let us know so we may rectify in any future reprint.

Except as permitted under U.S. Copyright Law, no part of this book may be reprinted, reproduced, transmitted, or utilized in any form by any electronic, mechanical, or other means, now known or hereafter invented, including photocopying, microfilming, and recording, or in any information storage or retrieval system, without written permission from the publishers.

For permission to photocopy or use material electronically from this work, please access www.copyright.com (http://www.copyright.com/) or contact the Copyright Clearance Center, Inc. (CCC), 222 Rosewood Drive, Danvers, MA 01923, 978-750-8400. CCC is a not-for-profit organization that provides licenses and registration for a variety of users. For organizations that have been granted a photocopy license by the CCC, a separate system of payment has been arranged.

Trademark Notice: Product or corporate names may be trademarks or registered trademarks, and are used only for identification and explanation without intent to infringe.

Library of Congress Cataloging-in-Publication Data

Names: Nicolaidou, Electra, editor. | Dessinioti, Clio, editor. | Katsambas, A. D. (Andreas D.), 1944- editor.
Title: Hypopigmentation / [edited by] Electra Nicolaidou, Clio Dessinioti, Andreas Katsambas.
Description: New York, NY : CRC Press/Taylor & Francis Group, [2020] |
Includes bibliographical references and index.
Identifiers: LCCN 2019015583| ISBN 9781138505230 (hardback : alk. paper) | ISBN 9781315146454 (ebook)
Subjects: | MESH: Hypopigmentation | Vitiligo | Skin Diseases
Classification: LCC RL790 | NLM WR 265 | DDC 616.5/5--dc23
LC record available at https://lccn.loc.gov/2019015583

Visit the Taylor & Francis Web site at
http://www.taylorandfrancis.com

and the CRC Press Web site at
http://www.crcpress.com

Contents

Preface		vii
Contributors		ix
1	Basic concepts on melanocyte biology	1
	Mauro Picardo and Daniela Kovacs	
2	Approach to hypopigmentation	13
	Clio Dessinioti and Andreas D. Katsambas	
3	Historical review of vitiligo	21
	Maja Kovacevic, Nika Franceschi, Mirna Situm, Andy Goren, Andrija Stanimirovic, Yan Valle, and Torello Lotti	
4	Epidemiology and classification of vitiligo	27
	Serena Gianfaldoni and Torello Lotti	
5	Pathophysiology of vitiligo	35
	Alexandra Miniati	
6	Segmental vitiligo	39
	Christina Bergqvist and Khaled Ezzedine	
7	Childhood versus post-childhood vitiligo	43
	Electra Nicolaidou and Styliani Mastraftsi	
8	Pharmacological therapy of vitiligo	49
	Ivana Binić and Andrija Stanimirović	
9	Surgical treatment of vitiligo	69
	Muhammed Razmi T., T. P. Afra, and Davinder Parsad	
10	Phototherapy and lasers in the treatment of vitiligo	79
	Viktoria Eleftheriadou	
11	Emerging treatments for vitiligo	85
	Angelo Massimiliano D'Erme and Giovanni Bagnoni	
12	Tuberous sclerosis complex	89
	Vesna Pljakoska, Katerina Damevska, and Natasa Teovska Mitrevska	
13	Oculocutaneous albinism	93
	Mira Kadurina, Anastasiya A. Chokoeva, and Torello Lotti	
14	Hermansky-Pudlak syndrome, Chediak-Chigasi syndrome, and Griscelli syndrome	97
	Vesna Pljakoska, Silvija Duma, and Andrej Petrov	
15	Piebaldism	101
	Jovan Lalošević and Miloš Nikolić	
16	Waardenburg syndrome	107
	Carmen Maria Salavastru, Stefana Cretu, and George Sorin Tiplica	
17	Alezzandrini syndrome, Margolis syndrome, Cross syndrome, and other rare genetic disorders	113
	Athanasios I. Pavlidis and Andreas D. Katsambas	
18	Mosaic hypopigmentation	117
	Irene Latour-Álvarez and Antonio Torrelo	
19	Skin disorders causing post-inflammatory hypopigmentation	127
	Polytimi Sidiropoulou, Dimitrios Sgouros, and Dimitris Rigopoulos	
20	Infectious and parasitic causes of hypopigmentation	133
	Serena Gianfaldoni, Aleksandra Vojvodic, Nooshin Bagherani, Bruce R. Smoller, Balachandra Ankad, Leon Gilad, Arieh Ingber, Fabrizio Guarneri, Uwe Wollina, and Torello Lotti	
21	Melanoma leukoderma	145
	Alexander J. Stratigos, Polytimi Sidiropoulou, and Dorothea Polydorou	
22	Halo nevi	149
	Christina Stefanaki	
23	Drug-induced hypopigmentation	153
	Katerina Damevska, Suzana Nikolovska, Razvigor Darlenski, Ljubica Suturkova, and Torello Lotti	

vi   Contents

24   Hypopigmentation from chemical and physical agents   159
         Katerina Damevska, Igor Peev, Ranthilaka R. Ranawaka, and Viktor Simeonovski
25   Guttate hypomelanosis and progressive hypomelanosis of the trunk (progressive macular hypomelanosis)   165
         Alexander Katoulis and Efthymia Soura

Index   177

Preface

The skin is the most visible organ, and dyschromias and disorders of pigmentation may be a common cause of significant psychological burden in affected individuals. Hypopigmentation of the skin is characterized clinically by areas of "off-white" color that is lighter compared to the surrounding normal skin, or by areas of complete loss of pigmentation characterized by absolute white color. Hypopigmentation may reflect cutaneous diseases such as vitiligo or mosaic or post-inflammatory hypopigmentation, or be a marker of underlying systemic disorders and complex genetic syndromes including tuberous sclerosis, albinism, piebaldism, Waardenburg syndrome, and other rare disorders. Moreover, hypopigmentation may be a sign of cutaneous T-cell lymphoma or be induced by drugs, including cancer immunotherapy such as anti-PD-1 agents.

This comprehensive illustrated text from international experts aims to enable clinicians to diagnose and treat the full range of these conditions in children and in adults by discussing detailed clinical clues and presenting signs and explaining the approach to management.

We want to thank all our co-authors for their work and CRC Press/Taylor & Francis and Robert Peden, for their support.

This book is dedicated by all three of us to our families for their patience, support, and thoughtfulness.

Electra Nicolaidou

Clio Dessinioti

Andreas D. Katsambas
Athens, Greece

Contributors

T. P. Afra
Department of Dermatology
IQRAA International Hospital and Research Centre
Calicut, India

Balachandra Ankad
Rajiv Gandhi University of Health Sciences
Bengaluru, India

Nooshin Bagherani
Dermatologist and Lawyer
Nooshin Bagherani' Office
Arak, Iran

and

Department of Molecular Medicine
Tehran University of Medical Sciences
Tehran, Iran

Giovanni Bagnoni
Unit of Dermatology
Melanoma & Skin Cancer Unit—AVNO
Livorno Hospital
Livorno, Italy

Christina Bergqvist
Department of Dermatology
University Hospital Henri Mondor
Créteil, France

Ivana Binić
University Clinical Centre
Medical School University of Niš
Niš, Serbia

Anastasiya A. Chokoeva
"Pro Art "—Clinic for Dermatology
 and Aesthetics
Plovdiv, Bulgaria

Stefana Cretu
Second Clinic of Dermatology
"Colentina" Clinical Hospital
Bucharest, Romania

Katerina Damevska
University Clinic of Dermatology
St. Cyril and Methodius University
Skopje, Republic of North Macedonia

Razvigor Darlenski
Department of Dermatology and Venereology
Trakia University
Stara Zagora, Bulgaria

and

Department of Dermatology and Venereology
Acibadem City Clinic Tokuda Hospital
Sofia, Bulgaria

Angelo Massimiliano D'Erme
Unit of Dermatology
Melanoma & Skin Cancer Unit—AVNO
Livorno Hospital
Livorno, Italy

Clio Dessinioti
1st Department of Dermatology and Venereology
National and Kapodistrian University of Athens
"Andreas Sygros" Hospital for Skin and Venereal Diseases
Athens, Greece

Silvija Duma
University Clinic of Dermatology
St. Cyril and Methodius University
Skopje, Republic of North Macedonia

Viktoria Eleftheriadou
Dermatology
Leicester Royal Infirmary
Leicester, United Kingdom

Khaled Ezzedine
Department of Dermatology
University Hospital Henri Mondor
Créteil, France

Nika Franceschi
Department of Dermatology and Venereology
University Hospital Center Sestre Milosrdnice
Zagreb, Croatia

Serena Gianfaldoni
Department of Dermatology
Guglielmo Marconi University
Rome, Italy

Leon Gilad
Department of Dermatology
Hebrew University of Jerusalem
Jerusalem, Israel

x Contributors

Andy Goren
Department of Dermatology and Venereology
Guglielmo Marconi University
Rome, Italy

Fabrizio Guarneri
Department of Clinical and Experimental
 Medicine—Dermatology
University of Messina
Messina, Italy

Arieh Ingber
Department of Dermatology
Hadassah University Hospital
Hebrew University of Jerusalem
Jerusalem, Israel

Mira Kadurina
Department of Dermatology
Guglielmo Marconi University
Rome, Italy

Alexander Katoulis
2nd Department of Dermatology and Venereology
National and Kapodistrian University of Athens
"Attikon" University General Hospital
Athens, Greece

Andreas D. Katsambas
Dermatology and Venereology
National and Kapodistrian University of Athens
Head
Dermatology Clinic
Hygeia Hospital
Athens, Greece

Maja Kovacevic
Department of Dermatology and Venereology
University Hospital Center Sestre Milosrdnice
Zagreb, Croatia

Daniela Kovacs
Cutaneous Physiopathology and Integrated
 Center of Metabolomics Research
San Gallicano Dermatological Institute
IRCCS
Rome, Italy

Jovan Lalošević
Clinic of Dermatovenereology
Clinical Center of Serbia
Belgrade, Serbia

Irene Latour-Álvarez
Department of Dermatology
University Children's Hospital Niño Jesús
Madrid, Spain

Torello Lotti
Department of Dermatology and Venereology
and
Department of Education Sciences
Guglielmo Marconi University
Rome, Italy

Styliani Mastraftsi
1st Department of Dermatology and Venereology
National and Kapodistrian University of Athens
"Andreas Sygros" Hospital for Skin and Venereal
 Diseases
Athens, Greece

Alexandra Miniati
Department of Adult Internal Medicine
Lowell General Hospital
Lowell, Massachusetts

Natasa Teovska Mitrevska
Department of Dermatology and Venereology
ReMedika Hospital
Skopje, Republic of North Macedonia

Electra Nicolaidou
1st Department of Dermatology and Venereology
National and Kapodistrian University of Athens
"Andreas Sygros" Hospital for Skin and Venereal
 Diseases
Athens, Greece

Miloš Nikolić
Department of Dermatovenereology
University of Belgrade School of Medicine
Belgrade, Serbia

Suzana Nikolovska
University Clinic of Dermatology
St. Cyril and Methodius University
Skopje, Republic of North Macedonia

Davinder Parsad
Department of Dermatology, Venereology,
 and Leprology
Postgraduate Institute of Medical Education
 and Research
Chandigarh, India

Athanasios I. Pavlidis
Department of Dermatology
Errikos Dunant Hospital Center
Athens, Greece

Igor Peev
University Clinic of Plastic and Reconstructive Surgery
St. Cyril and Methodius University
Skopje, Republic of North Macedonia

Andrej Petrov
Department of Dermatology and Venereology
Acibadem Sistina Hospital
Skopje, Republic of North Macedonia

and

Faculty of Medicine
Goce Delcev University
Shtip, Republic of North Macedonia

Mauro Picardo
Cutaneous Physiopathology and Integrated Center of
  Metabolomics Research
San Gallicano Dermatological Institute
IRCCS
Rome, Italy

Vesna Pljakoska
Department of Dermatology and Venereology
Acibadem Sistina Hospital
Skopje, Republic of North Macedonia

Dorothea Polydorou
Department of Dermatology and Venereology
"Andreas Sygros" Hospital for Skin and Venereal Diseases
Athens, Greece

Ranthilaka R. Ranawaka
Dermatology Clinic
General Hospital Kalutara
Sri Lanka

Muhammed Razmi T.
Department of Dermatology
IQRAA International Hospital and Research Centre
Calicut, India

Dimitris Rigopoulos
1st Department of Dermatology and Venereology
National and Kapodistrian University of Athens
"Andreas Sygros" Hospital for Skin and Venereal Diseases
Athens, Greece

Carmen Maria Salavastru
Paediatric Dermatology Discipline
"Carol Davila" University of Medicine and Pharmacy
Bucharest, Romania

Dimitrios Sgouros
1st Department of Dermatology and Venereology
National and Kapodistrian University of Athens
"Andreas Sygros" Hospital for Skin and Venereal Diseases
Athens, Greece

Polytimi Sidiropoulou
1st Department of Dermatology and Venereology
National and Kapodistrian University of Athens
"Andreas Sygros" Hospital for Skin and Venereal
  Diseases
Athens, Greece

Viktor Simeonovski
University Clinic of Dermatology
St. Cyril and Methodius University
Skopje, Republic of North Macedonia

Mirna Situm
Department of Dermatology and Venereology
University Hospital Center Sestre Milosrdnice
Zagreb, Croatia

Bruce R. Smoller
Department of Pathology
and
Department of Dermatology
University of Rochester
Rochester, New York

Efthymia Soura
1st Department of Dermatology and Venereology
National and Kapodistrian University of Athens
"Andreas Sygros" Hospital for Skin and Venereal Diseases
Athens, Greece

Andrija Stanimirovic
Department of Clinical Medicine
University of Applied Health Sciences
Zagreb, Croatia

Christina Stefanaki
1st Department of Dermatology and Venereology
National and Kapodistrian University of Athens
"Andreas Sygros" Hospital for Skin and Venereal Diseases
Athens, Greece

Alexander J. Stratigos
1st Department of Dermatology and Venereology
National and Kapodistrian University of Athens
"Andreas Sygros" Hospital for Skin and Venereal Diseases
Athens, Greece

Ljubica Suturkova
Faculty of Pharmacy
St. Cyril and Methodius University
Skopje, Republic of North Macedonia

xii Contributors

George Sorin Tiplica
Second Clinic of Dermatology
"Colentina" Clinical Hospital
and
Second Dermatology Discipline
"Carol Davila" University of Medicine
 and Pharmacy
Bucharest, Romania

Antonio Torrelo
Department of Dermatology
University Children's Hospital Niño Jesús
Madrid, Spain

Yan Valle
Vitiligo Research Foundation
New York, New York

Aleksandra Vojvodic
Department of Dermatology and Venereology
Military Medical Academy
Belgrade, Serbia

Uwe Wollina
Department of Dermatology and Venereology
Stadtisches Klinicum Dresden
Dresden, Germany

Basic concepts on melanocyte biology

MAURO PICARDO and DANIELA KOVACS

CONTENTS

Evolution/adaptation of human pigmentation and its heterogeneity — 1
Melanocytes and melanin synthesis — 3
Melanosome transport inside melanocytes and melanosome transfer to keratinocytes — 4
Cell–cell crosstalk in the control of melanocyte functionality — 7
Extracellular matrix microenvironment and melanocyte homeostasis — 9
Concluding remarks — 9
References — 9

EVOLUTION/ADAPTATION OF HUMAN PIGMENTATION AND ITS HETEROGENEITY

Melanocytes participate as the major performers in the complex scenario of biological components regulating the process of pigmentation. These cells are specialized in the synthesis of melanin pigments inside membrane-bound organelles, the melanosomes. Along with hemoglobin and carotenoids, melanin is the main pigment responsible for the color variations of our skin and hair. Differences in skin and hair color are considered to be adaptive responses and to be highly related to ultraviolet (UV) exposure and latitude. During evolution, human ancestors living in equatorial Africa were probably characterized by light pigmentation of the body, which was, however, covered by dark hair. The gradual loss of body hair paralleled the increase in the epidermal and stratum corneum thickness and in dark-photoprotective eumelanin pigmentation to prevent the damages of ultraviolet radiation (UVR) near the equator. Under intense UVR exposure, dark skin developed as a protective mechanism to limit destruction of cutaneous and systemic folate. Folate regulates important biological processes such as DNA synthesis, repair, methylation, and maintenance of active spermatogenesis, as well as melanin production. Folate deficiency has been linked to pregnancy complications and severe fetal abnormalities in neural tube development. The sensitivity of folate and of its main serum form, 5-methyltetrahydrofolate, to be degraded by UVR and reactive oxygen species (ROS) supports the hypothesis according to which the increased pigmentation occurring in high UVR-exposed terrestrial areas evolved to prevent fertility reduction caused by folate photodegradation. As hominins gradually moved outside of tropical latitudes, toward Eurasia, the Americas, and nonequatorial Africa, the intensity and duration patterns of UV exposure decreased together with a reduced potential for vitamin D production, thus favoring the promotion of depigmentation. Therefore, the wide array of pigmentation characterizing modern humans seems to be guided on the one hand by the need to promote photoprotection near the equator (stimulating the dark constitutive pigmentation) and on the other to promote the ultraviolet B (UVB)-induced photosynthesis of vitamin D at the poles (stimulating light constitutive pigmentation).[1–3] On the other hand, the evolution of epidermal pigmentation has been also proposed as a protective strategy against UV-mediated damages to the skin permeability barrier and as a defense against the high water loss occurring in dessicating external environments such as the sub-Saharan African regions. In support of this hypothesis, in comparison to lightly pigmented individuals, darkly skinned people show a more acidic pH of the stratum corneum, which is further acidified by the slow and delayed degradation/extrusion of melanin. It has been also theorized that the melanocytes of darkly skinned people secrete paracrine mediators able to stimulate epidermal differentiation and the production of lipids positively involved in the constitution of the skin barrier, thus efficiently improving barrier competence in dark skin. Moreover, a pigmented epidermis displays enhanced antimicrobial defense, a property strictly co-regulated and interconnected with permeability barrier homeostasis.[4–6]

Melanocytes originate from neural crest multipotent precursors and after steps of migration, proliferation, and differentiation finally settle into epidermis and hair follicles as well as extracutaneous sites, for example, mucosa, cardiovascular system, adipose tissue, cochlea, and choroid.[7–9] In the skin, they differentiate into dentritic pigment-producing melanocytes (Figure 1.1) and are distributed among keratinocytes of the epidermal basal layer and in hair follicles (Figure 1.2). Synthesized melanin primarily aims at protecting from the harmful effects of UV radiation derived from sunlight as well as, nowadays, from indoor tanning apparatuses, thanks to its ability to absorb UVR and damaging free radicals. The tanning response and the resulting promotion of pigmentation constitute the main protective mechanisms activated following acute and chronic UV exposure by melanocytes and the skin in its entirety.

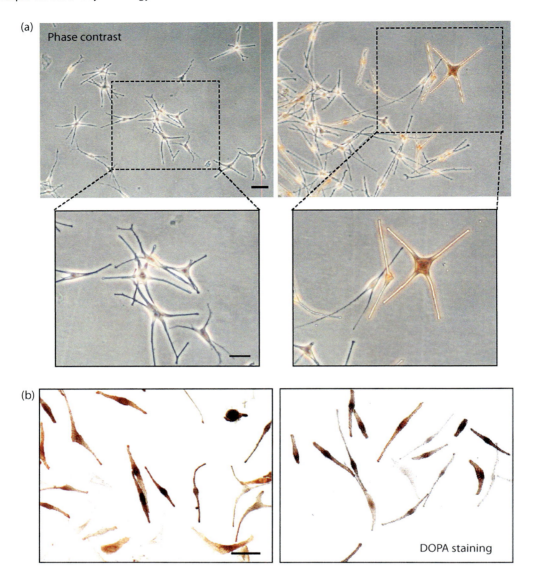

Figure 1.1 (a) Phase contrast microscopic analysis of primary cultures of normal human melanocytes showing the typical dendritic shape. (b) DOPA staining of human primary melanocytes displaying the cellular brown/black appearance due to the activity of tyrosinase on DOPA substrate. Scale bar: a, b: 50 μm.

Melanocytes actively interact with both epidermal and dermal compartments. Each melanocyte, through its dendrites, is in mutual connection with about 30–40 keratinocytes, constituting the epidermal melanin unit (Figure 1.3), and with dermal fibroblasts, thus establishing a finely balanced network of cell–cell crosstalk, ultimately influencing the color of the skin. Differentiated melanocytes display a low growth rate and elevated resistance to apoptosis as a result of their high intrinsic expression of the anti-apoptotic protein Bcl-2.[10] Despite variations in the density of melanocytic cells in diverse body areas, their overall number appears constant among human populations. Differences in ethnic color are rather related to the type and quantity of produced melanin and to its transfer, distribution pattern, and degradation into neighboring keratinocytes. There are two main types of melanin synthesized through the multistep process of melanogenesis: red/yellow pheomelanin and brown/black or dark eumelanin, which are both produced in different ratios. In light-skinned people, the predominant melanin type is usually pheomelanin, the melanosomes are smaller and less condensed, and they are transferred to keratinocytes grouped in membrane-bound clusters containing four to eight melanosomes.[11,12] As light keratinocytes terminally differentiate, melanosome structures are fully degraded in the upper epidermal layers.[11] Differently, in dark-skinned people, eumelanin is the main produced melanin type, and melanosomes are larger and more copious but singularly packaged and transferred into the surrounding keratinocytes, where their degradation and disappearance are slower[13] (Figure 1.4).

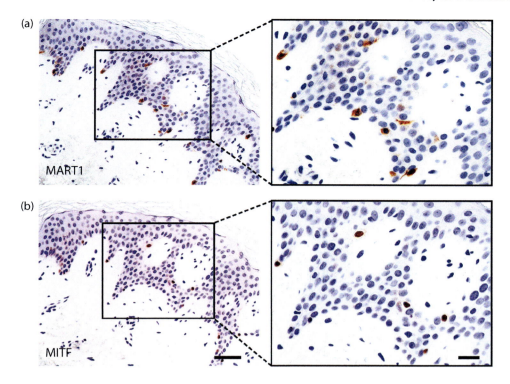

Figure 1.2 Serial sections of a skin specimen showing the presence of melanocytes identified using the melanocyte markers MART1 (melanoma antigen recognized by T cells 1) (melanosome structural protein) (a), and MITF (microphtalmia-associated transcription factor) (b). Nuclei are counterstained with hematoxylin. Right panels represent higher-magnification images of the black boxed areas. Scale bar: Left panels: 50 μm; higher-magnification images on the right panels: 20 μm.

MELANOCYTES AND MELANIN SYNTHESIS

A decisive aspect in determining skin color is the type of melanin synthesized by melanocytes. Melanin synthesis occurs within specialized membrane-bound organelles, the melanosomes, through four stages of maturation. Melanin arrangement inside melanosomes guarantees the protection of other cell compartments from oxidative stress produced during pigment synthesis and, at the same time, condensates melanin for its transfer to kertinocytes.[14] While maturing, melanosomes progressively acquire structural and enzymatic proteins, allowing them to produce pigment. At stage I, melanosomes appear as round vesicles without structural constituents. Progressing to stage II, they assemble into elongated fibrillar organelles containing structural (e.g., Pmel17—melanosomal matrix protein 17, also known as PMEL, SILV, gp100) and enzymatic proteins (tyrosinase), but they still lack pigment. Then, melanin synthesis begins and the produced pigment is placed on internal fibrils (stage III). At stage IV, melanosomes are mature and fully melanized. They are deprived of tyrosinase activity and are transferred along dendrites and then to the surrounding keratinocytes.[12] Within melanosomes, melanin synthesis occurs through a sequence of reactions guided by the coordinate actions of crucial enzymes, namely tyrosinase, tyrosinase-related protein 1 (TYRP-1),

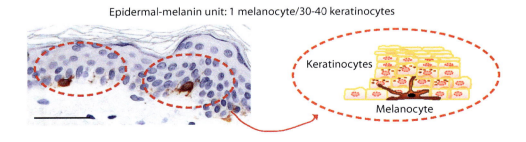

Figure 1.3 The epidermal-melanin unit showing the interactions between melanocytes and the surrounding keratinocytes. Left panel: Detection of melanocytes on a section of a skin specimen by immunohistochemical analysis of the expression of MART1. Scale bar: 50 μm.

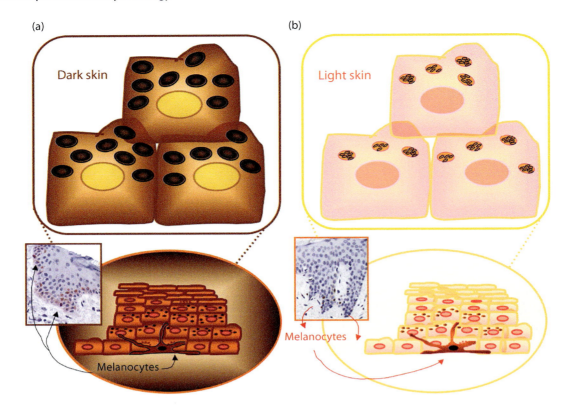

Figure 1.4 Pigmentation in dark and light skin. In dark-skinned people (left panel, a), melanosomes are large, abundant, and transferred to keratinocytes as singly packaged organelles. In light-skinned individuals (right panel, b), melanosomes are small, less matured, and transferred to keratinocytes as clusters in membrane-bound organelles, encompassing more melanosomes. Insert in a: immunohistochemical analysis of the expression of the melanocyte marker MITF in a darkly pigmented skin specimen. Arrows indicate stained melanocytes. Melanin pigment is observable inside basal and suprabasal keratinocytes. Insert in b: immunohistochemical analysis of the expression of the melanocyte marker MITF in a lightly pigmented skin specimen. Arrows indicate stained melanocytes.

and tyrosinase-related protein 2/dopachrome tautomerase (TYRP-2, DCT). The cooperation of these three enzymes leads to the production of two main melanin-type biopolymers: red-yellow pheomelanin and brown-black eumelanin. Melanogenic enzyme functionality and substrate obtainability drive the type of melanins produced. Tyrosinase governs the initial synthesis steps, hydroxylating L-tyrosine to L-3,4-dihydroxyphenylalanine (L-DOPA) (the earliest melanogenesis rate restricting step) and subsequently oxidizing DOPA to DOPAquinone. At this point, when sulfhydryl groups such as L-cysteine are available, dopaquinone reacts with them, forming cysteinylDOPA isomers, including 5-S-cysteinylDOPA and 2-S-cysteinylDOPA. They are hence oxidized and polymerize, producing pheomelanins via benzothiazine intermediates. As sulfhydryl groups are not available, dopaquinone is spontaneously subjected to cyclization and rearrangement to DOPAchrome. DOPAchrome spontaneously decarboxylates into 5, 6 dihydroxyindole (DHI), forming, by rapid oxidation and polymerization, dark brown-black insoluble DHI-melanin. In the presence of the enzymatic protein dopachrome tautomerase (TYRP2, DCT), dopachrome will generate DHI-2-carboxylic-acid (DHICA). TYRP1 catalyzes further DHICA oxidation and polymerization, leading to light-brown, fairly soluble DHICA eumelanin[15] (Figures 1.5 and 1.6). Eumelanin is prevalent in dark-skinned/black-haired individuals and protects from UV damage. Pheomelanin, which is higher in people with fair skin and red hair, generates an increased amount of free radicals, thus inducing more harmful effects. Several genes involved in melanin synthesis and melanosome formation, as well as in pigment trafficking inside melanocytes and melanin transfer to keratinocytes, decisively influence the variations in pigmentation observed among human populations. Multiple genes are known to directly or indirectly impact pigmentation, and mutations of many of these genes may lead to pigmentary disorders, either as hyper- or hypopigmentation.[16,17]

MELANOSOME TRANSPORT INSIDE MELANOCYTES AND MELANOSOME TRANSFER TO KERATINOCYTES

As melanosomes differentiate, they progressively move from the melanocyte perinuclear area to the dendrite tips. Melanosome intracellular movement occurs both antero- and retrogradely, toward microtubule proteins belonging to the kinesin and dynein/dynein-associated protein superfamilies, respectively. In the dendrites,

Melanosome transport inside melanocytes and melanosome transfer to keratinocytes   5

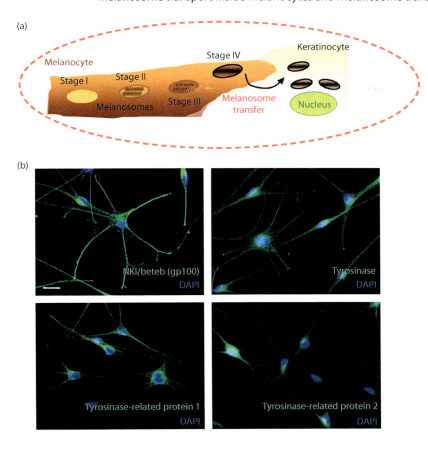

Figure 1.5 (a) Cartoon depicting the four stages of melanosome maturation within melanocytes. While maturing, melanosomes acquire the structural and enzymatic components necessary to produce melanin. (b) Immunofluorescence analysis of the expression of the structural melanosome-associated protein NKIbeteb/gp100 and of the enzymatic proteins tyrosinase, tyrosinase-related protein 1, and tyrosinase-related protein 2 in human primary melanocytes. Nuclei are counterstained with 4′,6′-diamidino-2 phenylindole (DAPI). Scale bar: 20 μm.

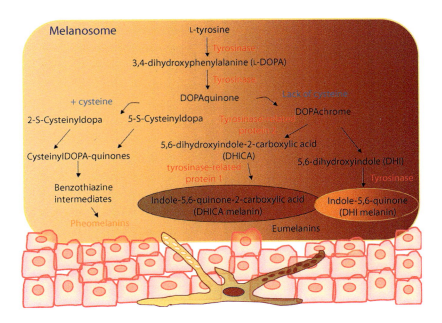

Figure 1.6 Melanin biosynthetic pathway. Two major melanin forms are synthesized within melanosomes: red-yellow pheomelanin and brown-black eumelanin.

melanosomes are then connected with peripheral actin filaments by a tripartite complex composed of the small GTPase Rab27a, its effector protein melanophillin, and the actin motor myosin Va, allowing their detachment from the microtubules and their settling close to the plasma membrane.[18,19] From the tips of the dendrites, fully melanized melanosomes are transferred to the neighboring keratinocytes, where they distribute as a supra-nuclear cap, aiming at protecting cell nuclei from the damaging effects of UV. Based on *in vitro* and ultrastructural studies, different models of melanosome intercellular transfer, which are not incompatible with each other, have been hypothesized: (i) Exocytosis of naked melanin (also referred to as melanocore) into the extracellular areas through the fusion of the melanocyte plasma- and melanosome membranes. The pigment particles are then taken up by the surrounding keratinocytes via phagocytosis. (ii) Cytophagocytosis: keratinocytes internalize melanocyte dendrite tips via phagocytosis. Subsequent fusion of lysosomes and dissolution of the melanosome membrane lead to the formation of phagolysosomes. The latter are then gradually degraded in vesicles containing melanin granules spread in the cytoplasm of keratinocytes. Filopodial phagocytosis, in which melanocyte filopodia containing melanosomes are phagocitosed by keratinocytes, has been also reported. (iii) Membrane fusion: melanosomes proceed via a thin, transient channel derived from the fusion of melanocyte-keratinocyte plasma membranes. Melanosome transfer by the fusion model has been also suggested to occur via melanocyte filopodia united with keratinocyte plasma membrane to form a tubular structure of actin filaments. (iv) Transfer through membrane-bound vesicles: melanocytes release membrane vesicles containing melanosomes, which are then phagocytosed by keratinocytes.[20–22]

Keratinocytes, for their part, actively participate in regulating the process of melanosome uptake. The expression of specific receptors on keratinocytes, but not on melanocytes, positively controls melanosome internalization. Among them, the G-protein-coupled protease-activated receptor 2 (PAR-2) is decisive in melanosome uptake by stimulating the process of phagocytosis. PAR-2 receptors are activated by proteolytic cleavage of their extracellular *N*-terminal domain via serine proteases. The cleavage discloses tethered ligands that bind the receptor, thus inducing its activation. Once activated, PAR-2 increases melanosome internalization by a Rho-dependent mechanism.[23,24] PAR-2 expression and activity are upregulated following UV[25] and are also correlated with skin color, showing more elevated levels with respect to lightly pigmented skin.[26] Melanosome transfer is also stimulated by the expression and activation of the keratinocyte growth factor receptor (KGFR) in early differentiated keratinocytes, where the levels of the receptor are increased. KGFR directly promotes the phagocytic process[27,28] (Figure 1.7).

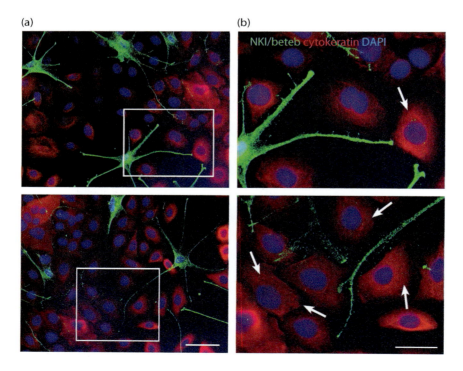

Figure 1.7 Double immunofluorescence staining of human primary melanocyte-keratinocyte co-cultures with anti-NKI-beteb antibody (green signal) to stain melanosomes and with anti-cytokeratin antibody (red signal) to detect keratinocytes. Intracytoplasmic dots positively stained for NKI-beteb are detectable in keratinocytes (white arrows), evidencing melanosome transfer. The images in (b) represent higher magnification of the boxed areas in (a). Scale bar: 50 μm.

CELL–CELL CROSSTALK IN THE CONTROL OF MELANOCYTE FUNCTIONALITY

Melanocyte homeostasis is guided by the active signaling crosstalk established with the surrounding epidermal and dermal microenvironment via secreted factors and intercellular connections.

Melanocyte-keratinocyte interactions

Keratinocytes impact melanocyte functions through adhesion molecules and an inter/intracellular network of paracrine/autocrine bioactive messengers, whose physiological release is upregulated in response to external triggers, first UV exposure and/or also inflammatory stimuli. Binding to their specific receptors, keratinocyte-derived mediators activate intracellular signaling pathways controlling the growth, survival, differentiation, and pigment synthesis of melanocytic cells.

Among these growth factor/receptor axes, the pro-opiomelanocortin (POMC) cleavage peptides alpha-melanocyte stimulating hormone (α-MSH) and adrenocorticotropic hormone (ACTH), via signaling through the G protein-coupled receptor melanocortin 1 receptor (MC1R), are key players in the induction of melanocyte differentiation and melanin synthesis. Activation of MC1R through cAMP-dependent signaling promotes the upregulation of the transcription factor microphtalmia-associated transcription factor (MITF). MITF is considered a crucial transcription factor for melanocyte functions (Figure 1.8), regulating the transcription of pigmentation-related genes (e.g., tyrosinase, TYRP-1, TYRP-2, PMEL, MART1), thus promoting melanocyte differentiation, as well as genes linked to survival (e.g., Bcl-2), cell cycle, and metabolism (e.g., CDK2).[29] Through the induction of MITF and, consequently, the pigmentation-related genes, MC1R regulates the production of eu- versus pheomelanin. Activating the receptor by agonists such as α-MSH or ACTH, the production of eumelanin is stimulated. Differently, the action of an antagonist, for example, Agouti signaling protein, may lead to the synthesis of pheomelanin. MC1R variants with a weak functionality are observed in fair-skinned/red-haired people, who are characterized by a prevalence of pheomelanin, a feeble potential for tanning, and increased risk for melanoma and nonmelanoma skin cancers.[30] Upon UV exposure, direct transcriptional activation of POMC/alpha-MSH occurs in keratinocytes by the tumor-suppressor protein p53,[31] thus promoting melanocyte functions. Besides its central role in regulating pigmentation, MC1R influences several other processes, not only in melanocytes but also in the skin microenvironment in its entirety, maintaining genomic integrity, controlling oxidative stress, and promoting the antioxidant defense system.[32] Recently, a connection between MC1R and nuclear receptor activation has been described, further underlying the multitude of functions guided by MC1R in cells and tissues. α-MSH has been shown to activate the nuclear receptor peroxisome proliferator-activated receptor-γ (PPAR-γ) through the induction of the phosphatidylinositol [PI(4,5)P2/PLCβ] signal pathway, demonstrating how MC1R has a role in controlling extrapigmentary functions such as proliferation via lipid mediators.[32,33]

Many other melanocyte mitogen and melanogen factors are produced by keratinocytes, for example, stem cell factor (SCF), endothelin-1 (ET-1), basic fibroblast growth factor (bFGF/FGF2), granulocyte-macrophage colony-stimulating factor (GM-CSF), and hepatocyte growth factor (HGF). As for α-MSH, the synthesis of most of them is significantly increased following UV irradiation. ET-1 acts, binding to endothelin receptor type B (EDNRB), promoting melanocyte growth and melanogenesis.[34] The SCF/c-kit tyrosine kinase receptor axis favors melanocyte survival and melanin production.[35] Comparable to POMC, the transcription and synthesis of both ET-1 and SCF are stimulated by p53.[36] Along with growth factors, other mediators released by keratinocytes in the course of biological processes such as inflammation or wound healing may function as activators of melanocytes. Among them, the arachidonic acid–derived lipid molecules prostaglandins E2 and F2a stimulate melanocyte dendricity and melanogenesis.[37] Keratinocytes secrete also nerve growth factor (NGF), which is implicated in melanocyte dendrite formation and melanin synthesis, survival, and migration.[38] In

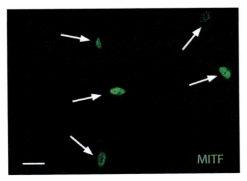 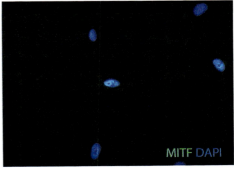

Figure 1.8 Immunofluorescence analysis of MITF expression (white arrows) in primary cultures of human melanocytes. Nuclei are counterstained with DAPI. Scale bar: 20 μm.

8 Basic concepts on melanocyte biology

the finely balanced crosstalk between keratinocytes and melanocytes, alongside messengers acting as positive inducers of the functionality of the latter, keratinocytes also release some inhibiting factors. TGF-β inhibits melanocyte proliferation, differentiation, and melanin synthesis. The production of TGF-β in keratinocytes is suppressed upon UV exposure, and such an event allows the upregulation of the transcription factor SOX3 in melanocytes, thus stimulating the pigmentation process.[39] Keratinocytes, as well as melanocytes themselves, express bone morphogenic proteins (BMPs), signaling molecules belonging to the TGFβ1 superfamily. Among them, BMP-4 is able to inhibit melanogenesis, decreasing tyrosinase expression. On the contrary, BMP-6 acts in the opposite way, stimulating melanin synthesis through the induction of tyrosinase expression and activity, together with melanin transfer from melanocytes to keratinocytes.[40,41] Following UV exposure, keratinocytes are also stimulated to synthesize the cytokine interferon gamma (IFN-γ), which exerts an inhibitory effect on pigmentation, decreasing the expression of enzymes deputed to melanin biosynthesis, thus impeding melanosome maturation.[42] Additional keratinocyte-derived cytokines with downregulating effects on melanization and melanocyte proliferation are interleukin 6 (IL-6), interleukin 1 alpha (IL-1α), and tumor necrosis factor alpha (TNF-α)[43] (Figure 1.9a).

Melanocyte-fibroblast interactions

Dermal fibroblasts play an active role in modulating melanocyte homeostasis through the secretion of growth factors and cytokines, which act both in a synergistic and sometimes overlapping fashion with respect to the keratinocyte-mediated signaling network. Additionally, some paracrine messengers released by fibroblasts can indirectly target melanocyte functions, inducing the production of biofactors able to either block or stimulate melanocyte activities in keratinocytes. Similar to growth factors and cytokines synthesized by keratinocytes, in this intricate epithelial-mesenchymal interaction, some fibroblastic bioactive messengers act as melanocyte activators, others as inhibitors. The physiological hypopigmented phenotype of the palms and soles has been attributed to increased expression of the Wnt pathway antagonist dickkopf1 (DKK1) in these body areas. This site-specific fibroblast-derived factor exerts a dual action: on the one hand, it suppresses melanocyte growth and melanin synthesis, and on the other, it acts on keratinocytes, decreasing the expression of the proteinase-activated receptor 2 actively involved in the process of melanosome transfer.[44] Furthermore, fibroblasts share with keratinocytes the production of TGF-β, with repressive properties on melanocytes.[39] However, the largest number of fibroblast-derived messengers exert a positive action on melanocyte activities, acting on their growth, survival, migration, and pigment production. Some of these pro-pigmenting mediators are also produced by epidermal cells, for example, SCF, HGF, and bFGF;

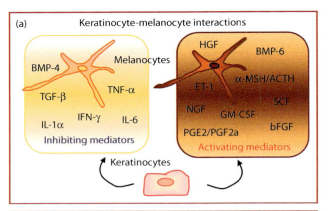

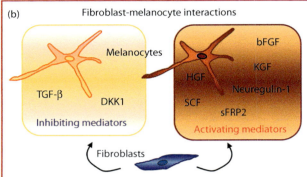

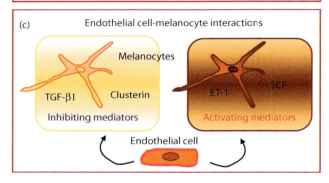

Figure 1.9 Summary of the stimulating and inhibiting bioactive mediators involved in the regulation of melanocyte functionalities. (a) Keratinocyte-derived messengers. (b) Fibroblast-derived messengers. (c) Endothelial cell-derived messengers.

others are exclusively of fibroblastic origin. Among the latter, neuregulin-1 has been demonstrated to be highly expressed in fibroblasts of type VI skin, where it positively participates in the regulation of constitutive pigmentation of darker skin.[45] Keratinocyte growth factor (KGF) belongs to the family of fibroblast growth factors and represents a further mesenchymal-specific pro-pigmenting paracrine mediator. KGF directly promotes melanosome transfer via activation of its receptor KGFR in keratinocytes. Additionally, it upregulates the synthesis and release of SCF from keratinocytes, thus indirectly promoting melanocyte pro-pigmenting and pro-growing activities. It has been also demonstrated that the treatment with KGF alone or in combination with IL-1α increases melanin production and deposition in pigmented epidermal equivalents and human skin explants.[27,46,47] The Wnt modulator secreted frizzled-related protein 2 (sFRP2) has been recently discovered as a further fibroblast-secreted stimulating factor, thanks to its ability to increase the expression levels of MITF and tyrosinase through beta catenin signaling[48] (Figure 1.9b).

Melanocyte-endothelial cell interactions

In the complex scenario of the epidermal-dermal interactions emerging as crucially involved in mediating melanocyte homeostasis under both physiological and pathological conditions, several reports have now been focused on the epithelial/endothelial cell–cell interplay. However, contradictory effects are reported in the literature, showing both positive and negative regulatory abilities of vascular endothelial cells on the process of pigmentation. A stimulatory effect of endothelial cell-derived ET-1 on melanogenesis, via the signaling pathway of the EDNRB on melanocytes, has been reported.[49] On the other hand, subsequent studies demonstrated the ability of endothelial cells to inhibit pigmentation via the secretion of high amounts of TGF-β1 and/or clusterin, which downregulate MITF and tyrosinase, thus keeping the level of produced pigment low.[50,51] Interestingly, upon UV irradiation, endothelial cells are activated to secrete increased levels of SCF, responsible for the paracrine stimulation of melanocytes and consequently increasing skin pigmentation[52] (Figure 1.9c).

EXTRACELLULAR MATRIX MICROENVIRONMENT AND MELANOCYTE HOMEOSTASIS

The epidermal and dermal extracellular matrix (ECM) microenvironment influences a large number of skin functions, for example, cell–cell crosstalk, adhesion, support, and migration. Dynamic interplays among extracellular matrix proteins, cells, and bioactive mediators are also critical regulators of melanocyte activities and cutaneous pigmentation. Early studies demonstrated the ability of several ECM proteins derived from dermal fibroblasts and endothelial cells (e.g., collagen I, collagen IV, fibronectin) to increase proliferation and tyrosinase activity in melanocytes cultured in media lacking mitogens.[53] More recently, the keratinocyte-derived ECM factor laminin-332 has been shown to promote the adhesion and migration of melanocytes,[54] as well as the synthesis of melanin by stimulating the extracellular uptake of the pigment precursor tyrosine.[55] ECM components also constitute a reservoir for cytokines and growth factors, thus regulating their local amount and activity. For instance, an uncontrolled degradation of heparan sulfate at the dermal-epidermal junction, as happens for the activation of heparanase following UV exposure, may result in excessive diffusion through the basement membrane of heparin-binding growth factors, such as the pro-pigmenting factors HGF and FGFs. Consequently, the uncontrolled propagation of growth factors and cytokines among the epidermis and dermis may inappropriately activate melanocytes.[56]

CONCLUDING REMARKS

Despite the relatively low number of melanocytes distributed throughout the epidermis in comparison to their neighboring keratinocytes, these cells represent intriguing and master players in the control of a multitude of cutaneous biological functions. Melanocyte homeostasis has been guided, over time, by both intrinsic and extrinsic factors (above all, UV exposure) that have contributed and are still contributing to the development and evolution of the pigmentary system. All these influences create an intricate and finely balanced signaling crosstalk, in which melanocytes exert a central and dynamic role in controlling the equilibrium and protection of the skin in its entirety. On the other hand, the network of bioactive messengers acts bidirectionally to and from the melanocytes toward the other dermal and epidermal cells. As a result, this mutual interaction confers on the whole cutaneous microenvironment the ability to strongly influence melanocytes themselves and therefore to contribute to both constitutive pigmentation and, whenever altered, to the onset and persistence of pigmentary disorders.

REFERENCES

1. Jablonski NG, Chaplin G. Colloquium paper: Human skin pigmentation as an adaptation to UV radiation. *Proc Natl Acad Sci USA*. 2010;107(Suppl 2):8962–8968.
2. Jablonski NG, Chaplin G. The colours of humanity: The evolution of pigmentation in the human lineage. *Philos Trans R Soc Lond B Biol Sci*. 2017;372(1724).
3. Jones P, Lucock M, Veysey M, Beckett E. The vitamin D–folate hypothesis as an evolutionary model for skin pigmentation: An update and integration of current ideas. *Nutrients*. 2018;10:554.
4. Gunathilake R, Schurer NY, Shoo BA et al. pH-regulated mechanisms account for pigment-type differences in epidermal barrier function. *J Invest Dermatol*. 2009;129:1719–1729.
5. Elias PM, Williams ML. Re-appraisal of current theories for the development and loss of epidermal pigmentation in hominins and modern humans. *J Hum Evol*. 2013;64:687–692.
6. Elias PM, Williams ML. Basis for the gain and subsequent dilution of epidermal pigmentation during human evolution: The barrier and metabolic conservation hypotheses revisited. *Am J Phys Anthropol*. 2016;161:189–207.
7. Lin JY, Fisher DE. Melanocyte biology and skin pigmentation. *Nature*. 2007;445:843–850.
8. Kawakami A, Fisher DE. Key discoveries in melanocyte development. *J Invest Dermatol*. 2011;131(E1):E2–E4.
9. Plonka PM, Passeron T, Brenner M et al. What are melanocytes really doing all day long…? *Exp Dermatol*. 2009;18:799–819.
10. McGill GG, Horstmann M, Widlund HR et al. Bcl2 regulation by the melanocyte master regulator MITF modulates lineage survival and melanoma cell viability. *Cell*. 2002;109:707–718.

11. Thong HY, Jee SH, Sun CC, Boissy RE. The patterns of melanosome distribution in keratinocytes of human skin as one determining factor of skin colour. *Br J Dermatol.* 2003;149:498–505.

12. Costin GE, Hearing VJ. Human skin pigmentation: Melanocytes modulate skin color in response to stress. *FASEB J.* 2007;21:976–994.

13. Ebanks JP, Koshoffer A, Wickett RR et al. Epidermal keratinocytes from light vs. dark skin exhibit differential degradation of melanosomes. *J Invest Dermatol* 2011;131:1226–1233.

14. Denat L, Kadekaro AL, Marrot L et al. Melanocytes as instigators and victims of oxidative stress. *J Invest Dermatol* 2014;134:1512–1518.

15. Nguyen NT, Fisher DE. MITF and UV responses in skin: From pigmentation to addiction. *Pigment Cell Melanoma Res.* 2019;32:224–236.

16. Sturm RA. Molecular genetics of human pigmentation diversity. *Hum Mol Genet.* 2009;18:R9–17.

17. Yamaguchi Y, Hearing VJ. Melanocytes and their diseases. *Cold Spring Harb Perspect Med.* 2014;4:pii: a017046.

18. Barral DC, Seabra MC. The melanosome as a model to study organelle motility in mammals. *Pigment Cell Res.* 2004;17:111–118.

19. Wasmeier C, Hume AN, Bolasco G, Seabra MC. Melanosomes at a glance. *J Cell Sci.* 2008; 121:3995–3999.

20. Van Den Bossche K, Naeyaert JM, Lambert J. The quest for the mechanism of melanin transfer. *Traffic.* 2006;7:769–778.

21. Singh SK, Kurfurst R, Nizard C et al. Melanin transfer in human skin cells is mediated by filopodia—A model for homotypic and heterotypic lysosome-related organelle transfer. *FASEB J.* 2010;24:3756–3769.

22. Tadokoro R, Takahashi Y. Intercellular transfer of organelles during body pigmentation. *Curr Opin Genet Dev.* 2017;45:132–138.

23. Seiberg M. Keratinocyte-melanocyte interactions during melanosome transfer. *Pigment Cell Res.* 2001;14:236–242.

24. Scott G, Leopardi S, Parker L et al. The proteinase-activated receptor-2 mediates phagocytosis in a Rho-dependent manner in human keratinocytes. *J Invest Dermatol.* 2003;121:529–541.

25. Scott G, Deng A, Rodriguez-Burford C et al. Protease-activated receptor 2, a receptor involved in melanosome transfer, is upregulated in human skin by ultraviolet irradiation. *J Invest Dermatol.* 2001;117:1412–1420.

26. Babiarz-Magee L, Chen N, Seiberg M, Lin CB. The expression and activation of protease-activated receptor-2 correlate with skin color. *Pigment Cell Res.* 2004;17:241–251.

27. Cardinali G, Ceccarelli S, Kovacs D et al. Keratinocyte growth factor promotes melanosome transfer to keratinocytes. *J Invest Dermatol.* 2005;125:1190–1199.

28. Belleudi F, Purpura V, Scrofani C et al. Expression and signaling of the tyrosine kinase FGFR2b/KGFR regulates phagocytosis and melanosome uptake in human keratinocytes. *FASEB J.* 2011;25:170–181.

29. Kawakami A, Fisher DE. The master role of microphthalmia-associated transcription factor in melanocyte and melanoma biology. *Lab Invest.* 2017;97:649–656.

30. Yamaguchi Y, Brenner M, Hearing VJ. The regulation of skin pigmentation. *J Biol Chem.* 2007;282:27557–27561.

31. Cui R, Widlund HR, Feige E et al. Central role of p53 in the suntan response and pathologic hyperpigmentation. *Cell.* 2007;128:853–864.

32. Maresca V, Flori E, Picardo M. Skin phototype: A new perspective. *Pigment Cell Melanoma Res.* 2015;28:378–389.

33. Flori E, Rosati E, Cardinali G et al. The α-melanocyte stimulating hormone/peroxisome proliferator activated receptor-γ pathway down-regulates proliferation in melanoma cell lines. *J Exp Clin Cancer Res.* 2017;36:142.

34. Imokawa G, Yada Y, Miyagishi M. Endothelins secreted from human keratinocytes are intrinsic mitogens for human melanocytes. *J Biol Chem.* 1992;267:24675–24680.

35. Slominski A, Tobin DJ, Shibahara S, Wortsman J. Melanin pigmentation in mammalian skin and its hormonal regulation. *Physiol Rev.* 2004; 84:1155–1228.

36. Murase D, Hachiya A, Amano Y et al. The essential role of p53 in hyperpigmentation of the skin via regulation of paracrine melanogenic cytokine receptor signaling. *J Biol Chem.* 2009;284:4343–4353.

37. Scott G, Leopardi S, Printup S et al. Proteinase-activated receptor-2 stimulates prostaglandin production in keratinocytes: Analysis of prostaglandin receptors on human melanocytes and effects of PGE2 and PGF2alpha on melanocyte dendricity. *J Invest Dermatol.* 2004;122:1214–1224.

38. Truzzi F, Marconi A, Pincelli C. Neurotrophins in healthy and diseased skin. *Dermatoendocrinol.* 2011;3:32–36.

39. Yang G, Li Y, Nishimura EK et al. Inhibition of PAX3 by TGF-beta modulates melanocyte viability. *Mol Cell.* 2008;32:554–563.

40. Yaar M, Wu C, Park HY et al. Bone morphogenetic protein-4, a novel modulator of melanogenesis. *J Biol Chem.* 2006;281:25307–25314.

41. Singh SK, Abbas WA, Tobin DJ. Bone morphogenetic proteins differentially regulate pigmentation in human skin cells. *J Cell Sci.* 2012;125:4306–4319.

42. Natarajan VT, Ganju P, Singh A et al. IFN g signaling maintains skin pigmentation homeostasis through regulation of melanosome maturation. *Proc Natl Acad Sci USA.* 2014;111:2301–2306.

43. Swope VB, Abdel-Malek Z, Kassem LM, Nordlund JJ. Interleukins 1 alpha and 6 and tumor necrosis factor-alpha are paracrine inhibitors of human melanocyte proliferation and melanogenesis. *J Invest Dermatol.* 1991;96:180–185.

44. Yamaguchi Y, Morita A, Maeda A, Hearing VJ. Regulation of skin pigmentation and thickness by Dickkopf 1 (DKK1). *J Investig Dermatol Symp Proc.* 2009;14:73–75.

45. Choi W, Wolber R, Gerwat W et al. The fibroblast-derived paracrine factor neuregulin-1 has a novel role in regulating the constitutive color and melanocyte function in human skin. *J Cell Sci.* 2010;123(Pt 18):3102–3111.

46. Kovacs D, Cardinali G, Aspite N et al. Role of fibroblast-derived growth factors in regulating hyperpigmentation of solar lentigo. *Br J Dermatol.* 2010;163:1020–1027.

47. Chen N, Hu Y, Li WH et al. The role of keratinocyte growth factor in melanogenesis: A possible mechanism for the initiation of solar lentigines. *Exp Dermatol.* 2010;19:865–872.

48. Kim M, Han JH, Kim JH et al. Secreted frizzled-related protein 2 (sFRP2) functions as a melanogenic stimulator; the role of sFRP2 in UV-induced hyperpigmentary disorders. *J Invest Dermatol.* 2016; 136:236–244.

49. Regazzetti C, De Donatis GM et al. Endothelial cells promote pigmentation through endothelin receptor B activation. *J Invest Dermatol.* 2015;135:3096–3104.

50. Park JY, Kim M, Park TJ, Kang HY. TGFb1 derived from endothelial cells inhibits melanogenesis. *Pigment Cell Melanoma Res.* 2016;29:477–480.

51. Kim M, Lee J, Park TJ, Kang HY. Paracrine crosstalk between endothelial cells and melanocytes through clusterin to inhibit pigmentation. *Exp Dermatol.* 2018;27:98–100.

52. Kim M, Shibata T, Kwon S et al. Ultraviolet-irradiated endothelial cells secrete stem cell factor and induce epidermal pigmentation. *Sci Rep.* 2018;8:4235.

53. Hedley S, Gawkrodger DJ, Weetman AP, MacNeil S. Investigation of the influence of extracellular matrix proteins on normal human melanocyte morphology and melanogenic activity. *Br J Dermatol.* 1996;135:888–897.

54. Chung H, Suh EK, Han IO, Oh ES. Keratinocyte-derived laminin-332 promotes adhesion and migration in melanocytes and melanoma. *J Biol Chem.* 2011;286:13438–13447.

55. Chung H, Jung H, Lee JH et al. Keratinocyte-derived laminin-332 protein promotes melanin synthesis via regulation of tyrosine uptake. *J Biol Chem.* 2014; 289:21751–21759.

56. Iriyama S, Ono T, Aoki H, Amano S. Hyperpigmentation in human solar lentigo is promoted by heparanase-induced loss of heparan sulfate chains at the dermal-epidermal junction. *J Dermatol Sci.* 2011;64:223–228.

Approach to hypopigmentation

2

CLIO DESSINIOTI and ANDREAS D. KATSAMBAS

CONTENTS

Introduction	13
Diagnostic approach to hypopigmentation	13
Congenital hypopigmentation or not?	14
Special considerations based on the distribution of hypopigmentation	14
Congenital hypopigmentation	14
Noncongenital hypopigmentation	17
References	19

INTRODUCTION

Cutaneous pigmentation is a complex human trait, influenced by melanin, capillary blood flow, cutaneous chromophores (lycopene, carotene), and collagen in the dermis. The synthesis and type of melanin and its distribution within melanosomes are genetically regulated by a number of genes, such as *MC1R, TYR, OCA2, SLC24A5, MATP,* and *ASIP*.[1]

Disorders of hypopigmentation may be linked to a variety of causal factors, including genetic defects or acquired conditions such as vitiligo or contact with topical environmental agents, as a sequel to another inflammatory skin disease, or due to systemic drug intake leading to hypopigmentation.

DIAGNOSTIC APPROACH TO HYPOPIGMENTATION

The diagnostic approach to patients with cutaneous hypopigmentation requires an understanding of the types of hypopigmentation disorders. Hypopigmentation disorders are classified as hypomelanotic/amelanotic and hypomelanocytic/amelanocytic, which are due to melanin deficiency and reduction or absence of melanocyte number, respectively. For the diagnostic approach, a further categorization that distinguishes cutaneous hypopigmentation disorders into congenital or acquired, and circumscribed, mixed, or generalized may be extremely helpful.[2,3]

The approach to the patient presenting with hypopigmentation is based on a thorough understanding of the possible causes of hypopigmentation and the clinical presentation of each condition. A diagnostic approach includes:

- *Family history of hypopigmentation*
- *Medical history to ask the patient for*:
  1. A known history of other skin diseases that may result in temporary hypopigmentation during the resolution of their primary lesions, such as psoriasis. The characteristic primary or secondary lesions of these skin diseases may also be present.
  2. Infectious or parasitic skin diseases (leprosy, treponematoses), sarcoidosis, and mycosis fungoides may present with hypopigmentation or hypopigmented lesions. The characteristic primary or secondary lesions of these skin diseases are also usually present to guide the diagnosis. Morphea, discoid lupus, lichen sclerosus, and scleroderma may present hypopigmented/depigmented lesions with concomitant induration or epidermal atrophy that will guide correct diagnosis.[4]
  3. The use of systemic drugs or topical agents should be investigated as a possible cause of hypopigmentation/depigmentation.
  4. Ask about traveling to endemic regions for endemic treponematosis.

- *History of hypopigmentation*: Age at onset (congenital or later in life), stable or increasing in size
- *Complete physical examination*: Distribution and extent of hypopigmentation (widespread or circumscribed), presence of hair hypopigmentation, other skin lesions, palpation of lymph nodes
- *Wood's light examination*:
  - Accentuates (increases contrast) depigmented (chalk-white) skin and may differentiate from hypopigmented (off-white) skin. In depigmented skin, there is absence of epidermal melanin, and the underlying fluorescent compounds of the skin give a characteristic chalky bluish-white appearance. On the contrary, hypopigmented skin shows an off-white accentuation without fluorescence.[4]
  - Punctiform red to orange fluorescence may be seen in the follicles in progressive macular hypomelanosis of the trunk.[5]
- *Further evaluations depending on suspected condition may include*:
  - *For tuberous sclerosis complex (TSC)*: Genetic testing, renal ultrasound, cardiac echocardiogram, ophthalmologic evaluation, neuroimaging
  - *For suspected hypopigmentation due to gene defects in the pigmentation pathway*: Hearing screening, ophthalmologic evaluation
  - *For hypopigmented mycosis fungoides, sarcoidosis, leprosy*: Cutaneous biopsy and histopathologic examination to establish diagnosis

14 Approach to hypopigmentation

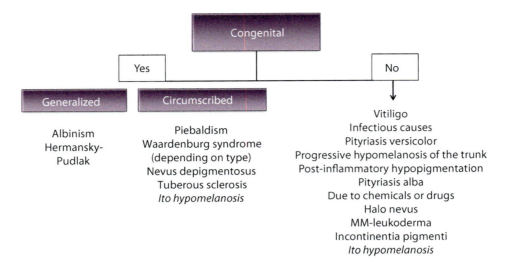

Figure 2.1 Diagnostic approach to hypopigmentation. (Hypopigmented lesions of Ito hypomelanosis may be recognized at birth or become visible during the neonatal period or early childhood.)

CONGENITAL HYPOPIGMENTATION OR NOT?

An important step in the diagnostic ladder of hypopigmentation is answering the question of whether the hypopigmentation is congenital (i.e., present at birth) (Figure 2.1). A basic classification of hypopigmentation is summarized below:

a. *Congenital hypopigmentation*
   - Due to defects in the pigmentation pathway: widespread or circumscribed
   - Nevus depigmentosus
   - Ito hypomelanosis
   - Tuberous sclerosis

b. *Not congenital hypopigmentation*
   - Incontinentia pigmenti
   - Acquired hypopigmentation
     - Vitiligo
     - Pityriasis versicolor
     - Progressive hypomelanosis of the trunk
     - Pityriasis alba
     - Post-inflammatory hypopigmentation
     - Melanoma leukoderma
     - Due to chemicals or drugs

SPECIAL CONSIDERATIONS BASED ON THE DISTRIBUTION OF HYPOPIGMENTATION

The distribution of hypopigmentation may assist in the diagnostic approach (Figure 2.2). Examples of characteristic distribution in disorders of hypopigmentation include:

- *Following Blaschko lines*: Incontinentia pigmenti, linear hypomelanosis (congenital, stable)
- *Bilateral, symmetric distribution of white patches that may progress over time*: Nonsegmental vitiligo
- *Segmental*: Vitiligo

- *Conditions with discrete hypopigmented macules*: Tuberous sclerosis complex, idiopathic guttate hypomelanosis, post-inflammatory hypopigmentation
- *Conditions with discrete depigmented macules*: Vitiligo, drug- or chemical-induced leukoderma

CONGENITAL HYPOPIGMENTATION

Human congenital disorders of hypopigmentation may originate from mutations affecting the complex pathway of melanocyte development and function. The distinction

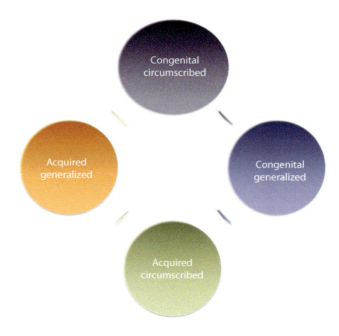

Figure 2.2 The distribution of hypopigmentation assists in the diagnostic approach.

of a genetic disorder of hypopigmentation is important, as genetic defects in the migration of melanoblasts, or the formation of melanin pathways or melanosome formation and transfer, as presented above, are not expected to improve/repigment with systemic or topical treatments or phototherapy.

Further disorders of hypopigmentation that may be congenital (i.e., present at birth), but are not caused by specific gene defects, are Ito hypomelanosis and nevus depigmentosus, which are due to cutaneous mosaicism. Also, tuberous sclerosis complex is a multisystem disease that may present with characteristic hypopigmented lesions. It may be familial or sporadic. Among sporadic cases, most (over 70%) are due to defects in the tuberous sclerosis complex genes *TSC1* and *TSC2*. However, these genes do not regulate in the pigmentation pathway, but are involved in cell growth and proliferation.[6] There are cases of hypopigmented lesions, such as nevus depigmentosus or hypopigmented lesions of tuberous sclerosis, that may be congenital but are not noticed until infancy when the child is exposed to the sun, especially in very light-colored skin.

Disorders of hypopigmentation due to gene defects in the pigmentation pathway

Genetic disorders of hypopigmentation are typically present at birth. They are caused by an inherited genetic defect in a particular step in the pigmentation pathway. The cutaneous pigmentation is a multistep process regulated by various signaling pathways and transcription factors and includes the following major steps (Figure 2.3)[1,7]:

1. Melanoblast migration from the neural crest to the skin (Waardenburg syndrome type 1–4/WS1-WS4, piebaldism, Tietz syndrome). Melanoblasts, the precursors of melanocytes, migrate, proliferate, and differentiate on their way to the basal epitheium of the epidermis and hair bulbs of the skin, the uveal tract of the eye, the stria vascularis, the vestibular organ and the endolymphatic sac of the ear, and the leptomeninges of the brain.[8] So, genetic disorders of hypopigmentation due to genetic defects of melanoblast migration may be accompanied by extracutaneous findings such as deafness and eye disorders.
2. Melanin synthesis in the melanosome (oculocutaneous albinism type 1–4/OCA1-4).
3. Melanosome formation in the melanocytes (Hermansky-Pudlak syndrome type 1–7/HPS1-7, Chediak-Higashi syndrome/CHS1).
4. Mature melanosome transfer to the tips of the dendrites (Griscelli syndrome type 1–3/GS1-3).

The basic differentiating characteristics of congenital disorders of hypopigmentation caused by gene defects in the pigmentation pathway are summarized in Table 2.1.

Piebaldism and Waardenburg and Tietz syndromes represent disorders of melanoblast migration or proliferation during embryonic development and are characterized by stable congenital white patches of the skin (leukoderma) and hair (poliosis or white forelock).[1]

Piebaldism: Rare autosomal dominant disorder with congenital depigmented patches of the midforehead, chest, abdomen, and extremities, where no melanocytes are found. These patches may sometimes contain hyperpigmented macules. Cutaneous depigmentation ranges from only a

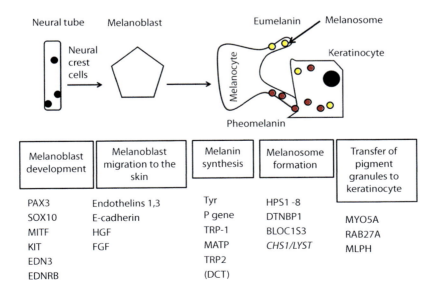

Figure 2.3 Biologic function of melanocytes and genes that control the pigmentary pathway. MATP, membrane-associated transporter protein; MITF, microphthalmia transcription factor; TRP, tyrosinase-related protein; BLOC3, biogenesis of lysosome-related organelle complex; HPS, Hermansky-Pudlak syndrome; CHS, Chediak-Higashi syndrome; MYO5A, myosin 5A; MLPH, melanophilin; DCT, dopachrome tautomerase; EDN3, endothelin 3; EDNRB, endothelin receptor B. (From Dessinioti C et al. *Exp Dermatol* 2009;18:741–749, with permission.)

Table 2.1 Basic useful characteristics for the differential diagnosis of disorders of depigmentation caused by gene defects in the pigmentation pathway

	Albinism	Hermansky-Pudlak syndrome	Chediak-Higashi syndrome	Griscelli syndrome	Piebaldism	Waardenburg syndrome
Etiology	Genetic	Genetic	Genetic	Genetic	Genetic	Genetic
Inherited or sporadic	Inherited	Inherited	Inherited	Inherited	Inherited	Inherited
Age at onset of depigmentation	Congenital	Congenital	Congenital	Congenital	Congenital	Congenital
Distribution of depigmentation	Generalized	Generalized or circumscribed	Generalized Silvery sheen to the hair and skin	Pigmentary dilution of skin, hair	Circumscribed	Circumscribed
Type of disorder of depigmentation	Normal melanocytes, no melanin	Normal melanocytes, no melanin	Disorder of melanosome formation and transfer	Disorder of melanosome formation and transfer	No melanocytes in white lesions	No melanocytes in white lesions
Clinical findings	Depending on type Skin, hair, eyes Photophobia, nystagmus, decreased visual acuity, cutaneous sensitivity to UVR, increased risk for NMSC	Depending on type Ocular/cutaneous albinism Platelet disorders: bleeding diathesis, ceroid storage disease resulting in pulmonary fibrosis, kidney failure, granulomatous colitis	Decreased iris pigmentation, strabismus, nystagmus, severe immunodeficiency, pancytopenia, bleeding, bruising, hepatosplenomegaly, neurological disorders	Depending on type Immune defects, neurological manifestations	White forelock White patches may contain hyperpigmented macules	Depending on type White patches of skin and hair Heterochromia irides, dystopia canthorum, congenital deafness, limb anomalies, Hirschsprung disease
Course of depigmentation	Stable	Stable	Stable	Stable	Stable	Stable

white forelock with minimal ventral depigmentation to almost entire body and hair depigmentation.[9,10]

Waardenburg syndrome (WS): Autosomal dominant genetic disorder characterized by piebaldism and sensorineural deafness. The disease is commonly classified into four clinical types with possible extracutaneous findings.[1,11,12]

Tietz syndrome: Rare autosomal dominant disorder, characterized by generalized depigmentation, blue eyes, and congenital deafness.[13]

Most forms of congenital hypopigmentation that are caused by defects in melanin synthesis are types of oculocutaneous albinism (OCA) and affect ocular as well as cutaneous melanocytes.[1]

Hermansky-Pudlak syndrome: Rare, albinism with extrapigmentary disorders. Platelet storage pool deficiency resulting in bleeding diathesis, ceroid storage disease resulting in pulmonary fibrosis, kidney failure, granulomatous colitis.[14]

Chediak-Higashi syndrome: Rare autosomal recessive disorder characterized by oculocutaneous albinism, neutropenia, recurrent infections, thrombocytopenia, bleeding diathesis, neurologic defects. Fatal in the first decade of life from infections or bleeding.[6] Most cases are fatal unless treated by bone marrow transplantation.

Griscelli syndrome (GS): Rare autosomal recessive disorder characterized by oculocutaneous albinism, severe immunodeficiency, neurologic defects.[1]

NONCONGENITAL HYPOPIGMENTATION

The basic differentiating characteristics of disorders with hypopigmentation/depigmentation that typically appear later in life are summarized in Table 2.2.

Incontinentia pigmenti (IP) is a rare, hereditary, X-linked dominant disorder that may present with hypopigmentation in adult life. IP is usually lethal in males, so female patients are almost exclusively recognized (92%). *IKBKG* (previously *NEMO*) is the gene known to be associated with IP.[15] Stages of skin changes in IP include stage 1 (vesiculo-bullous stage), stage 2 (verrucous stage), and stage 3 (hyperpigmented stage). The fourth stage (atrophic/hypopigmented stage) may present in approximately 13% of patients with IP. Hypopigmentation presents as swirls of atrophic hypopigmented or depigmented bands of streaks along the Blaschko lines, which are also hypohydrotic and hairless. Reduction of melanin in the epidermis has been described. The hypopigmented lesions present in adult life. Extracutaneous abnormalities are frequent[3] (Table 2.2). Diagnostic criteria have been proposed.[15]

Acquired disorders of hypopigmentation

Vitiligo is a common disorder of hypopigmentation.[3] It may appear at any age, but usually presents during childhood or young adulthood, while it is rarely described in newborns and infants.[3] Vitiligo may be classified on the basis of the extension and distribution of lesions into nonsegmental vitiligo (NSV, including acrofacial, mucosal, generalized, universal, mixed, and rare variants) and segmental vitiligo

(SV).[16] NSV presents with amelanotic lesions on various body areas with a bilateral and symmetrical distribution that may spread or repigment over time, showing an unpredictable course. SV is characterized by an early age of onset; rapid stabilization; and unilateral, segmental distribution (Table 2.2).[3]

Acquired diseases that may present with hypopigmented skin lesions include sarcoidosis, pityriasis versicolor, leprosy, syphilis (leukoderma syphiliticum), and hypopigmented mycosis fungoides.[5,10]

Furthermore, post-inflammatory hypopigmentation may be caused by various skin diseases during the resolution of their primary skin lesions, as is the case with psoriasis. A thorough medical history is essential for the diagnostic approach to the patient, as hypopigmentation may be due to topical agents or systemic drug intake. Melanoma-associated leukoderma may appear in patients with melanoma treated with immunotherapy and is a reported marker of favorable prognosis.[4,17]

Idiopathic guttate hypomelanosis presents with sharply demarcated, hypopigmented to depigmented macules, mainly in adults of more advanced age, and shows a predilection for the lower, or more rarely, the upper extremities.[5]

Progressive macular hypomelanosis of the trunk presents with hypopigmented macules or patches on the trunk. There is characteristic punctiform red to orange fluorescence in the follicles under Wood's lamp light.[5]

Tuberous sclerosis complex

Tuberous sclerosis complex is a genetic disease that may be caused by inherited or sporadic mutations and leads to hamartomatous lesions in many organs that appear in different periods of life.[6] Patients with TSC often seek medical attention due to skin lesions or for seizures. TSC may be diagnosed by positive genetic testing and with clinical diagnostic criteria (two major or one major with two or more minor for definite diagnosis, and either one major or two or more minor for possible diagnosis). Negative genetic testing does not exclude TSC diagnosis.[18] A complete skin examination should be performed to evaluate for the number of hypopigmented macules; the presence of angiofibromas on the face; "confetti" skin lesions; and a shagreen patch, most commonly on the lower back, that may present from an early age. The characteristic hypopigmented macules (ash leaf) were first described by Fitzpatrick in 1968.[19] They may appear at birth or present within the first few years of life.[19,20] Wood's lamp examination to accentuate hypomelanotic macules is beneficial in the detection of these macules in infants (Table 2.2). The number of melanocytes is not decreased in TSC hypopigmented lesions, in contrast with the lesions of vitiligo.[21] There is decreased melanization of melanosomes.[3] In older patients, dental pits and ungual fibromas may be clinically detected. Clinical suspicion of TSC will prompt further evaluations and follow-up.[18] Improvement of hypomelanotic macules has been reported with topical rapamycin in a small number of patients[21–23] and with topical sirolimus in a patient with TSC.[24]

Table 2.2 Basic useful characteristics for the differential diagnosis of disorders of hypopigmentation/depigmentation

	Vitiligo	Ito hypomelanosis	Nevus depigmentosus	Incontinentia pigmenti	Tuberous sclerosis
Etiology	Acquired	Cutaneous mosaicism	Cutaneous mosaicism	Genetic	Genetic
Inherited or sporadic	Sporadic or familial (heritable)	Sporadic or inherited	Nonhereditary	Inherited	Sporadic or inherited
Age at onset of hypopigmentation	Any age; Childhood or young adulthood; Very rarely congenital	Congenital; Neonatal; Early infancy	Congenital, rarely early childhood	Usually only females; Adults	Hypopigmented (off-white) macules may be present at birth or within the first years of life
Distribution of hypopigmentation	Generalized or circumscribed; Symmetrical	Circumscribed; Unilateral or bilateral, following Blaschko lines	Unilateral off-white lesions; May be solitary	Circumscribed, following Blaschko lines	Discrete hypopigmented macules
Type of disorder of hypopigmentation	Normal melanocytes, no melanin	Decreased number of melanocytes	Normal number of melanocytes, decrease of melanin	Reduction of melanin in the epidermis	Decreased melanization of melanosomes
Clinical findings	White, depigmented patches of skin and hair; Chalky bluish-white appearance with Wood's light	Linear whorled hypomelanosis; Disorders of central nervous system, eyes, teeth	Hypomelanotic lesion, does not cross the midline; Off-white with Wood's lamp	In 13%, whorled hypomelanosis. Linear, atrophic, hypohidrotic hypomelanosis; Loss of hair in lesions; Disorders of central nervous system, eyes, teeth, hair	Hypopigmented off-white skin macules; Confetti-like macules; Epilepsy, angiofibromas, retinal hamartomas, renal angiomyolipoma, cardiac rhabdomyoma (diagnostic criteria apply)
Course of hypopigmentation	Unpredictable for NSV. May progress or repigment with treatment	Stable	Stable	Stable	Repigmentation with treatment has been reported in a small number of patients

REFERENCES

1. Dessinioti C, Stratigos AJ, Rigopoulos D, Katsambas AD. A review of genetic disorders of hypopigmentation: Lessons learned from the biology of melanocytes. *Exp Dermatol.* 2009;18(9):741–749.

2. Mollet I, Ongenae K, Naeyaert JM. Origin, clinical presentation, and diagnosis of hypomelanotic skin disorders. *Dermatol Clin.* 2007;25(3):363–371, ix.

3. Ortonne JP, Bahadoran P, Fitzaptrick TB et al. Hypomelanoses and hypermelanoses. In: Freedberg IM, Eisen AZ, Woff K. et al., eds. *Fitzpatrick's Dermatology in General Medicine.* New York: McGraw-Hill; 2003:836–881.

4. Saleem MD, Oussedik E, Schoch JJ, Berger AC, Picardo M. Acquired disorders with depigmentation: A systematic approach to vitiliginoid conditions. *J Am Acad Dermatol.* 2018.

5. Saleem MD, Oussedik E, Picardo M, Schoch JJ. Acquired disorders with hypopigmentation: A clinical approach to diagnosis and treatment. *J Am Acad Dermatol.* 2018.

6. Narayanan V. Tuberous sclerosis complex: Genetics to pathogenesis. *Pediatr Neurol.* 2003;29(5):404–409.

7. Tomita Y, Suzuki T. Genetics of pigmentary disorders. *Am J Med Genet C Semin Med Genet.* 2004;131C(1):75–81.

8. Lin JY, Fisher DE. Melanocyte biology and skin pigmentation. *Nature.* 2007;445(7130):843–850.

9. Giebel LB, Spritz RA. Mutation of the KIT (mast/stem cell growth factor receptor) protooncogene in human piebaldism. *Proc Natl Acad Sci USA.* 1991;88(19):8696–8699.

10. Dessinioti C, Stratigos AJ. Piebaldism. https://www.dermatologyadvisor.com/dermatology/piebaldism/article/691421/. Accessed January 2, 2019.

11. Zazo Seco C, Serrao de Castro L, van Nierop JW et al. Allelic mutations of KITLG, encoding KIT ligand, cause asymmetric and unilateral hearing loss and Waardenburg syndrome type 2. *Am J Hum Genet.* 2015;97(5):647–660.

12. Liu XZ, Newton VE, Read AP. Waardenburg syndrome type II: Phenotypic findings and diagnostic criteria. *Am J Med Genet.* 1995;55(1):95–100.

13. Smith SD, Kelley PM, Kenyon JB, Hoover D. Tietz syndrome (hypopigmentation/deafness) caused by mutation of MITF. *J Med Genet.* 2000;37(6):446–448.

14. Wei ML. Hermansky-Pudlak syndrome: A disease of protein trafficking and organelle function. *Pigm Cell Res.* 2006;19(1):19–42.

15. Minic S, Trpinac D, Obradovic M. Incontinentia pigmenti diagnostic criteria update. *Clin Genet.* 2014;85(6):536–542.

16. Ezzedine K, Lim HW, Suzuki T et al. Revised classification/nomenclature of vitiligo and related issues: The Vitiligo Global Issues Consensus Conference. *Pigment Cell Melanoma Res.* 2012;25(3):E1–E13.

17. Gogas H, Ioannovich J, Dafni U et al. Prognostic significance of autoimmunity during treatment of melanoma with interferon. *N Engl J Med.* 2006;354(7):709–718.

18. Northrup H, Krueger DA, International Tuberous Sclerosis Complex Consensus Group. Tuberous sclerosis complex diagnostic criteria update: Recommendations of the 2012 International Tuberous Sclerosis Complex Consensus Conference. *Pediatr Neurol.* 2013;49(4):243–254.

19. Fitzpatrick TB, Szabo G, Hori Y, Simone AA, Reed WB, Greenberg MH. White leaf-shaped macules. Earliest visible sign of tuberous sclerosis. *Arch Dermatol.* 1968;98(1):1–6.

20. Teng JM, Cowen EW, Wataya-Kaneda M et al. Dermatologic and dental aspects of the 2012 International Tuberous Sclerosis Complex Consensus statements. *JAMA Dermatol.* 2014;150(10):1095–1101.

21. Arbiser JL. Efficacy of rapamycin in tuberous sclerosis-associated hypopigmented macules: Back to the future. *JAMA Dermatol.* 2015;151(7):703–704.

22. Wataya-Kaneda M, Tanaka M, Yang L et al. Clinical and histologic analysis of the efficacy of topical rapamycin therapy against hypomelanotic macules in tuberous sclerosis complex. *JAMA Dermatol.* 2015;151(7):722–730.

23. Jozwiak S, Sadowski K, Kotulska K, Schwartz RA. Topical use of mammalian target of rapamycin (mTOR) inhibitors in tuberous sclerosis complex-A comprehensive review of the literature. *Pediatr Neurol.* 2016;61:21–27.

24. Malissen N, Vergely L, Simon M, Roubertie A, Malinge MC, Bessis D. Long-term treatment of cutaneous manifestations of tuberous sclerosis complex with topical 1% sirolimus cream: A prospective study of 25 patients. *J Am Acad Dermatol.* 2017;77(3):464–472. e463.

Historical review of vitiligo

3

MAJA KOVACEVIC, NIKA FRANCESCHI, MIRNA SITUM, ANDY GOREN,
ANDRIJA STANIMIROVIC, YAN VALLE, and TORELLO LOTTI

CONTENTS

Introduction	21	Treatment of vitiligo through the ages	22
Perception of vitiligo from ancient times to the modern period	21	Prognosis	24
		References	24
Social stigmatization of patients from ancient times to the modern period	22		

INTRODUCTION

Vitiligo, as well as other pigmentation disorders, has been observed throughout history. These disorders causing white, light, or dark spots have caused distress and rejection and have led to the isolation of affected people for thousands of years. Until the invention of the microscope and biopsy and the discovery of histochemical stains, skin color was a mystery and the mechanism for skin color production was based on myths, folklore, and religious theories.[1] Over the years, various theories have been proposed regarding the etiology of vitiligo, while the most accepted theories include the genetic, autoimmune, neurogenic, and melanocyte self-destruction hypotheses.[2] Treatments for this disorder have been investigated since ancient times and various remedies have been suggested in medical literature over the years. Although great progress has recently been achieved regarding this depigmentation disorder, a long history of difficult management and the still perplexing etiology of the disease, as well as ill treatment of patients suffering from this disorder, indicate the importance of further scientific research, along with education of the public and patients concerning this disease. First, however, as Hippocrates declared, "The physician must know what his predecessors have known if he does not wish to deceive both himself and others."[3]

PERCEPTION OF VITILIGO FROM ANCIENT TIMES TO THE MODERN PERIOD

From ancient times, depigmenting disorders altered the quality of a patient's life. The earliest descriptions of these disorders were found in Iranian literature, *Tarkh-e-Tibble*, in 2200 BC,[4] while the *Ebers Papyrus* from 1500 BC observes two types of disorders that affect skin color, probably both vitiligo and leprosy.[5] Various terms describing white spots such as "Kilas," "Palita," "Sveta Khista," and "Charak" were found in Indian sacred books, *Atharva Veda* (1400 BC), and the Buddhist sacred book *Vinay Pitak* (224–544 BC).[6] Some of the terms, such as "Sveta Khista," were used to describe leprosy, so it is not surprising that vitiligo was often confused with this disease. White skin was also mentioned in literature from the Far East dating from 1200 BC, in prayers known as Makatominoharai where the "shira bito" or white man is described (Kopera). In his book *Clio*, Greek historian Herodotus (484–425 BC) notices white spots on foreigners and considers them a sign of sin against the sun.[7]

Several religious books also mention vitiligo. In the Old Testament of the Holy Bible, the Hebrew word "Zora'at" includes five groups of depigmenting disorders combined with other entities such as inflammation, scaling, atrophy, white hairs, and "white spots" per se, interpreted as vitiligo or post-inflammatory leukoderma.[6] In the Greek version of the Bible, Leviticus 13, the word "Zora'at" was translated as "white leprosy," which enhanced the prejudices toward the disease. In the Koran, the Arabic name for vitiligo, "alabras," is mentioned and was also translated as "leprosy" in several languages. Taking into consideration all mistranslations, it is not surprising that even Hippocrates (460–355 BC) included vitiligo, leprosy, lichen, and psoriasis in the same category of diseases.

The term "vitiligo" was most probably first used by Celsus in the first century BC in his medical publication *De Medicina* and may have been derived from the Latin word "vitium" meaning defect or blemish, or "vitulum" meaning small blemish.[8] Others, however, suggest that the term may have been derived from the Latin word "vitelius," meaning calf, referring to the skin of this animal.[8]

European descriptions of vitiligo date from the Early Modern age. In the sixteenth century, Italian physician Hieronymus Mercurialis elucidated the pathogenesis of vitiligo in his book *De morbus cutaneis* (Mercurialis). According to his explanation, accumulated phlegm under the skin results in the appearance of leukoderma, and as a confirmation of his theory, he uses the ancient writings of the Greek philosopher Plato.[1] In the seventeenth century, Korean authors described certain hypopigmented and depigmented entities such as vitiligo, naevus depigmentosus, tinea versicolor, naevus anemicus, and albinism in *Doney Bogam*, Eastern medical writing from the Yi dynasty.[9] Proposed therapeutic options included arsenic, mercury, and sulfur ointments. The importance of the disease was further emphasized by the portrait of an eminent official of the Korean Yi dynasty whose face was painted with vitiligo lesions.[10] Interestingly, with this artwork, Korean society showed acceptance of the patients and not discrimination, contrary to many other civilizations at that time and also today.

In the nineteenth century, Louis Brocq introduced the term "dyschromy," defined by the lack of pigmentation (achromy) in vitiliginous skin combined with an increase of pigmentation at the periphery of the lesion (hyperchromy).[11] In the same century, histopathologic characteristics of vitiligo were described by Moritz Kaposi as lack of pigment granules in deep rete cells and increase of pigmentation on the periphery.[12] The etiology of the disease remained questionable from ancient times to the modern period. From the nineteenth century, the role of triggering factors has been suggested in vitiligo onset, with emotional stress and stimulation of the nervous system being predominant.[11] A definition of vitiligo was finally established in the twentieth century: "Vitiligo can be described as an acquired, primary, usually progressive, melanocyte loss of still mysterious etiology, clinically characterized by circumscribed achromic macules often associated with leucotrichia, and progressive disappearance of melanocytes in the involved skin."[6,13]

SOCIAL STIGMATIZATION OF PATIENTS FROM ANCIENT TIMES TO THE MODERN PERIOD

Social stigmatization of patients with vitiligo has been described alongside the first writings about the disease itself. Buddhist literature indicates that patients with Kilasa were not able to become priests, while Indian Rigveda literature considers patients with Switra, as well as their offspring, unsuitable for marriage.[6] Herodotus believed that vitiligo patients were sinners against the sun, and, interestingly, his hypothesis included animals as well, mainly white pigeons. In Leviticus (13:34), descriptions of patients with white spots include torn clothes, untidy hair, and covering of their upper lip due to the belief that they are unclean and have sinned against the God.[14] In order to reduce social stigmatization of vitiligo patients, the Catholic church added in 1943 the following note with reference to Leviticus 13: "Various kinds of skin blemishes are treated here, which were not contagious but simply disqualified their subjects from associations with others, until they were declared ritually clean. The Hebrew term used does not refer to Hansen disease, currently called leprosy."[6]

According to Islamic theologians, if the husband or wife had baras, it was a legitimate reason for divorce. Harrith bin Hilliza, an Arabic poet, states that vitiligo patients were able to receive emperors' messages only if they were behind a screen, in order to avoid direct contact. Stigmatization and disfigurement of vitiligo patients were also present in the nineteenth century. In his writings, Brito describes the disfigurement of vitiligo patients: "The appearance of the unfortunate victims of vitiligo is striking, and scarcely fails to evoke a feeling of horror and pity for the afflicted. The picture of otherwise dark person, marked with spots perfectly white, even to eyes familiarized to the sight, appears repugnant."[15]

Due to the long-lasting misleading association of contagion with vitiligo, stigmatization of vitiligo patients is still present nowadays. Modern life dictates perfection in different contexts; imperfection in skin appearance due to evident contrast of depigmented patches causes emotional devastation in many patients. Any condition that impairs skin appearance might have different consequences in the sense of normal social life, work opportunities, and emotional bonding as well. Despite global progress in modern times, vitiligo still remains a disease that leads to low self-esteem, depression, self-consciousness, isolation, and stigmatization in many countries worldwide.

TREATMENT OF VITILIGO THROUGH THE AGES

Treatment of white spots or vitiligo has been sought since the disorder was first observed, attesting to the significance of the disease in all cultures and societies. In Table 3.1, a partial list of treatment modalities tried throughout history is presented.

The *Ebers Papyrus* (c. 1550 BC), the *Atharva Veda*, (c. 1400 BC), other Indian and Buddhist medical literature (c. 200 AC), and Chinese literature from the Sung period (c. 700 AC) mention herbal remedies for the treatment of vitiligo.[6]

According to Indian medical literature, "Malapu" (*Ficus hispida*) and "Babchi" (*Psoralea corylifolia*) administered orally or topically were the most effective remedies.[16] In the "Charaka Samhita," juice of the fruit "Malapu" is recommended followed by exposure to sunlight. Subsequently developed blisters should be ruptured, after which repigmentation occurs. Other recommendations for curing "Svitra" in the "Charaka Samhita" include preparations with seeds of radish and Babchi seeds rubbed in cow's urine; a plaster prepared of redwood fig, Babchi seeds, and white flowered leadwort in cow's urine; red arsenic prepared with peacock's bile; seeds of Babchi, lac, or ox-bile; and extracts of Indian berberry, antimony, long pepper, and iron powder.[17,18] *Psoralea corylifolia*, called "Pu Ku Chih," is also mentioned in the ancient Chinese literature as a method for treating leukoderma.[19] It was later established that both of these herbs, "Malapu" and "Babchi," contain psoralens, demonstrating that photochemotherapy was also practiced in ancient times.[17] The *Atharva Veda* mentions two drugs, "asikni" and "shyama," that lead to repigmentation of the skin when applied topically. These medicines were praised in poems in an attempt to even skin color.[16]

Seeds of the plant *Ammi majus* that grows as a weed in the Nile Delta were used by Egyptians. The Arabic pharmaceutical encyclopedia *Mofradat Al Adwiya* (*The Book of Medicinal and Nutritional Terms*) written by Ibn El-Bitar (c. 1200 BC) first documented the use of *Ammi majus*. Exposure to sunlight followed the administration of the remedy. The usefulness of this plant was also known

Table 3.1 Partial list of treatments for vitiligo throughout history

Topical and oral treatments	• Rose-flavored honey • Bitter almonds in vinegar • Babchi seeds • Bergamot • Ginkgo biloba • Anapsos • Agaric • Turpeth • Colocynth • Khellin • Tincture of nux vomica • Syrup of betony • Oxymel • Mustard • Copper • Iron • Zinc • Manganese • Nickel • Cobalt • Calcium • Arsenic • Silver nitrate • Dopa • ACTH • Metharmon-F • α-MSH • Melagenina • Vitamins: B_6, B_{12}, C, D, E • Prostaglandin analogue • Ascorbic acid • Folic acid • Hydrochloric acid • Hydrogen peroxide • Pseudocatalase • Steroids • Calcineurin inhibitors • Methotrexate • Levamisole • Tretinoin • Carmustine (BCNU) • Clofazimine • Antimalarials: Chloroquine, quinacrine, mefloquine • Thiambutosine • Cyclosporine • Dapsone • Fluorouracil • Fluphenazine enanthate • Mechlorethamine • Aspirin • Isoprinosine • Cyclophosphamide • Resorcin paste

(Continued)

Table 3.1 (Continued) Partial list of treatments for vitiligo throughout history

	• Lithium salts • Pentoxifylline • Minoxidil • Monoamine oxidase inhibitors • Monobenzyl ether of hydroquinone • Vesicants • Escharotics • Corrosive sublimate • Cantharidin • Byzantine syrup • Crude coal tar • Anthralin • Anapsos
Procedures and phototherapy	• Cryotherapy • Dermabrasion • Surgical excision • Minigrafting autografts • Thermal and caustic blistering • Vibrapuncture • Finsen lamp • Phenylalanine-UVA • Psoralens + sunlight • Psoralen + UVA • Narrowband UVB
Other	• Cosmetics • Diets • Tattooing

Source: Adapted from Montes LF. *Vitiligo: Current Knowledge and Nutritional Therapy.* 3rd ed. Buenos Aires: Westhoven Press; 2006; Sehgal VN, Srivastava G. *J Dermatolog Treat.* 2006; 17(5):262–275.

to a Berberian tribe living in northwestern Africa under the name Aatrillal.[6,17]

In ancient Korea, sulfur and various arsenic or mercury ointments were applied locally following exposure to sunlight. Another topically applied remedy combined the juice of fig fruit and leaves, unripe walnut shells, moss, Japanese parsley, buttercups, and rice bran followed by exposure to sunlight. However, patients were frequently overexposed to sunlight, resulting in extreme sunburn and worsening of depigmented lesions. Other methods included the use of garlic, ginger, or vinegar to induce skin irritation. Herbal remedies containing ginseng, black sesame, white peony, sweet flag plant, barberry root, and chaulmoogra seeds were administered orally and depended on the type of vitiligo. It was suggested that they normalized the immune imbalance of the body. Medicine consisting of parsley and angelica induced photosensitization following exposure to sunlight, as they contain furocoumarins. Other treatments included acupuncture along with topically applied herbs, while red bean powder was used as cosmetic camouflage.[9]

In the beginning of the nineteenth century, systemic application of bromides, iodides, valerianates, mercury, antimony, and arsenic was used, as well as subcutaneous injection of pilocarpine, saline, or bromoiodic baths. Different mixtures containing croton oil, iodine, sublimate, and naphtol have been suggested for topical use; however, all these recommendations showed limited to no effect.[20] In his work, Brito listed possible treatment options such as the use of silver nitrate; excision, which may be succeeded by grafts; dermal injections of silver nitrate solutions followed by exposure to sunlight; tattooing; and internal administration of silver salts for treating vitiligo.[15]

Photo(chemo)therapy

In the beginning of the twentieth century, Nils Ryberg Finsen, the founder of modern phototherapy, developed the Finsen light, a source of short ultraviolet (UV) waves produced by a carbon or mercury arc. Finsen was awarded the Nobel Prize in Medicine in 1903 for his contribution to the treatment of lupus vulgaris with concentrated light radiation, starting a whole new era in the treatment of dermatologic diseases. Subsequently, patients with vitiligo were exposed to such UV light and, in certain patients, visible improvement was seen after a series of treatments.[20,21]

The basis for future development of phototherapy occurred in the 1940s when the active ingredients of *Ammi majus*, 8-methoxypsoralen (8-MOP) and 5-methoxypsoralen (5-MOP), were isolated. The first studies with 8-MOP followed by sun exposure were performed in vitiligo patients by the Egyptian physician Abdel Moneim El-Mofty, showing promising results.[22–24] Subsequent studies in patients with vitiligo confirmed the good safety profile and efficacy of these psoralens.[25,26]

In the 1970s, ultraviolet irradiators emitting high-intensity ultraviolet A (UVA) radiation were invented that were designed for oral psoralen photochemotherapy to deliver uniform high doses of UVA irradiation. This approach was much more effective and represented the real start of psoralen plus ultraviolet A (PUVA) photochemotherapy, a term introduced by Fitzpatrick and Parrish.[27,28] PUVA became the treatment of choice for a wide variety of skin disorders. The use of PUVA has recently declined due to evidence of photodamage and photocarcinogenesis and the development of narrowband ultraviolet light B (311 nm) irradiation devices, shown to be as efficacious as PUVA for vitiligo with fewer side effects.[29–32]

Topical corticosteroids

The first study involving a topical corticosteroid was conducted in the 1970s with betamethasone 17-valerate in flexible collodion by Kandil, applied once daily on localized vitiligo macules with more or less satisfactory results, depending on the duration of the disease and disease stage.[33] Other studies involving betamethasone 17-valerate soon followed.[34,35] Additionally, studies involving clobetasol propionate 0.05% cream[36–39] and later fluticasone propionate and mometasone were also conducted.[40]

Topical calcineurin inhibitors

In 2002, the first studies with tacrolimus ointment 0.03% and 0.1% were conducted in patients with vitiligo. Findings showed that tacrolimus ointment was an effective and safe treatment modality.[41–43] A case report involving a 19-year-old patient with vitiligo on the face treated with pimecrolimus cream followed.[44]

PROGNOSIS

The prognosis of vitiligo has also been documented in ancient literature. In a compilation of ancient Indian medicine, *Ashtanga Hridaya* (600 AD), written by Vagbhata, "Svitra can be cured if the hair over these patches has not turned white; if the patches are not numerous; if the patches are not connected with each other; if the patches have freshly occurred; and if the patches are not caused by burns." The condition termed "kilāsa," a variety of leukoderma, was regarded as being "incurable if the patches were present in the genital and anal regions, palms and lips, even if these patches were fresh. Such patients should never be treated if the physician desired to have success in life."[17,45] In the work "Prognostic," Hippocrates also made similar observations that "these complaints (vitiligo) are the more easily cured the more recent they are, and the younger the patients, and the more the soft and fleshy the parts of the body in which they occur."[14,17]

REFERENCES

1. Nordlund JJ. The medical treatment of vitiligo: An historical review. *Dermatol Clin.* 2017;35(2):107–116.
2. Koranne RV, Sachdeva KG. Vitiligo. *Int J Dermatol.* December 1988;27(10):676–681.
3. Adams, F. (Trans.-Ed.). *The Genuine Works of Hippocrates.* London: The Sydenham Society, 1848.
4. Najamabadi M. *Tarikh-e-Tibbe-Iran*, Volume I. Teheran, Iran: Shamsi, 1934.
5. Ebbel B. *The Papyrus Ebers.* Copenhagen: Levin and Munskgaard, 1937.
6. Gauthier Y, Benzekri L. Historical aspects. In: Picardo M, Taieb A, eds. *Vitiligo.* Berlin, Heidelberg: Springer-Verlag; 2010:3–9.
7. Kopera D. History and cultural aspects of vitiligo. In: Hann S-K, Nordlund J, eds. *Vitiligo: A Monograph on the Basic and Clinical Science.* Oxford, UK: Blackwell Scientific Publishers; 2000:13–17.
8. Panda AK. The medicohistorical perspective of vitiligo. *Bull Ind Hist Med* 2005;25:41–46.
9. Hann SK, Chung HS. Historic view of vitiligo in Korea. *Int J Dermatol* 1997;36:313–315.
10. Lee S. Vitiligo auf einem historischen Portrait. *Hautarzt* 1982;33:335–336.
11. Brocq L, ed. *Traitment des Maladies de la Peau.* Paris: Doin, 1892:853–855.
12. Kaposi M, ed. *Pathologie and Therapie der Hautkrankheiten.* 5th ed. Berlin/Wien: Urban and Schwarzenberg, 1st ed, 1879:703–707.

13. Prasad PV, Bhatnagar VK. Medico-historical study of "Kilasa" (vitiligo/leucoderma) a common skin disorder. *Bull Ind Inst Hist Med* 2003;33:113–127.

14. Goldman L, Richard S, Moraites R. White spots in biblical times. *Arch Derm* 1966;93:744–753.

15. Brito PS. On leucoderma, vitiligo, ven kuttam (Tamil) or cabbare (Singhalese), and several new methods of treatment. *Br Med J* 1885;1(1269):834–835.

16. Singh G, Ansari Z, Dwivedi RN. Letter: Vitiligo in ancient Indian medicine. *Arch Dermatol.* 1974; 109(6):913.

17. Nair BK. Vitiligo—A retrospect. *Int J Dermatol.* 1978;17(9):755–917.

18. Shree Gulabkunverba Ayurvedic Society, ed. *Charaka Samhita.* Jamnagar, India: Shree Gulabkunverba Ayurvedic Society, 1949.

19. Khushboo PS, Jadhav VM, Kadam VJ, Sathe NS. *Psoralea corylifolia* Linn.—"*Kushtanashini.*" *Pharmacogn Rev.* 2010;4(7):69–76.

20. Hann SK, Nordlund JJ, editors. *Vitiligo: A Monograph on the Basic and Clinical Science.* New York: John Wiley & Sons, 2008.

21. Menon AN. Ultra-violet therapy in cases of leucoderma. *Ind Med Gaz* 1945;80:612–614.

22. Fahmy IR, Abu-Shady H, Schönberg AA. Crystalline principle from *Ammi majus* L., *Nature* 1947;160(4066):468.

23. Fahmy IR, Abu-Shady H. *Ammi majus* Linn: The isolation and properties of ammoidin, ammidin and majudin, and their effect in the treatment of leukoderma. *QJ Pharm Pharmacol.* 1948;21(4): 499–503.

24. El-Mofty AM. A preliminary clinical report on the treatment of leukoderma with *Ammi majus* Linn, *J Egypt Med Assoc.* 1948;31:651–665.

25. Lerner AB, Denton CR, Fitzpatrick TB. Clinical and experimental studies with 8-methoxypsoralen in vitiligo. *J Invest Dermatol.* 1953;20(4):299–314.

26. Pathak MA, Mosher DB, Fitzpatrick TB. Safety and therapeutic effectiveness of 8-methoxypsoralen, 4,5′,8-trimethylpsoralen, and psoralen in vitiligo. *Natl Cancer Inst Monogr.* 1984;66:165–173.

27. Parrish JA, Fitzpatrick TB, Tanenbaum L, Pathak MA. Photochemotherapy of psoriasis with oral methoxsalen and longwave ultraviolet light. *N Engl J Med.* 1974;291(23):1207–1211.

28. Pathak MA, Fitzpatrick TB. The evolution of photochemotherapy with psoralens and UVA (PUVA): 2000 BC to 1992 AD. *J Photochem Photobiol B.* 1992;30(14):3–22.

29. Parsad D, Kanwar AJ, Kumar B. Psoralen-ultraviolet A vs. narrow-band ultraviolet B phototherapy for the treatment of vitiligo. *J Eur Acad Dermatol Venereol.* 2006;20(2):175–177.

30. Westerhof W, Nieuweboer-Krobotova L. Treatment of vitiligo with UV-B radiation vs topical psoralen plus UV-A. *Arch Dermatol.* 1997;133(12):1525–1528.

31. Scherschun L, Kim JJ, Lim HW. Narrow-band ultraviolet B is a useful and well-tolerated treatment for vitiligo. *J Am Acad Dermatol.* 2001;44(6):999–1003.

32. Whitton ME, Pinart M, Batchelor J, Leonardi-Bee J, González U, Jiyad Z, Eleftheriadou V, Ezzedine K. Interventions for vitiligo. *Cochrane Database Syst Rev.* 2015;(2):CD003263.

33. Kandil E. Vitiligo: Response to 0.2% betamethasone 17-valerate in flexible collodion. *Dermatologica.* 1970;141:277–81.

34. Kandil E. Treatment of vitiligo with 0.1% betamethasone 17-valerate in isopropyl alcohol: A double blind trial. *Br J Dermatol.* 1974;91:457–460.

35. Koopmans-van DB, Goedhart-van DB, Neering H, van Dijk E. The treatment of vitiligo by local application of betamethasone 17-valerate in a dimethyl sulfoxide cream base. *Dermatologica.* 1973;146:310–314.

36. Bleehen SS. The treatment of vitiligo with topical corticosteroids. Light and electronmicroscopic studies. *Br J Dermatol.* March 1976;94(Suppl 12):43–50.

37. Clayton R. A double-blind trial of 0%–05% clobetasol proprionate in the treatment of vitiligo. *Br J Dermatol.* 1977;96(1):71–73.

38. Kumari J. Vitiligo treated with topical clobetasol propionate. *Arch Dermatol.* 1984;120(5):631–635.

39. Liu XQ, Shao CG, Jin PY, Wang HQ, Ye GY, Yawalkar S. Treatment of localized vitiligo with ulobetasol cream. *Int J Dermatol.* May 1990;29(4):295–297.

40. Westerhof W, Nieuweboer-Krobotova L, Mulder PG, Glazenburg EJ. Left-right comparison study of the combination of fluticasone propionate and UV-A vs. either fluticasone propionate or UV-A alone for the long-term treatment of vitiligo. *Arch Dermatol.* 1999;135(9):1061–1066.

41. Grimes PE, Soriano T, Dytoc MT. Topical tacrolimus for repigmentation of vitiligo. *J Am Acad Dermatol.* 2002;47(5):789–791.

42. Smith DA, Tofte SJ, Hanifin JM. Repigmentation of vitiligo with topical tacrolimus. *Dermatology.* 2002;205(3):301–303.

43. Grimes PE, Morris R, Avaniss-Aghajani E, Soriano T, Meraz M, Metzger A. Topical tacrolimus therapy for vitiligo: Therapeutic responses and skin messenger RNA expression of proinflammatory cytokines. *J Am Acad Dermatol.* 2004;51(1):52–61.

44. Mayoral FA, Gonzalez C, Shah NS, Arciniegas C. Repigmentation of vitiligo with pimecrolimus cream: A case report. *Dermatology.* 2003;207(3):322–323.

45. Dash B, Kashyap L, eds. *Diagnosis and Treatment of Diseases in Ayurveda*, Volume 5. New Delhi, India: Concept Publishing Company, 1991.

Epidemiology and classification of vitiligo

4

SERENA GIANFALDONI and TORELLO LOTTI

CONTENTS

Introduction	27	Classification and clinical features	28
Epidemiology	27	References	32

INTRODUCTION

Vitiligo is an acquired, chronic, pigmentary disorder characterized by the progressive loss and dysfunction of the melanocytes from epidermis and epidermal appendages, which results in hypopigmented cutaneous areas that progressively become amelanotic.

In the last decades, several theories about its etiopathogenesis (e.g., genetic, neuronal, autoimmune, biochemical hypotheses), have been proposed, but none of them is strongly supported (Table 4.1) and the exact nature of the disease is still unclear.[1] Nevertheless, recent data indicate that vitiligo is a T-cell–mediated autoimmune disorder, maybe triggered by oxidative stress, associated with an underlying genetic predisposition.[2]

EPIDEMIOLOGY

Vitiligo is a quite common skin disease. Its worldwide prevalence has been estimated to be 0.5%–1.0%.[3] However, a recent review of vitiligo's epidemiology, conducted by Krüger and Schallreuter on more than 50 studies, reports a greater general prevalence, ranging between 0.5% and 2.0%.[4]

The incidence of vitiligo varies in different countries, ranging from 0.1% to over 8.8%.[5] The highest rates of incidence have been recorded in India, Mexico, and Japan,[6] while the lowest rates are reported in Caucasians of Finland, England, and Denmark.[4–5,7] Apart from a real difference in vitiligo's incidence, the data are partially conditioned by the different modalities in collecting data, sometimes limited to a small sample of the population,[4] and by the different psychological impact of the disease in patients of

Table 4.1 Etiopathophysiological theories for vitiligo

- Autocytotoxic theory
- Autoimmune theory
- Biochemical theory
- Inflammatory theory
- Melanocytorrhagy theory
- Neurohumoral theory
- Oxidative stress theory
- Theory of decreased melanocyte lifespan

different races.[8,9] It is possible that the major color contrast between healthy pigmented skin and vitiliginous skin (leopard-like skin appearance) observed in dark-skinned people leads to a deep stigma and forces patients to seek dermatological consultation.[5]

Males and females are equally affected.[10,11] Only two studies report a higher prevalence of vitiligo in males than in females, with a ratio of about 1.6:1.[12,13] In contrast, other epidemiological studies record that females are more affected than males. However, this result seems to be related only to a greater negative psychological effect of the disease in women than in men, so that they present for treatment more frequently.[14]

Vitiligo may develop at all ages, but it is rarely described in newborns and infants.[5] Most patients (79%–80%) present the disease before 30 years of age.[6,15,16] Childhood-onset vitiligo (before age 12 years) is common, affecting about 32%–37% of all patients.[16,17] Recent studies underline how vitiligo prevalence progressively increases with age.[4,18]

It is well known that the prevalence of the disease varies in different countries and races.[12] Apart from differences due to nonunified methods in collecting epidemiological data, it is clear that vitiligo incidence has fluctuations that seem to be related to both genetic and environmental factors.

Nowadays, vitiligo is considered to be inherited in a non-Mendelian, multifactorial, and polygenic pattern.[2,20] Its heritability ranges from 46% to 16%[21]; close relatives of vitiligo patients have increased risk of vitiligo and other autoimmune diseases, which are about 6–18-fold elevated.[22,23]

To date, more than 30 loci for vitiligo susceptibility have been identified. Among these, only 10% of genes encode for molecules relevant to normal melanogenesis (e.g., TYR, which encodes for tyrosinase, and MC1R, which encodes for melanocortin receptor and regulates melanogenesis), while 90% of them encode for HLA haplotypes (e.g., HLAs-A2, -DR4, -DR7, -DQB1*0303) and other immunoregulatory proteins, which are implicated in both cellular and humoral immunity (Table 4.2).[21,24,25]

From genetic studies on vitiligo, two interesting data points have emerged. The first is that genetic alterations in vitiligo patients may lead to the onset of comorbidities

Table 4.2 Some of the genes that may be implicated in vitiligo pathogenesis

Gene	Protein	Function
BACH2	BTB and CNC homology 1, basic leucine zipper	B-cell transcriptional repressor
CCR6	Chemokine receptor type 6	Regulation of B-cell differentiation
CD 44	CD44 antigen	T-cell regulator
CD80	B-cell activation antigen B7-1	T-cell priming by B cells, T cells, and dendritic cells
CLNK	Mast cell immunoreceptor signal transducer	Immunoreceptor signaling
CTLA4B	Cytotoxic T lymphocytes antigen 4	Inhibition of T cells
FOXD3	Forkhead box D3	Transcriptional regulator of neuronal crest
FOXP1	Forkhead box P1	Regulation of lymphoid cell development
FOXP3	Forkhead box p3	Transcriptional regulator of T reg cell function and development
GZMB	Granzyme B	Mediator of T-cell and NK apoptosis
HLA A-B-C	Leukocyte antigen B or C α chain	Presentation of peptide antigen
HLA-A	Leukocyte antigen A α chain	Presentation of peptide antigen
HLA-DRB1-DQA1	Major histocompatibility complex class II	Presentation of peptide antigen
IFIH1	Interferon-induced RNA helicase	Regulation of innate antiviral immune responses
IL2RA	Interleukin 2 receptor	Regulation of lymphocyte response to bacteria
PTPN22	Lymphoid-specific protein tyrosinase phosphatase nonreceptor 22	Regulation of T-cell receptor signaling
RERE	Atrophin-like protein 1	Regulation of apoptosis
TG/SLA	Tyroglobulin SRC-like adaptor isoform C	Regulation of antigen receptor signaling in T and B cells
TICAM1	Toll-like receptor adaptor molecule 1	Innate antiviral immune responses
TSLP	Thymic stromal lymphoprotein	Regulation of T-cell and DC maturation
UBASH3A	Ubiquitin associated and SH3 domain containing	Regulation of T-cell signaling
XBP1	X-box binding protein 1	Transcriptional regulator of MHC class II

(Table 4.3), such as autoimmune and endocrine diseases.[26] Among these, the association with autoimmune thyroid disorders is the more commonly described.[27] Other endocrinological disorders that may be associated with vitiligo are hypoparathyroidism, Addison's disease, polyglandular syndrome type I and type II, and diabetes mellitus. Vitiligo has been also described in association with numerous autoimmune diseases, such as hematologic disorders and several skin diseases (Table 4.4),[28,29] and, more recently, with systemic inflammatory disorders like obesity and metabolic syndrome.[30]

Another interesting finding is the correlation between vitiligo and melanoma. Some of the genes expressed by melanocytes in vitiligo have been observed to be involved in susceptibility to malignant melanoma with an opposite role. The development of depigmentary disorders in melanoma patients seems to lead to a more favorable prognosis, maybe as sign of an active immune response directed against melanocytes.[31]

Apart from a genetic background, many data support the important role of environmental trigger factors in the development of vitiligo[32] (Table 4.5). First, there is evidence of a variable prevalence of the disease in different countries. Also suggestive are the data about the incidence of vitiligo among families. In fact, while up to 20% of patients have an affected relative, the majority of vitiligo cases are sporadic. Finally, the incidence of concordance of pigmentary disease

Table 4.3 Examples of genetic alterations detected in vitiligo patients with comorbidities

Gene	Protein	Comorbidities
PTPN22	Lymphoid-specific protein tyrosinase phosphatase nonreceptor 22	Type 1 DM, Graves' disease, RA, Addison disease, psoriasis, IBD
CTLA4B	Cytotoxic T lymphocytes antigen 4	Type 1 DM, Graves' disease, Hashimoto thyroiditis, IBD, SLE
CCR6	Chemokine receptor type 6	IBD, AR, Graves' disease
IL2RA	Interleukin 2 receptor	Type 1 DM, Graves' disease, RA, multiple sclerosis, SLE

in monozygotic twins is approximately 23%.[23] Although the exact mechanism of action of the different trigger factors is still unclear, their role in vitiligo pathobiology is well known, such as the importance of recognizing them to limit the incidence and progression of the disease.

CLASSIFICATION AND CLINICAL FEATURES

Clinically, vitiligo is characterized by asymptomatic, milk-white macules and patches, with well-defined borders

Table 4.4 Common autoimmune diseases associated with vitiligo

- Alopecia areata
- Atopic dermatitis
- Autoimmune hemolytic anemia
- Autoimmune thyroid disease
- Diabetes mellitus
- Guillain-Barré syndrome
- Inflammatory bowel disease
- Myasthenia gravis
- Morphea
- Multiple sclerosis
- Pemphigus vulgaris
- Pernicious anemia
- Psoriasis
- Rheumatoid arthritis
- Sjögren syndrome
- Systemic lupus erythematosus
- Others

Table 4.5 Trigger factors that may be involved in vitiligo onset

- Physical stress: major illness, surgical operations, accidents
- Intercurrent infections and repeated antibiotic intake
- UVR and sunburns
- Chemical factors: thiols, phenols, catechols, mercaptoamines, quinones and their derivatives
- Endocrine factors: pregnancy
- Malnutrition: malnutritional habits; intake of preserved, stale, or junk food
- Psychosocial insecurity/shocks

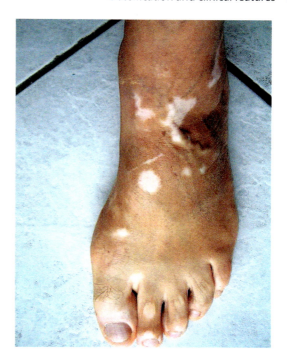

Figure 4.1 White macules of vitiligo. (Courtesy Dermatologic Clinic, University of Parma.)

Table 4.6 Clinical variants of vitiligo

Type of vitiligo	Characteristics
Punctata vitiligo	Small, punctuate-like, depigmented macules
Follicular vitiligo	Vitiligo involving the follicular reservoir with poor cutaneous lesions
Inflammatory vitiligo	Erythematous halo surrounding the white patches
Trichrome vitiligo	Hypopigmented area between the central amelanotic zone and the peripheral normal skin
Quadrichrome vitiligo	Variant of trichrome vitiligo with foci of repigmentation at the follicular osti
Pentachrome vitiligo	Lesions show the occurrence of five shades of color, white to black
Blue vitiligo	Bluish appearance of skin color

(Figure 4.1). Lesions may vary in number, form, and distribution, and may affect skin, mucous membranes, and hair. Characteristic is Koebner's phenomenon, consisting of the development of new lesions at sites of skin trauma.

In some cases, vitiligo patients may also show different clinical variants of the disease (Table 4.6)[33,34] and abnormalities of the melanocytes localized in different organs (e.g., eyes and ears).[35,36] Not rarely, nail abnormalities (e.g., longitudinal ridging, leukonychia, absent lunula, onycholysis, and others) may also be detected.[37]

Classically, vitiligo may be classified, on the basis of the extension of the disease, into localized, generalized, or universalis forms (Table 4.7).

More recently, the Vitiligo Global Issues Consensus Conference proposed another classification for the disease, which is based on the clinical features and natural history of vitiligo (Table 4.8).[38] The new classification recognizes three main types of vitiligo: nonsegmental vitiligo (NSV), segmental vitiligo (SV), and indeterminate forms.

NSV is the most commonly described. Even if it can occur at any age, it usually develops in young people between the ages of 10 and 30 years. Clinically, it is characterized by a heterogeneous group of types, in which amelanotic lesions usually involve different parts of the body with a bilateral and symmetrical distribution. Typical of all the types are the unpredictable course and the possible association with comorbidities. In NSV, the most commonly described type is generalized vitiligo (also known as vitiligo vulgaris), characterized by multiple lesions that usually involve the face, trunk, and upper and lower limbs, especially on trauma-exposed areas (Figures 4.2 and 4.3). Another common type of NSV is acrofacial, characterized by white patches limited to the face and distal end of extremities, but it can later progress to widespread forms.

Table 4.7 Classification of vitiligo on the basis of the extent of the disease

Localized	Generalized	Universalis
• *Focal:* One or more macules in one area but not clearly in a segmental distribution • *Unilateral/segmental:* One or more macules involving a unilateral segment of the body—lesions stop abruptly at the midline • *Mucosal:* Lesions limited to mucous membranes	• *Vulgaris:* Scattered patches that are widely distributed • *Acrofacialis:* White patches on the distal extremities and face • *Mixed:* Vitiligo acrofacialis and vulgaris	• Complete or nearly complete depigmentation

Table 4.8 Classification of vitiligo based on the clinical features and natural history of the disease

Types	Characteristics	Subtypes
Segmental vitiligo (SV)	One or more vitiliginous patches, in a linear or flag-like pattern of mosaicism, with a unilateral dermatomal distribution	Unisegmental Bisegmental Multisegmental
Nonsegmental vitiligo (NSV)	Heterogeneous group of clinical subtypes with multifocal localization, usually in a symmetric pattern	Acrofacial Mucosal (more than one site affected) Generalized Universal Mixed (associated with segmental vitiligo) Rare forms
Unclassified or indeterminate		Focal Mucosal (only one site)

In some cases, mixed vitiligo may be also be described. Clinically, it is characterized by the combination of segmental and nonsegmental vitiliginous lesions.[39] Recently, a particular subtype of mixed vitiligo has been described. It consists of segmental and nonsegmental vitiligo following Blaschko lines.[40]

Rarer variants of NSV are universal and mucosal vitiligo. The first consists of complete or nearly complete skin depigmentation (80%–90% of the body's surface), often associated with mucosal and scalp hair involvement. The second is characterized by acromic lesions localized on the oral and genital mucosa, sometimes associated with more common cutaneous lesions.

Finally, there are rarer variants of NSV: punctata, minor, and follicular. The first is characterized by punctuate-like, depigmented macules; the second by a partial defect in pigmentation, which seems to be limited to dark-skinned individuals; and the third by poor cutaneous lesions involving the follicular reservoir.

SV is less common than nonsegmental vitiligo, representing about 5%–16% of overall vitiligo cases.[41] Differently from NSV, SV is characterized by an early age of onset, rapid stabilization, and less common association with comorbidities.[19]

Clinically, it is characterized by one or more vitiliginous macules, with a typical unilateral and segmental or band-shaped distribution, usually respecting the midline (Figure 4.4). On the basis of the lesions' localization, SV may be further classified as unisegmental, bisegmental, or multisegmental. Among these, the unisegmental type is the most commonly described.

A particular manifestation of SV is poliosis, which is characterized by a patch of white hair.[1]

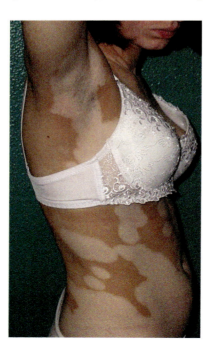

Figure 4.2 Generalized nonsegmental vitiligo. (Courtesy Dermatologic Clinic, University of Parma.)

Classification and clinical features 31

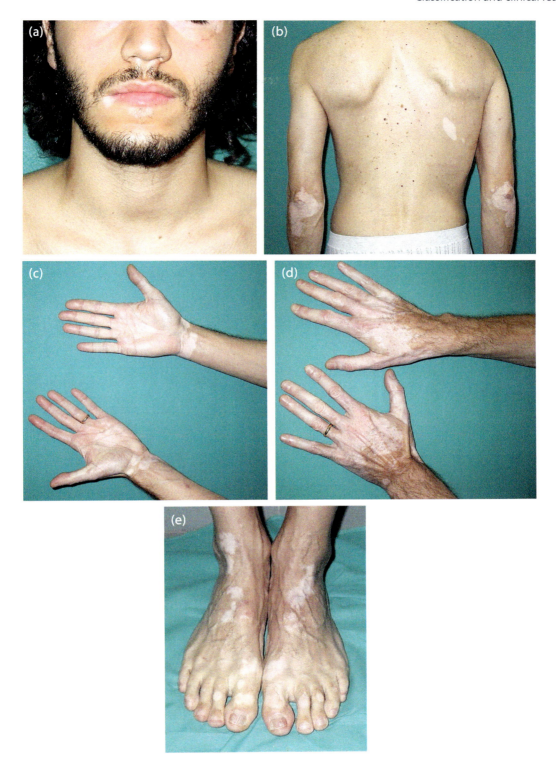

Figure 4.3 (a–e) Generalized nonsegmental vitiligo. (Courtesy Dermatologic Clinic, University of Parma.)

Finally, there is indeterminate vitiligo, which comprises forms with isolated mucosal involvement and focal forms. While the first is characterized by lesions affecting only one mucosa, focal vitiligo is characterized by small isolated macules without segmental distribution, which does not evolve to NSV after a period of at least 2 years.

Despite the possibility of classifying vitiligo on the basis of different parameters (e.g., morphology, extension, natural history), the classification of the disease remains a challenging endeavor and each patient should be considered individually for proper management and treatment.[42]

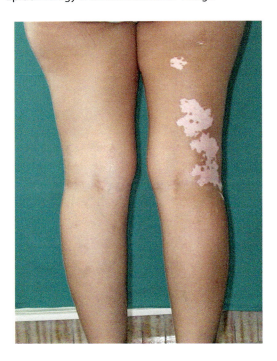

Figure 4.4 Segmental vitiligo. (Courtesy Dermatologic Clinic, University of Parma.)

REFERENCES

1. Lotti T, Hautmann G, Hercogovà J. Vitiligo: Disease or symptom? From the confusion of the past to current doubts. In: Lotti T, Hercogovà J, eds. *Vitiligo. Problems and Solutions*. New York: Marcel Dekker; 2004:1–14.
2. Lee BW, Schwartz RA, Hercogová J, Valle Y, Lotti TM. Vitiligo road map. *Dermatol Ther*. 2012;25(Suppl C):S44–S56.
3. Taïeb A, Picardo M; VETF Members. The definition and assessment of vitiligo: A consensus report of the Vitiligo European Task Force. *Pigment Cell Res*. 2007;20:27–35.
4. Krüger C, Schallreuter KU. A review of the worldwide prevalence of vitiligo in children/adolescents and adults. *Int J Dermatol* 2012;51:1206–1212.
5. Alzolibani AA, Robaee AA, Zedan K. Genetic epidemiology and heritability of vitiligo. In: Dr. Hwa Park KK. ed. *Vitiligo—Management and Therapy*. 2011.
6. Sehgal VN, Srivastava G. Vitiligo: Compendium of clinico-epidemiological features. *Indian J Dermatol Venereol Leprol*. 2007;73:149–156.
7. Howitz J, Brodthagen H, Schwartz M et al. Prevalence of vitiligo. Epidemiological survey on the Isle of Bornholm, Denmark. *Arch Dermatol*. 1977;113:47–52.
8. Lotti T, Hanna D, Buggiani G, Urple M. The color of the skin: Psycho-anthropologic implications. *JCosmet Dermatol*. 2005;4(3):219–220.
9. Ahmed I, Ahmed S, Nasreen S. Frequency and pattern of psychiatric disorders in patients with vitiligo. *J Ayub Med Coll Abbottabad*. 2007;19(3):19–21.
10. Handa S, Kaur I. Vitiligo: Clinical findings in 1436 patients. *J Dermatol*. 1999;26:653–657.
11. Lotti TM, Berti SF, Hercogova J et al. Vitiligo: Recent insights and new therapeutic approaches. *G Ital Dermatol Venereol*. 2012;147(6):637–647.
12. Wang X, Du J, Tinglin Wang T et al. Prevalence and clinical profile of vitiligo in China: A community based study in six cities. *Acta Derm Venereol*. 2013;93:62–65.
13. McBurney E. Vitiligo: Clinical picture and pathogenesis. *Arch Intern Med*. 1979;139:1295–1297.
14. Alikhan A, Felsten LM, Daly M et al. Vitiligo: A comprehensive overview Part I. Introduction, epidemiology, quality of life, diagnosis, differential diagnosis, associations, histopathology, etiology, and work-up. *J Am Acad Dermatol*. 2011;65:473–491.
15. Behl PN, Kotia A, Sawal P. Vitiligo: Age group related trigger factor and morphological variants. *Indian J Dermatol Venereol Lepr*. 1994;60:275–279.
16. Nicolaidou E, Antoniou C, Miniati A et al. Childhood- and later-onset vitiligo have diverse epidemiologic and clinical characteristics. *J Am Acad Dermatol*. 2012;66:954–958.
17. Ezzedine K, Diallo A, Léauté-Labrèze C et al. Pre- vs. post-pubertal onset of vitiligo: Multivariate analysis indicates atopic diathesis association in pre-pubertal onset vitiligo. *Br J Dermatol*. 2012;167:490–495.
18. Al-Refu K. Vitiligo in children: A clinical-epidemiologic study in Jordan. *Pediatr Dermatol*. 2012;29:114–115.
19. van Geel N, Mollet I, Brochez L et al. New insights in segmental vitiligo: Case report and review of theories. *Br J Dermatol*. 2012;166:240–246.
20. Sun XK, Xu AE, Meng W et al. Study on genetic epidemiology on 815 patients with vitiligo in the Zhejiang area. *Zhonghua Liu Xing Bing Xue Za Zhi*. 2005;26:911–914.
21. Spritz RA. Modern vitiligo genetics sheds new light on an ancient disease. *J Dermatol*. 2013;40(5): doi:10.1111/1346-8138.12147.
22. Laberge G, Mailloux CM, Gowan K et al. Early disease onset and increased risk of other autoimmune diseases in familial generalized vitiligo. *Pigment Cell Res*. 2005;18:300–305.
23. Alkhateeb A, Fain PR, Thody A et al. Epidemiology of vitiligo and associated autoimmune diseases in Caucasian probands and their families. *Pigment Cell Res*. 2003;16:208–214.
24. Jin Y, Ferrara T, Gowan K et al. Next-generation DNA re-sequencing identifies common variants of TYR and HLA-A that modulate the risk of generalized vitiligo via antigen presentation. *J Invest Dermatol*. 2012;132(6):1730–1733.
25. Zhang XJ, Chen JJ, Liu JB. The genetic concept of vitiligo. *J Dermatol Sci*. 2005;39(3):137–146.
26. Lotti T, D'Erme AM. Vitiligo as a systemic disease. *Clin Dermatol*. 2014;32(3):430–434.

27. Nejad SB, Qadim HH, Nazeman L et al. Frequency of autoimmune diseases in those suffering from vitiligo in comparison with normal population. *Pak J Biol Sci.* 2013;16(12):570–574.

28. Gill L, Zarbo A, Isedeh P et al. Comorbid autoimmune diseases in patients with vitiligo: A cross-sectional study. *J Am Acad Dermatol.* 2016;74(2):295–302.

29. Chen YT, Chen YJ, Hwang CY et al. Comorbidity profiles in association with vitiligo: A nationwide population-based study in Taiwan. *J Eur Acad Dermatol Venereol.* 2015;29(7):1362–1369.

30. Pietrzak A, Bartosińska J, Hercogová J et al. Metabolic syndrome in vitiligo. *Dermatol Ther.* 2012;(25 Suppl 1):S41–S43.

31. Spritz RA. The genetics of generalized vitiligo: Autoimmune pathways and an inverse relationship with malignant melanoma. *Genome Med.* 2010;2:78.

32. Silverberg JI, Reja M, Silverberg NB. Regional variation of and association of US birthplace with vitiligo extent. *JAMA Dermatol.* 2014;150(12):1298–305.

33. Lee DY, Kim CR, Lee JH. Trichrome vitiligo in segmental type. *Photodermatol Photoimmunol Photomed.* 2011;27(2):111–112.

34. Chandrashekar L. Dermatoscopy of blue vitiligo. *Clin Exp Dermatol.* 2009;34(5):e125–e126.

35. Huggins RH, Janusz CA, Schwartz RA. Vitiligo: A sign of systemic disease. *Indian J Dermatol Venereol Leprol.* 2006;72:68–71.

36. Akay BN, Bozkir M, Anadolu Y et al. Epidemiology of vitiligo, associated autoimmune diseases and audiological abnormalities: Ankara study of 80 patients in Turkey. *J Eur Acad Dermatol Venereol.* 2010;24(10):1144–1150.

37. Anbar T, Hay RA, Abdel-Rahman AT et al. Clinical study of nail changes in vitiligo. *J Cosmet Dermatol.* 2013;12:67–72.

38. Ezzedine K, Lim HW, Suzuki T et al. Revised classification/nomenclature of vitiligo and related issues: The Vitiligo Global Issues Consensus Conference. *Pigment Cell Melanoma Res.* 2012;25(3):E1–13.

39. Ezzedine K, Gauthier Y, Léauté-Labrèze C et al. Segmental vitiligo associated with generalized vitiligo (mixed vitiligo): A retrospective case series of 19 patients. *J Am Acad Dermatol.* 2011;65:965–971.

40. Kovacevic M, Stanimirovic A, Vucic M et al. Mixed vitiligo of Blaschko lines: A newly discovered presentation of vitiligo responsive to combination treatment. *Dermatol Ther.* 2016;29(4):240–243.

41. Hann SK, Lee HJ. Segmental vitiligo: Clinical findings in 208 patients. *J Am Acad Dermatol.* 1996;35:671–674.

42. Hercogová J, Schwartz RA, Lotti TM. Classification of vitiligo: A challenging endeavor. *Dermatol Ther.* 2012;25(Suppl 1):S10–S16.

Pathophysiology of vitiligo

5

ALEXANDRA MINIATI

CONTENTS

Genetic predisposition	35	Neuroendocrine phenomena	36
Oxidative stress	35	Conclusion	37
Autoimmunity	36	References	37

Vitiligo is an acquired chronic cutaneous disorder of depigmentation, characterized by the absence of functional melanocytes,[1] with an estimated prevalence of 0.5%–2% of the general population.[2] Clinically, it consists of well-demarcated, white macules and papules of varying size and distribution. Despite the ease of clinical diagnosis, the exact pathophysiological mechanisms that lead to hypopigmentation are still unresolved. Several theories are involved in melanocyte disappearance, namely genetic predisposition, environmental triggers, metabolic abnormalities, and impaired inflammatory and immune responses leading to apoptosis.[3]

GENETIC PREDISPOSITION

The genetic etiology of vitiligo appears to be multifactorial, following a non-Mendelian pattern. HLA class I molecules present peptide antigens on the surface of almost all cells, whereas HLA class II molecules present antigens on the surface of antigen-presenting cells, such as dendritic cells, mononuclear phagocytes, and B cells. Autoimmune vitiligo is strongly associated with the MHC class II region and is associated with the production of cytokines that contribute to immune responses targeting different pathogens.[4] A total of 23 new risk susceptibility loci have recently been identified using genome-wide association studies of autoimmune vitiligo, encoding for immunomodulatory proteins that participate in melanocyte apoptosis.[5]

An interesting genetic fact was the identification of a polymorphism for the thymic stromal lymphopoietin (TSLP) gene −847C > T, which was found to increase susceptibility to generalized vitiligo by decreasing TSLP mRNA expression levels.[6] Moreover, a recent comprehensive association analysis of candidate genes for generalized vitiligo showed strong evidence of primary genetic association with vitiligo for TSLP,[7] suggesting the important role of this gene in disease pathogenesis. TSLP is a cytokine structurally and functionally similar to interleukin 7 (IL-7) and has been implicated in conditions like asthma, allergic rhinitis, and atopic dermatitis, based on its ability to maintain immune homeostasis.[8]

OXIDATIVE STRESS

Oxidative stress has been historically suggested as the initial event in vitiligo pathogenesis, causing lethal effects on melanocytes through the production of free radicals.[9] This hypothesis was based on the fact that some intermediates generated during melanin synthesis, such as dopaquinones and indoles, are toxic to melanocytes.[9] In addition, an imbalance in enzymatic and nonenzymatic antioxidant systems may also contribute in oxidative stress theory.[9] Low levels of catalase have been implicated in oxidative stress in segmental vitiligo, whereas the generation of oxidative stress in nonsegmental vitiligo may be attributed to low levels of glutathione peroxidase and reduced glutathione.[9] In response to prolonged hydrogen peroxide (H_2O_2) exposure, the function of several proteins is affected, including stress proteins such as heat shock protein 70 (Hsp70), which normally prevent degradation of cellular proteins.[10] Once released into the extracellular environment, these stress proteins are very immunogenic, serving as autoantigens. The intracellular production of H_2O_2 in the epidermis is associated with the defective recycling of the tetrahydropterins $6BH_4$ and $7BH_4$. In particular, $6BH_4$ serves as the cofactor for both phenylalanine hydroxylase (PAH) and tyrosine hydroxylase (TH). Once formed, it is recycled by the enzyme 4α-hydroxy-$6BH_4$-dehydratase (DH). DH activity is decreased in melanocytes of vitiligo patients, leading to the defective recycling of $6BH_4$, which in turn promotes the formation of $7BH_4$.[9] The latter can then inhibit PAH, causing the formation of free radicals. Increased $6BH_4$ levels can also inhibit tyrosinase, leading to defective melanin production.[9]

Under the condition of altered redox status in vitiligo epidermis, keratinocytes undergo vacuolar degeneration, secondary to apoptosis, resulting in their inability to produce an adequate amount of melanocyte growth factors, such as stem cell factor (SCF), leading to melanocyte apoptosis.[11] SCF, released by keratinocytes, is essential for the survival of melanocytes, and binds to the c-kit receptor on melanocytes. Mutant alleles at the SCF/c-kit locus can lead to dysregulation of the expression of tyrosinase mRNA.[12] Oxidative stress can trigger the loss of dendrites of melanocytes, thus affecting melanosome transfer to surrounding keratinocytes.[9] Oxidative stress can also induce apoptosis in melanocytes[9] by releasing caspase-activating cytochrome c from mitochondria, a mechanism that involves the imbalance between Bax (pro-apoptotic protein) and Bcl-2 (anti-apoptotic protein) levels.[9]

AUTOIMMUNITY

Most recent evidence suggests that autoimmune-based melanocyte damage is the main etiologic pathway in vitiligo pathogenesis.[3] Both cell-mediated and humoral immunity participate in melanocyte destruction. Histopathological evidence of the perilesional skin of vitiligo have suggested the involvement of T lymphocytes, mainly CD4+ and CD8+ T cells, in the disease process.[13] Interferon-gamma (IFN-γ) produced by Th-1 cells increases angiogenesis through the expression of VEGF by both Th-1 cells and keratinocytes.[14] VEGF, in turn, further induces angiogenesis and vascular permeability, along with polarization of TH-1 cells, and increases the secretion of IFN-γ.[14] High levels of cytotoxic CD8+ T lymphocytes against tyrosinase antigens have been detected in HLA-positive vitiligo patients.[15] The release of inflammatory cytokines, especially interleukin-1 (IL-1), interleukin-6 (IL-6), tumor necrosis factor (TNF), and IFN-γ after skin trauma (known as the Koebner phenomenon) might be an essential trigger that recruits T cells in the skin and exposes them to new antigen-expressing melanocytes.[16] Autoreactive T cells kill melanocytes in experiments in which T cells isolated from perilesional vitiligo skin are co-incubated with autologous uninvolved skin.[17] Labeled T cells isolated from vitiligo lesions infiltrated the normal skin, migrated to the epidermal-dermal junction, and were found in close association with dying melanocytes.[17] Depletion of CD8+ T cells prevented melanocyte destruction, whereas enrichment for these cells enhanced it,[17] supporting the key role of CD8+ T cells in vitiligo. Recent evidence has also shown that IFN-γ-derived chemokine CXCL10 is essential for driving vitiligo pathogenesis through the recruitment of autoreactive CD8+ T cells to the epidermis, and autoreactive T cells depend upon the chemokine receptor of CXCL10, CXCR3, to transfer to the skin to kill melanocytes.[18] IFN-γ signals through the IFN-γ receptor, which in turn recruits Janus kinases (JAKs) to transduce the signal intracellularly. JAKs phosphorylate STAT1, a transcription factor that then translocates to the nucleus to induce transcription of IFN-γ-inducible genes, including CXCL10.[18] Blocking CXCL10 in diseased mice can prevent vitiligo and restore pigmentation.[18]

Antibodies binding to melanocyte antigens induce melanocyte necrosis *in vitro* through antibody-dependent cellular cytotoxicity (ADCC) and complement activation.[19] Such antibodies mainly belong to the IgG and IgA classes,[19] and the serum levels of these autoantibodies seem to correlate with the extent of vitiligo.[19] Recently, several B-cell autoantigens have been identified using phage display methodology in patients with particularly nonsegmental vitiligo and include antigens to γ-enolase, α-enolase, heat shock protein 90, osteopontin, ubiquitin-conjugating enzyme, translation initiation factor 2, and GTP protein Rab38.[20] Tyrosine hydroxylase is another recently identified B-cell–dependent autoantigen involved in both segmental and nonsegmental vitiligo,[21] autoantibody levels of which were more frequent in patients with active disease.[21]

TNF is released in response to skin trauma,[16] and it has been shown to induce IL-8 (CXCL8) mRNA expression in a melanoma cell line;[22] it can also upregulate IL-8 receptor expression in normal melanocytes.[23] IL-8 is a chemokine important in inflammatory skin diseases and is produced by monocytes, mast cells, fibroblasts, endothelial cells, dendritic cells, and keratinocytes.[24] IL-8 is also chemotactic to neutrophils, T lymphocytes, basophils, and keratinocytes.[24] IL-8 relative gene expression was shown to be significantly higher (p=0.01) in lesional vitiligo skin than in control skin,[25] and human melanocytes stimulated by TNF and IL-1 showed increased release of IL-8.[25] It was recently also reported that chemically induced vitiligo led to increased production of IL-6 and IL-8.[26] These findings, along with the fact that IL-8 is a known chemokine to induce oxidative stress, leading indirectly to both keratinocyte and melanocyte apoptosis in vitiligo,[2] could suggest a possible pathophysiologic role of IL-8 in the disease process.

NEUROENDOCRINE PHENOMENA

Neuroimmune interactions are very important in mediating the effects of stress in the skin[27] and can also affect the vitiligo development process.[28] For instance, corticotropin-releasing hormone (CRH) increases skin inflammation,[29] and in the skin upregulates the synthesis and secretion of pro-opiomelanocortin (POMC) and its peptides, with POMC being an important regulator of melanogenesis.[28,30] Melanocortin-1, a product of POMC maturation, has a number of variants, including those of its receptor on melanocytes.[31] mRNA expression of POMC and its receptors, melanocortin receptor-1 (MC1R) and -4 (MC4R), is significantly decreased in lesional vitiligo skin and instead increased in nonlesional vitiligo skin compared to healthy controls.[32] Polymorphisms in the melanocortin system are associated with vitiligo.[33] Nevertheless, no autoantibodies were identified in the blood of vitiligo patients that could have interfered with the action of α-melanocyte-stimulating hormone (α-MSH) on MC1R.[34]

Neurochemical mediators that are secreted by cutaneous axon terminals, such as norepinephrine (NE) and acetylcholine (Ach), are toxic to melanocytes.[9] NE has direct melanocytotoxic effects by interfering with cellular sulfhydryl groups, impairing mitochondrial calcium uptake, and inhibiting melanogenesis. Elevated levels of NE-degrading enzyme monoamine oxidase (MAO) in both melanocytes and keratinocytes in vitiligo skin result in the accumulation of toxic levels of free radicals, promoting melanocyte destruction.[9]

CONCLUSION

Literature review shows that the pathogenesis of vitiligo typically involves more than one of the above-mentioned mechanisms, with immunological parameters, mainly cytotoxic T lymphocytes, cytokines, and regulatory T cells, influencing the outcome of different treatments for vitiligo. However, further scientific studies and efforts are needed, especially through clinical studies, to elucidate the complex mechanisms underlying vitiligo, leading to better therapeutic choices for the affected individuals.

REFERENCES

1. Tobin DJ, Swanson NN, Pittelkow MR et al. Melanocytes are not absent in lesional skin of long duration vitiligo. *J Pathol.* 2000;191(4):407–416.
2. Schallreuter KU, Bahadoran P, Picardo M et al. Vitiligo pathogenesis: Autoimmune disease, genetic defect, excessive reactive oxygen species, calcium imbalance, or what else? *Exp Dermatol.* 2008;17(2):139–140.
3. Boniface K, Seneschal J, Picardo M et al. Vitiligo: Focus on clinical aspects, immunopathogenesis and therapy. *Clin Rev Allergy Immunol.* 2018;54(1):52–67.
4. Cavalli G, Hayashi M, Jin Y et al. MHC class II super-enhancer increases surface expression of HLA-DR and HLA-DQ and affects cytokine production in autoimmune vitiligo. *Proc Natl Acad Sci USA.* 2016;113(5):1363–1368.
5. Jin Y, Andersen G, Yorgov D et al. Genome-wide association studies of autoimmune vitiligo identify 23 new risk loci and highlight key pathways and regulatory variants. *Nat Genet.* 2016;48(11):1418–1424.
6. Cheong KA, Chae SC, Kim YS et al. Association of thymic stromal lymphopoietin gene −847C>T polymorphism in generalized vitiligo. *Exp Dermatol.* 2009;18(12):1073–1075.
7. Birlea SA, Jin Y, Bennett DC et al. Comprehensive association analysis of candidate genes for generalized vitiligo supports *XBP1, FOXP3* and *TSLP. J Invest Dermatol.* 2011;131:371–381.
8. Ziegler SF, Artis D. Sensing the outside world: TSLP regulates barrier immunity. *Nat Immunol.* 2010;11(4):289–293.
9. Guerra L, Dellambra E, Brescia S et al. Vitiligo: Pathogenetic hypotheses and targets of current therapies. *Curr Drug Metab.* 2010;11(5):451–467.
10. Salem MM, Shalbaf M, Gibbons NC et al. Enhanced DNA binding capacity on up-regulated epidermal wild-type p53 in vitiligo by H_2O_2-mediated oxidation: A possible repair mechanism for DNA damage. *FASEB.* 2009;23(11):3790–3807.
11. Moretti S, Fabbri P, Baroni G et al. Keratinocyte dysfunction in vitiligo epidermis: Cytokine microenvironment and correlation to keratinocyte apoptosis. *Histol Histopathol.* 2009;24(7):849–857.
12. McGill GG, Horstmann M, Widlund HR et al. Bcl-2 regulation by the melanocyte master regulator MITF modulates lineage survival and melanoma cell viability. *Cell.* 2002;109:707–718.
13. Wańkowicz-Kalińska A, van de Wijngaard RM, Tigges BJ et al. Immunopolarization of CD4+ and CD8+ T cells to type-1-like is associated with melanocyte loss in human vitiligo. *Lab Invest.* 2003;83(5):683–695.
14. Aroni K, Voudouris S, Ioannidis E et al. Increased angiogenesis and mast cells in the center compared to the periphery of vitiligo lesions. *Arch Dermatol Res.* 2010;302:601–607.
15. Mandelcorn-Monson RL, Shear NH, Yay E et al. Cytotoxic T lymphocyte reactivity to gp100, MelanA/MART1 and tyrosinase in HLA-A2-positive vitiligo patients. *J Invest Dermatol.* 2003;121:550–556.
16. Van Geel N, Speeckaert R, Taieb A et al. on behalf of the other VETF members. Koebner's phenomenon in vitiligo: European position paper. *Pigment Cell Melanoma Res.* 2011;24(3):564–573.
17. Van den Boorn JG, Konijnenberg D, Dellemijn TA et al. Autoimmune destruction of skin melanocytes by perilesional T cells from vitiligo patients. *J Invest Dermatol.* 2009;129(9):2220–2232.
18. Rashighi M, Agarwal P, Richmond JM et al. CXCL10 is critical for the progression and maintenance of depigmentation in a mouse model of vitiligo. *Sci Transl Med.* 2014;6(223):223ra23.
19. Sandoval-Cruz M, Garcia-Carrasco M, Sánchez-Porras R et al. Immunopathogenesis of vitiligo. *Autoimmune Rev.* 2011;10(21):762–765.
20. Waterman EA, Gawkrodger DJ, Watson PF et al. Autoantigens in vitiligo identified by the serological selection of a phage-displayed melanocyte cDNA expression library. *J Invest Dermatol.* 2010;130(1): 230–240.
21. Kemp EH, Emhemad S, Akhtar S et al. Autoantibodies against tyrosinase hydroxylase in patients with non-segmental (generalized) vitiligo. *Exp Dermatol.* 2011;20(1):35–40.
22. Mohler T, Scheibenbogen C, Hafele J et al. Regulation of interleukin-8 mRNA expression and protein secretion in a melanoma cell line by tumour necrosis factor-alpha and interferon-gamma. *Melanoma Res.* 1996;6:307–311.
23. Norgauer J, Dichmann S, Peters F et al. Tumor necrosis factor alpha induces upregulation of CXC-chemokine receptor type II expression and magnifies the proliferative activity of CXC-chemokines in human melanocytes. *Eur J Dermatol.* 2003;13:124–129.
24. Luger TA, Schwarz T. Evidence of an epidermal cytokine network. *J Invest Dermatol.* 1990;95:100–14S.
25. Miniati A, Weng Z, Zhang B et al. Stimulated human melanocytes express and release interleukin-8, which is inhibited by luteolin: Relevance to early vitiligo. *Clin and Experimental Dermatol.* 2014;39:54–57.

26. Toosi S, Orlow SJ, Manga P. Vitiligo-inducing phenols activate the unfolded protein response in melanocytes resulting in upregulation of IL-6 and IL-8. *J Invest Dermatol.* 2012;132:2601–2609.
27. Arck PC, Slominski AT, Theoharides TC et al. Neuroimmunology of stress: Skin takes center stage. *J Invest Dermatol.* 2006;126(8):1697–1704.
28. Slominski AT, Wortsman J. Neuroendocrinology of the skin. *Endocr Rev.* 2000;21:457–487.
29. Donelan J, Boucher W, Papadopoulou N et al. Corticotropin-releasing hormone induces skin vascular permeability through a neurotensin-dependent process. *Proc Natl Acad Sci USA.* 2006;103(20):7759–7764.
30. Slominski AT, Tobin DJ, Shibahara S et al. Melanin pigmentation in mammalian skin and its hormone regulation. *Physiol Rev.* 2004;84:1155–1228.
31. Dessinioti C, Antoniou C, Katsambas A et al. Melanocortin 1 receptor variants: Functional role and pigmentary associations. *Photochem Photobiol.* 2011;87(5):978–987.
32. Kingo K, Aunin E, Karelson M et al. Gene expression analysis of melanocortin system in vitiligo. *J Dermatol Sci.* 2007;48(2):113–122.
33. Traks T, Keermann M, Karelson M et al. Polymorphism in melanocortin system and MYG1 genes are associated with vitiligo. *J Eur Acad Dermatol Venereol.* 2019;33(2):e65–e67.
34. Agretti P, De Marco G, Sansone D et al. Patients affected by vitiligo and autoimmune diseases do not show antibodies interfering with the activity of the melanocortin 1 receptor. *J Endocrinol Invest.* 2010;33(11):784–788.

Segmental vitiligo

6

CHRISTINA BERGQVIST and KHALED EZZEDINE

CONTENTS

Introduction	39	Mixed vitiligo	41
Pathogenesis	39	Classification of segmental vitiligo on the face	41
Epidemiology	39	Treatment overview	41
Clinical features	40	References	42
Differential diagnosis	41		

INTRODUCTION

Vitiligo is an acquired, chronic depigmenting disorder of the skin characterized by progressive loss of melanocytes. Segmental vitiligo (SV) is a distinct entity with distinctive clinical features. Indeed, the classification of segmental vitiligo as a separate entity from vitiligo was first suggested by Koga in 1977[1] according to results of a sweat gland secretion stimulation test and the distribution of the lesions (unilateral or bilateral). He referred to vitiligo distributed in a dermatomal fashion as Type B to differentiate it from the nondermatomal distribution of vitiligo referred to as type A. In 2011, an international consensus classified segmental vitiligo separately from all other forms of vitiligo, and the term "vitiligo" was defined to designate all forms of nonsegmental vitiligo (including acrofacial, mucosal, generalized, universal, mixed, and rare variants).[2] "Mixed vitiligo" (MV), in which segmental and nonsegmental vitiligo coexist in one patient, is classified as a subgroup of nonsegmental vitiligo. Distinguishing SV from other types of vitiligo was one of the most important decisions of the consensus, primarily because of its prognostic implications.

PATHOGENESIS

The pathophysiology of the segmental distribution remains highly controversial.[3,4] To date, there is no consensus concerning the mechanism underlying lesion distribution in SV. The basis for Koga's notion of differentiating SV from nonsegmental vitiligo was originally established on an etiologic basis.[1,5] Indeed, in 1977, Koga proposed that the pathogenesis of the two types differ: whereas he considered the nonsegmental type an immunologic disorder associated with autoimmune disease, he suggested the segmental type was the result of a dysfunction of the sympathetic nerves in the affected area.[1] In both types, however, acquired melanocyte loss is the common denominator. According to El Mofty, unlike in generalized vitiligo, the association with autoimmune diseases seems to be less significant in SV.[6] On the other hand, several reports have debated this concept. In the report of Hann and Lee, 6.7% of patients with SV had an associated allergic or autoimmune disease.[7]

However, given that allergic and autoimmune disorders are common in the general population, whether these associations are true or simply coincidental is controversial. Further and stronger epidemiological studies are needed to help elucidate this association.

Furthermore, halo nevus has been shown to be associated with SV nearly as frequently as with nonsegmental vitiligo (8.6% in nonsegmental vitiligo vs. 6.4% in SV),[8] and a family history of vitiligo has been found in approximately 12% of SV cases.[7–9] More recent clinical reports of nonsegmental and mixed vitiligo have questioned the notion that these forms of vitiligo are different and support the hypothesis that SV and nonsegmental vitiligo are parts of the same disease spectrum and that SV could have a polygenetic background as well.[10–15]

Early studies on SV have provided evidence that physiologic abnormalities associated with sympathetic nerve dysfunction play a role in the pathogenesis of SV. Wu et al. have demonstrated an increased cutaneous blood flow in segmental vitiligo lesions compared to the contralateral normal skin and a significantly increased a- and b-adrenoceptor response in those lesions.[16] However, Taieb et al. suggested that these sympathetic abnormalities found in SV may simply be a confounding factor associated with the absence of melanocytes, since these latter have the capacity to release several neuromediators in the skin. Moreover, they suggested the somatic mosaicism hypothesis of SV, and that SV and nonsegmental vitiligo are found along a continuum with shared predisposing genetic factors that would affect first the skin pigmentary system and secondarily activate skin immune/inflammatory responses, leading to a more severe expression of the disease.[4]

Moreover, evidence of inflammation has been reported in early cases of SV, further pointing toward the fact that both nonsegmental vitiligo and SV may have a related inflammatory or immune-related etiology.[3]

EPIDEMIOLOGY

Although the worldwide prevalence of vitiligo is 0.5%–1%,[2] the incidence of SV is not well established. Segmental vitiligo accounts for 5%–16% of overall vitiligo cases.[7,17]

In a study on an Egyptian population, El-Mofty et al. reported that only 5% (41 out of 821) of patients had segmental vitiligo.[6] Koga and Tango reported that 27.9% of their patients (134 out of 481) had SV (referred to as type B).[5] Several studies reported that the prevalence of SV in Korean vitiligo patients ranged from 5.5% to 29.6%.[7] On the contrary, a study done on a large number of Chinese vitiligo patients showed lower prevalence of the segmental form (2.5% of the total prevalence) and higher prevalence of focal vitiligo (36%) than reported in other studies.[18] This variability in epidemiological data could be accounted for by differences in disease classification due to the lack of consensus in previous years, inconsistent reporting by patients, and varied populations.

Segmental vitiligo tends to occur at a younger age than nonsegmental vitiligo,[19] before the age of 30 years in 87% of cases and before the age of 10 years in 41.3%.[7] In Hann and Lee's report, the mean age of onset was 15.6 years.[7] The earliest reported onset was immediately after birth, whereas the latest was 54 years. Most cases were less than 3 years in duration at referral, ranging from 2 months to 15 years.[7]

CLINICAL FEATURES

Segmental vitiligo refers to depigmented macules distributed in a segmental distribution, and typically it is associated with leukotrichia and a rapid onset (Figure 6.1). The characteristic lesion is clinically similar to the macule seen in nonsegmental vitiligo: a totally amelanotic, nonscaly, chalky-white macule with distinct margins. However, a less uniform depigmentation pattern has also been reported in SV compared to nonsegmental vitiligo. In fair-skinned patients, the lesions are not easily distinguishable under normal light, but can be discernible with Wood's light examination.

The depigmented patches are usually confined to a single dermatome, with partial or complete involvement. Indeed, monosegmental vitiligo is defined as one or more white depigmented macules distributed on one side of the body, usually respecting the midline with early leukotrichia, with a rapid onset over a few weeks or months and a rapid stabilization with an overall protracted course. They may sometimes cross the midline.

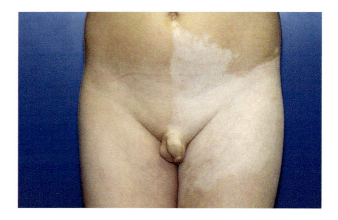

Figure 6.1 Large segmental vitiligo of the left hip and abdomen in a 5-year-old boy.

Monosegmental vitiligo is the most common form of SV;[7,20] however, other distribution patterns are possible whereby the depigmented patch overlaps several ipsi or contralateral dermatomes or occurs on large areas delineated by Blaschko lines. The onset may be simultaneous or not. An evident segmental distribution of the lesions with midline demarcation, along with the characteristic features of segmental vitiligo (protracted course, leukotrichia), help in distinguishing this diagnosis from nonsegmental vitiligo in bilateral cases. In Hann's report, 5 out of the 240 patients with SV had two different depigmented segments. The clinical course of bilateral SV seems similar to that of unilateral SV.

The head is involved in more than 50% of cases.[7,8] The most commonly involved dermatome is that of the trigeminal nerve.[7,9,21] The next common locations in decreasing order of frequency are: the trunk, the limbs, the extremities, and the neck.[6–9]

Early SV starts as an oval-shaped white macule or patch that is difficult to differentiate from focal vitiligo. Focal vitiligo refers to a small, isolated, depigmented lesion without an obvious distribution pattern. It can be a part of segmental or nonsegmental vitiligo; however, if after 1–2 years it still has not evolved into nonsegmental or segmental vitiligo, it is regarded as unclassifiable vitiligo.[2]

In SV, the depigmentation spreads within the segment over a period of 6–24 months. After initial rapid spreading in the affected dermatome, the SV patch most often remains stable.[7] Rarely, however, it can progress again after being quiescent for several years, and if does so, it usually spreads over the same dermatome. Disease recurrence can occur after years of stability.[22] However, in very rare cases, lesions may become generalized and become part of mixed vitiligo.[11,22]

Distinguishing features from nonsegmental vitiligo

It is important to distinguish SV from other types of vitiligo, principally because of its prognostic implications. In addition to its limited, segmental distribution, SV has other distinguishing characteristics as compared to nonsegmental vitiligo.

- Nonsegmental vitiligo can occur at any age, whereas SV typically has an earlier age of onset than nonsegmental vitiligo.[7,9,21]
- Segmental vitiligo typically has a rapidly progressive (over a period of 6–24 months) but limited course. Nonsegmental vitiligo typically evolves over time, in both distribution and extension patterns.
- SV has early involvement of melanocytes of hair follicles, with up to 50% of SV patients presenting poliosis in affected areas. In nonsegmental vitiligo, body hair remains pigmented, although hair depigmentation can occur in later stages with disease progression.
- Melanocyte autologous grafting typically yields a good long-term response in SV patients, with stable repigmentation, whereas nonsegmental vitiligo usually relapses within autologous grafting sites.

DIFFERENTIAL DIAGNOSIS

The most common differential diagnosis is nevus depigmentosus, also known as achromic nevus since it presents as a congenital hypomelanoses of segmental distribution. Indeed, it is usually congenital or seen within the first year of life and grows proportionally to the child's growth. The achromic nevus usually includes a normal number of melanocytes compared with perilesional skin; however, it is the production of melanin pigment that is reduced. In difficult cases, a biopsy is needed to differentiate nevus depigmentosus from SV.

MIXED VITILIGO

Mixed vitiligo refers to the concomitant occurrence of SV and nonsegmental vitiligo. In general, SV typically precedes nonsegmental vitiligo.

Mixed vitiligo was first reported in a child treated with UVB, which left a recalcitrant segmental lesion suggestive of preexisting SV.[23] The term "mixed vitiligo" as referring to the concomitant occurrence of SV and nonsegmental vitiligo was first coined by Mulekar et al. in 2006.[13] Ezzedine et al. subsequently proposed definition criteria in a case series.[11] These include:

- Absence of depigmented areas in a segmental distribution at birth and in the first year of life, and an examination by Wood's lamp that excludes nevus depigmentosus.
- SV followed by nonsegmental vitiligo with a delay of at least 6 months.
- SV affecting at least 20% of the theoretical distribution of a dermatomal segment or presenting a definite Blaschko linear distribution.
- Response to narrowband UVB treatment in between SV (poor response) and nonsegmental vitiligo (good response).

Leukotrichia and halo nevi at onset may be risk factors for developing MV in patients with SV.[10]

The co-occurrence of SV and nonsegmental vitiligo in the same patient has been viewed as a superimposed segmental manifestation of a generalized polygenic disorder, in which segmental involvement precedes disease generalization and is more resistant to therapy.[24,25]

CLASSIFICATION OF SEGMENTAL VITILIGO ON THE FACE

The progression of SV is usually limited to months or a few years. Since SV occurs most frequently on the face, understanding the precise spreading pattern is of interest for both patients and physicians, as it helps in predicting the prognosis.

Hann et al. classified patterns of SV distribution on the face:[21]

- Type 1a represents the lesion that originates from the right side of the forehead, crosses the midline of the face, and spreads down to the eyeball, nose, and cheek of the left side of the face.

- Type 1b is the mirror image of 1a. The lesion originates from the left side of the face and spreads down the right side of the face, crossing the midline.
- Type 2 represents the lesion that originates from the area between the nose and lip, then arches to the preauricular area.
- Type 3 represents the lesion that originates from the lower lip and spreads down to the chin and neck.
- Type 4 represents the lesion that originates from the right side of the forehead and spreads down to the eyeball, nose, and cheek areas without crossing the midline.
- Type 5 represents the lesion that is confined to the left cheek area.

In their study, type 1 was the most common and type 5 the least common.

Gauthier and Taïeb proposed a simplified classification of SV of the face based on studies comparing sites involved by herpes zoster and SV:[26]

- *Type I*: V1 ophthalmic branch (partial or total involvement)
- *Type II*: V2 maxillar branch (partial or total involvement)
- *Type III*: V3 mandibular branch (partial or total involvement)
- *Type IV*: Mixed distribution patterns on several dermatomes

$$IVa = V1 + V$$

$$IVb = V2 + V3$$

$$IVc = V1 + V2 + V3$$

- *Type V*: Cervicofacial distribution

In the majority of cases (64%), SV did not exactly follow some dermatomes and instead overlapped one, two, or three dermatomes. On the other hand, SV was distributed exactly to a trigeminal dermatome: ophthalmic (V1), maxillary (V2), and mandibular (V3) in 26% of cases.

TREATMENT OVERVIEW

Reliable data regarding the treatment of SV are limited given the fact that most studies did not differentiate between the types of vitiligo.

SV was long considered to be resistant to treatment. However, recent studies have been reporting promising results, especially when introduced at an early stage. Within the first 6 months, patients should be offered a treatment with potent topical corticosteroids or topical immune modulators combined with light therapy, such as narrowband UVB light or targeted excimer lamp or laser. Oral steroid mini-pulse therapy is also another option if the lesion is still in the active phase. In a recent retrospective study of 159 cases, the authors found that combination therapy with 308-nm excimer laser, topical tacrolimus, and short-term systemic corticosteroids were associated with good response in segmental vitiligo. In this study, prolonged disease duration, poliosis, and plurisegmental subtype were shown to be independent prognostic factors of poor response in patients with SV.[27]

On the other hand, if these medical therapies fail, or if the disease is at a later stage, surgery can be considered. Overall, stable SV is a good indication for epidermal grafting, especially given that the presence of leukotrichia in SV makes it more resistant to standard medical therapies.

The surgical techniques that are recommended by the European guidelines comprise tissue grafts (full-thickness punch, split-thickness, and suction-blister grafts) and cellular grafts (cultured melanocytes and noncultured epidermal cellular grafts). The three tissue grafting methods seem to have similar success rates of repigmentation.[28]

REFERENCES

1. Koga M. Vitiligo: A new classification and therapy. *Br J Dermatol.* 1977;97:255–261.
2. Ezzedine K, Lim HW, Suzuki T et al. Revised classification/nomenclature of vitiligo and related issues: The Vitiligo Global Issues Consensus Conference. *Pigment Cell Melanoma Res.* 2012; 25:E1–E13.
3. van Geel NA, Mollet IG, De Schepper S et al. First histopathological and immunophenotypic analysis of early dynamic events in a patient with segmental vitiligo associated with halo nevi. *Pigment Cell Melanoma Res.* 2010;23:375–384.
4. Taieb A, Morice-Picard F, Jouary T et al. Segmental vitiligo as the possible expression of cutaneous somatic mosaicism: Implications for common non-segmental vitiligo. *Pigment Cell Melanoma Res.* 2008;21:646–652.
5. Koga M, Tango T. Clinical features and course of type A and type B vitiligo. *Br J Dermatol.* 1988; 118:223–228.
6. el-Mofty AM, el-Mofty M. Vitiligo. A symptom complex. *Int J Dermatol.* 1980;19:237–244.
7. Hann SK, Lee HJ. Segmental vitiligo: Clinical findings in 208 patients. *J Am Acad Dermatol.* 1996;35:671–674.
8. Barona MI, Arrunategui A, Falabella R et al. An epidemiologic case-control study in a population with vitiligo. *J Am Acad Dermatol.* 1995;33:621–625.
9. Hann SK, Park YK, Chun WH. Clinical features of vitiligo. *Clin Dermatol.* 1997;15:891–897.
10. Ezzedine K, Diallo A, Leaute-Labreze C et al. Halo naevi and leukotrichia are strong predictors of the passage to mixed vitiligo in a subgroup of segmental vitiligo. *Br J Dermatol.* 2012; 166:539–544.
11. Ezzedine K, Gauthier Y, Leaute-Labreze C et al. Segmental vitiligo associated with generalized vitiligo (mixed vitiligo): A retrospective case series of 19 patients. *J Am Acad Dermatol.* 2011;65:965–971.
12. van Geel N, De Lille S, Vandenhaute S et al. Different phenotypes of segmental vitiligo based on a clinical observational study. *J Eur Acad Dermatol Venereol.* 2011;25:673–678.
13. Mulekar SV, Al Issa A, Asaad M et al. Mixed vitiligo. *J Cutan Med Surg.* 2006;10:104–107.
14. Schallreuter KU, Kruger C, Rokos H et al. Basic research confirms coexistence of acquired Blaschkolinear vitiligo and acrofacial vitiligo. *Arch Dermatol Res.* 2007;299:225–230.
15. Schallreuter KU, Kruger C, Wurfel BA et al. From basic research to the bedside: Efficacy of topical treatment with pseudocatalase PC-KUS in 71 children with vitiligo. *Int J Dermatol.* 2008;47:743–753.
16. Wu CS, Yu HS, Chang HR et al. Cutaneous blood flow and adrenoceptor response increase in segmental-type vitiligo lesions. *J Dermatol Sci.* 2000;23:53–62.
17. Silverberg NB. Update on childhood vitiligo. *Curr Opin Pediatr.* 2010;22:445–452.
18. Wang X, Du J, Wang T et al. Prevalence and clinical profile of vitiligo in China: A community-based study in six cities. *Acta Derm Venereol.* 2013;93:62–65.
19. Nicolaidou E, Antoniou C, Miniati A et al. Childhood- and later-onset vitiligo have diverse epidemiologic and clinical characteristics. *J Am Acad Dermatol.* 2012;66:954–958.
20. Lerner AB. Vitiligo. *J Invest Dermatol.* 1959;32:285–310.
21. Hann SK, Chang JH, Lee HS et al. The classification of segmental vitiligo on the face. *Yonsei Med J.* 2000;41:209–212.
22. Park JH, Jung MY, Lee JH et al. Clinical course of segmental vitiligo: A retrospective study of eighty-seven patients. *Ann Dermatol.* 2014;26:61–65.
23. Gauthier Y, Cario Andre M, Taieb A. A critical appraisal of vitiligo etiologic theories. Is melanocyte loss a melanocytorrhagy? *Pigment Cell Res.* 2003;16:322–332.
24. Happle R. [Segmental type 2 manifestation of autosome dominant skin diseases. Development of a new formal genetic concept]. *Hautarzt.* 2001;52:283–287.
25. Happle R. Superimposed segmental manifestation of polygenic skin disorders. *J Am Acad Dermatol.* 2007;57:690–699.
26. Gauthier Y, Taïb A. Proposal for a new classification of segmental vitiligo of the face. *Pigment Cell Melanoma Res.* 2006;19:515.
27. Bae JM, Yoo HJ, Kim H, Lee JH, Kim GM. Combination therapy with 308-nm excimer laser, topical tacrolimus, and short-term systemic corticosteroids for segmental vitiligo: A retrospective study of 159 patients. *J Am Acad Dermatol.* 2015;73:76–82.
28. Ezzedine K, Eleftheriadou V, Whitton M et al. Vitiligo. *Lancet.* 2015;386:74–84.

Childhood versus post-childhood vitiligo

7

ELECTRA NICOLAIDOU and STYLIANI MASTRAFTSI

CONTENTS

Introduction	43	The psychological burden of vitiligo	45
Epidemiology	43	Differential diagnosis	45
Clinical presentation	43	Treatment	45
Comorbidities	44	References	47
Halo nevi	44		

INTRODUCTION

Vitiligo is a chronic, difficult-to-manage, acquired disease characterized by the appearance of milk-white macules and patches of different shapes and sizes. It is a common disease, with a worldwide prevalence in the general population that ranges from 0.06% to 2.28%.[1]

Many different pathogenetic mechanisms have been proposed for vitiligo,[2] and the disease is characterized by various clinical types,[3] so it has been proposed that vitiligo may represent a heterogeneous group of disorders that present with the same phenotype.

Vitiligo may appear from shortly after birth to late adulthood. Childhood vitiligo (CV) is defined as disease onset before the age of 12 years. Studies from Greece,[4] France,[5] and India[6] report disease onset in childhood in 32%–40% of patients.

Several differences have been described in epidemiology and clinical presentation between CV and post-childhood vitiligo (PCV).[4–8] In this chapter, we will present recent data regarding CV with an emphasis on the differences between CV and PCV. Treatment options for CV will also be discussed.

EPIDEMIOLOGY

The prevalence of vitiligo in children and adolescents worldwide ranges from 0% to 2.16%.[1] A large study from Denmark[9] showed a prevalence of 0.09% in children up to 9 years of age and of 0.15% in children and adolescents from 10 to 20 years of age. A Chinese study[10] reported a prevalence of 0.1% in children 0 to 9 years of age, similar to the Danish study, but a higher prevalence of 0.36% in children and adolescents from 10 to 19 years of age.

Typically, vitiligo appears after the age of 4.[4,6,11–13] Two studies from India[6,11] and one from China[12] reported onset of vitiligo before the age of 4 in only 17% of affected children.

There seems to be no agreement among studies for the sex preference of CV. Studies from Greece,[4] France,[5] India,[6,11] Brazil,[13] and the United States[14] described a female predominance of 57%–66%. In contrast, studies from Korea,[8] China,[12] the United States,[15] and Jordan[16] reported equal numbers of boys and girls with the disease. Whether the male:female ratio is different between CV and

PCV is also unclear. Most studies reported no difference in the male:female ratio between CV and PCV,[4,5,8] but a female preponderance in CV compared to PCV has also been reported.[6]

CLINICAL PRESENTATION

The typical clinical lesion of vitiligo, which consists of well-demarcated milk-white macules and patches, is the same in both CV and PCV. The frequently affected sites (face, dorsal surface of the hands and feet, fingers, elbows, knees, shins, axillae, and anogenital region) are also the same.[17] Koebner phenomenon, characterized by the development of vitiligo lesions at sites of trauma, is also a feature of CV and has been observed in 11%[11]–24%[6] of children with vitiligo in India.

The sites of initial disease presentation seem to differ between CV and PCV. CV frequently appears initially on the head and neck area, especially on the eyelids.[4] Studies from Greece,[4] Korea,[8] and India[6,11] showed that, in 31%–59% of patients, the disease begins in the head and neck area. CV only rarely begins in the upper limbs.[4,6,8,11] The sites of initial disease presentation have been compared between CV and PCV in two studies[4,6] and have been found to be significantly different, with far more patients with PCV developing lesions initially in the upper limbs, especially the hands and fingers.[4]

Leukotrichia may be associated with CV due to the involvement of the melanocytic reservoir that exists in the hair follicles. Leukotrichia may be present both in vitiliginous areas and in areas with clinically normal-appearing skin.[18]

Even though vitiligo is usually asymptomatic, symptoms such as pruritus and burning sensation of the skin have been demonstrated in 30% of children and adolescents with the disease.[19]

According to the more recent classification system for vitiligo, the disease is divided into two major clinical forms, *vitiligo/nonsegmental vitiligo* (NSV) and *segmental vitiligo* (SV).[3]

In NSV, the depigmented lesions vary greatly in size and usually involve both sides of the body, with a symmetrical distribution (Figures 7.1 and 7.2). NSV is much more common than SV in both CV and PCV. In CV, 67%–95%

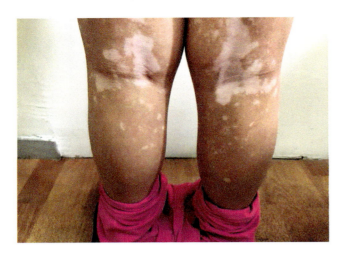

Figure 7.1 Nonsegmental CV.

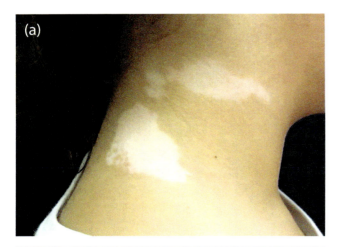

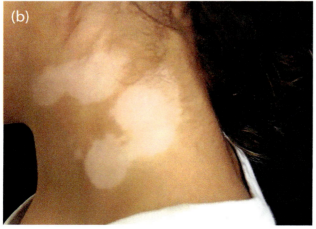

Figure 7.2 Nonsegmental CV: symmetrical lesions on the neck.

of patients present with NSV.[4,6,8,11,12] Segmental vitiligo is confined to a unilateral segment (Figure 7.3), and it is characterized by an early age of onset. SV typically progresses within the involved segment over a period of 6–24 months and then usually stabilizes. SV accounts for

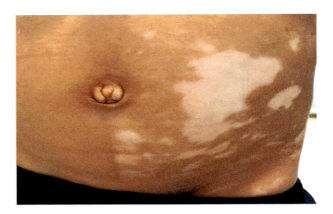

Figure 7.3 Segmental CV.

5%–33% of all forms of CV[4,6,8,11,12] and is more common in CV compared to PCV.[4,6,8]

COMORBIDITIES

NSV may be associated with several other autoimmune disorders, including autoimmune thyroid disease, rheumatoid arthritis, pernicious anemia, alopecia areata, psoriasis, adult-onset type 1 diabetes, and Addison disease.[17,20] Thyroid disorders are the most common comorbidity.[21] Thyroid dysfunction has been observed in several studies that included patients with CV.[22–25] Vitiligo usually precedes the development of thyroid dysfunction, and thyroid dysfunction can be subclinical.[23]

Comorbidities seem to differ between CV and PCV. In a cross-sectional study that included 233 patients, a significantly higher prevalence of thyroid disease was observed in patients with PCV compared to patients with CV.[4] Furthermore, in a prospective observational study that included 679 patients, thyroid disease or the presence of thyroid antibodies was independently associated with PCV compared to CV.[5] In contrast to thyroid disease, allergic diseases[4] and atopic dermatitis[5] have been reported more frequently in CV compared to PCV.

HALO NEVI

A halo nevus (Figure 7.4), also termed Sutton's nevus, is a melanocytic nevus that is surrounded by a depigmented

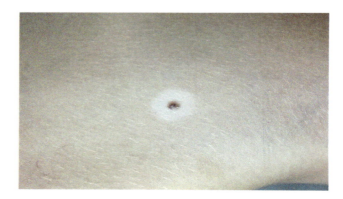

Figure 7.4 Halo nevus in CV.

rim. The presence of halo nevi in children with vitiligo varies greatly among different countries and races: 2.5% in a study from Korea,[8] 7.2% in a Chinese study,[12] 18.4% in a study from France,[26] and 26% in a study from the United States.[27] An Italian study that included 27 children with halo nevi and vitiligo reported that in 11 children (40.7%), the appearance of halo nevi and vitiligo was almost simultaneous; in 9 children (33.3%), halo nevi preceded vitiligo; while in 7 children (25.9%), halo nevi followed the onset of vitiligo.[28]

Halo nevi are more commonly found in patients with disease onset in childhood or adolescence. A positive association between age at vitiligo onset younger than 18 years and the appearance of halo nevi in vitiligo patients has been reported.[29] In another study, the presence of halo nevi were independently associated with CV compared to PCV.[5]

The significance of the presence of halo nevi in children has not been fully studied. In a study that followed 54 children with halo nevi for more than 5 years, 2 children, both with multiple halo nevi, developed vitiligo.[28] The same study concluded that in children with multiple halo nevi, the risk of vitiligo and other autoimmune diseases seemed to be higher compared to children with a single halo nevus.

THE PSYCHOLOGICAL BURDEN OF VITILIGO

Vitiligo may have significant psychological and emotional impact on both children and their parents, and it has been associated with impairment of quality of life, social stigmatization, emotional distress, anxiety, depression, embarrassment, low self-esteem, deterioration of self-confidence, and social isolation.[30–34] Teenagers seem to be affected to a greater extent compared to younger children.[19]

DIFFERENTIAL DIAGNOSIS

The differential diagnosis of nonsegmental CV includes a wide range of congenital and acquired disorders. For lesions appearing before the age of 2 years, congenital hypomelanoses[35] must be ruled out, including piebaldism, tuberous sclerosis, albinism, and Waardenburg syndrome. For acquired lesions appearing at a later age, several acquired hypomelanoses must be excluded. These include pityriasis versicolor, progressive macular hypomelanosis, atopic dermatitis, pityriasis alba, lichen sclerosus et atrophicus, morphea, and hypopigmented mycosis fungoides.

The differential diagnosis of childhood SV mainly includes the nevus depigmentosus/hypochromic nevus and the nevus anemicus. Nevus depigmentosus is usually a congenital lesion that is stable in shape, which grows in proportion to the child's growth. Nevus anemicus is a congenital solitary, hypopigmented lesion, which is caused by a localized hypersensitivity to catecholamines with resultant vasoconstriction. The lesional skin in nevus anemicus is characterized by a normal number of melanocytes and normal amount of melanin.

TREATMENT

Adequate sun protection should be recommended for children with vitiligo for the prevention of potential burning of vitiliginous skin as well as tanning of perilesional skin, which will increase the contrast with lesions. Cosmetic camouflage may be used to conceal visible affected areas. In case of recognized psychosocial impairment, psychological therapeutic interventions are recommended.

Annual thyroid screening is suggested for children with vitiligo, especially for those with nonsegmental disease.

Topical treatment and phototherapy are the main treatment modalities for children with vitiligo.

Topical treatment: Corticosteroids and calcineurin inhibitors

Topical corticosteroids (TCSs) and topical calcineurin inhibitors (TCIs) are the most commonly used topical agents for the treatment of vitiligo in children. Sun-exposed areas (face and neck), patients with dark skin, and recent lesions respond better to topical treatments, while acral lesions respond poorly.[36]

Topical corticosteroids have been found to offer benefits in both facial and nonfacial childhood vitiligo. Their effectiveness may be attributed to their anti-inflammatory and immunosuppressive effects. A retrospective study that included 101 children with vitiligo treated with moderate-to high-potency TCS reported repigmentation of lesions in 64% of children.[37] However, the long-term use of TCS is a concern due to local and systemic side effects. Ongoing usage of corticosteroids topically can result in skin atrophy, telangiectasias, hypertrichosis, acneiform eruptions, striae, glaucoma, systemic absorption, suppression of hypothalamic-pituitary-adrenal axis, Cushing syndrome, and growth retardation in children. Risk factors for systemic adverse effects are thought to include young age, extent of skin surface treated, frequency and length of treatment, potency of drug, and use of occlusion. In the previously mentioned retrospective study, children with vitiligo treated with TCS on the face and neck were 8.36 times more likely to have systemic absorption and abnormal cortisol levels compared with children treated on other body areas.[37]

Topical calcineurin inhibitors, tacrolimus and pimecrolimus, have showed good therapeutic efficacy in the management of CV without the side effects related to TCS use. However, up to now, their prescription for vitiligo is off label in most countries, as tacrolimus has been approved as a topical agent for moderate to severe atopic dermatitis and pimecrolimus for mild to moderate atopic dermatitis.

Tacrolimus and pimecrolimus inhibit the activation and proliferation of T cells and subsequently the production of cytokines, including TNF-α and IFN-γ, which have been found to be elevated in patients with vitiligo. These agents are not atrophogenic and can therefore be applied long-term on sensitive sites such as the face, intertriginous regions, and genitalia. In a prospective, randomized, double-blind, placebo-controlled study[38] that compared the efficacy of topical clobetasol propionate 0.05% and tacrolimus ointment 0.1% in 100 children with facial and nonfacial vitiligo, clobetasol propionate and tacrolimus were found to be equally effective in both facial and nonfacial lesions, with facial lesions responding faster than nonfacial ones.

Topical pimecrolimus has been also used with good results in vitiligo lesions, especially facial ones. In an open, comparative study that compared the efficacy of topical mometasone cream versus pimecrolimus cream in 40 children with localized vitiligo, the mean repigmentation rate, after 3 months of treatment, was 65% in the mometasone group and 42% in the pimecrolimus group, but the difference was not statistically significant.[39] Pimecrolimus was effective only on facial lesions.

Side effects of TCI are not common and include transient pruritus, burning sensation, and erythema. Both agents should be used in children older than 2 years of age. They also bear a black-box warning regarding a theoretical risk of malignancy.

Phototherapy

Psoralens plus ultraviolet A (PUVA) phototherapy is contraindicated in children, but narrowband (311 nm) ultraviolet B (NB-UVB) phototherapy has been extensively used in CV, resulting in stabilization and repigmentation of lesions in widespread and progressive disease.[40] Repigmentation may be initiated by activation, proliferation, and migration of melanocytes upward along the surface of the outer root sheath to the nearby epidermis, where they form perifollicular pigmentation islands.[41]

Response to treatment varies among studies.[42] Njoo et al., in an open, uncontrolled trial,[43] evaluated the efficacy and safety of NB-UVB in 51 children with generalized vitiligo (half with skin phototypes II to III and half with skin phototypes IV to V) treated with twice-weekly NB-UVB therapy for a maximum period of 1 year. Treatment resulted in >75% repigmentation in 53% of children and in stabilization of the disease in 80%, with limited and transient adverse events. The best repigmentation rate was achieved in lesions located on the face (72% of the lesions) and neck (74% of the lesions). In a recent retrospective study that included 71 Asian children with vitiligo, with skin phototypes of IV to VI, at least 50% repigmentation rate was achieved in 74% of children treated with NB-UVB phototherapy. Children with generalized vitiligo responded better (good response in 62%) than those with segmental vitiligo (good response in 44%).[44] Generally, lesions on the face and neck[43,45] and dark skin phototypes (IV to V) responded better to treatment in both adults and children.[42–47]

NB-UVB has also been used in combination with topical treatment. NB-UVB and TCI seem to act synergistically in both adults[48,49] and children.[50] One open-label, prospective study that evaluated the combined therapy of NB-UVB with topical tacrolimus 0.03% ointment in children with vitiligo 4–14 years of age reported >50% repigmentation in 60% of vitiligo patches treated with combination therapy and only in 20% of lesions treated with NB-UVB monotherapy. All patches on the face and trunk showed good to excellent response, compared to 33.3% of patches on the extremities.[50] Despite the satisfactory results that have been reported, the combination therapy of NB-UVB

with TCI gives rise to concerns about the possible increased risk of skin carcinogenesis.

In conclusion, NB-UVB has been reported to be an effective, safe, and well-tolerated treatment modality for childhood vitiligo, with no systemic effects. Acute adverse effects are mild and transient and include erythema, pruritus, and xerosis. However, long-term NB-UVB therapy carries the risk for photocarcinogenesis and photoaging.[51] Therefore, NB-UVB phototherapy should be used cautiously for periods longer than 12 months in children. In case of nonresponse after 6 months, discontinuation of treatment should be considered.

308-nm excimer laser

The 308-nm excimer laser has also been used as a targeted phototherapy modality for CV. The main advantage of the excimer laser is the selective, targeted treatment of lesional skin only. Thus, the risk of adverse effects associated with generalized phototherapy is reduced.[42] Furthermore, the excimer laser can reach lesions located on body areas hardly accessible by NB-UVB phototherapy, such as skin folds. However, the excimer laser may fail to stabilize vitiligo, since unlesional skin remains untreated.

The 308-nm excimer laser is indicated for macules and small patches of vitiligo. In a retrospective study that included children with vitiligo, 50% of 40 vitiligo patches treated twice weekly with the 308-nm excimer laser obtained an acceptable degree (>50%) of repigmentation, with lesions located on the face, neck, and trunk responding better to treatment.[52] Another retrospective study of Asian children with vitiligo demonstrated good response in 53% of children treated with the 308-nm excimer laser.[53] A synergistic effect between the excimer laser and pimecrolimus has also been described. In a randomized, single-blinded Chinese study,[54] 71% of childhood vitiligo lesions treated with excimer laser twice weekly combined with 1% topical pimecrolimus twice daily achieved >50% repigmentation, compared with 50% of lesions treated with excimer laser alone twice weekly. The excimer laser showed excellent therapeutic results on the face and trunk, while the combined therapy was superior to single laser treatment only for facial lesions.

Adverse effects of the excimer laser include mild to severe erythema, while pruritus and blistering might also be observed.[52–54] In case of nonresponse after 20–30 sessions (3–5 months of a twice-weekly treatment schedule), different therapeutic options should be considered.

Surgical treatment

Several surgical techniques that include tissue and cellular grafts have been developed for the treatment of recalcitrant vitiligo lesions in patients with stable disease (no new or expanding lesions for at least 1 year) and a negative history of Koebner phenomenon.

Skin grafting is not an ordinary treatment modality for childhood vitiligo. However, several techniques, including suction blister epidermal grafting,[55] noncultured cellular grafting,[56,57] and cultured melanocyte transplantation,[58,59] have been used in children with good results. Mottled repigmentation and irregular texture of repigmented skin can occur. Side effects include pain, infection, and scarring.

REFERENCES

1. Kruger C, Schallreuter KU. A review of the worldwide prevalence of vitiligo in children/adolescents and adults. *Int J Dermatol*. 2012;51:1206–1212.
2. Malhotra N, Dytoc M. The pathogenesis of vitiligo. *J Cutan Med Surg*. 2013;17:153–172.
3. Ezzedine K, Lim HW, Suzuki T et al. Revised classification/nomenclature of vitiligo and related issues: The Vitiligo Global Issues Consensus Conference. *Pigment Cell Melanoma Res*. 2012;25:E1–13.
4. Nicolaidou E, Antoniou C, Miniati A, Lagogianni E, Matekovits A, Stratigos A, Katsambas A. Childhood- and later-onset vitiligo have diverse epidemiologic and clinical characteristics. *J Am Acad Dermatol*. 2012;66:954–958.
5. Ezzedine K, Diallo A, Léauté-Labrèze C et al. Pre- vs. post-pubertal onset of vitiligo: Multivariate analysis indicates atopic diathesis association in pre-pubertal onset vitiligo. *Br J Dermatol* 2012;167:490–495.
6. Agarwal S, Gupta S, Ojha A, Sinha R. Childhood vitiligo: Clinicoepidemiologic profile of 268 children from Kumaun region of Uttarakhand, India. *Pediatr Dermatol* 2013;30:348–353.
7. Halder RM, Grimes PE, Cowan CA, Enterline JA, Chakrabarti SG, Kenney JA. Childhood vitiligo. *J Am Acad Dermatol*. 1987;16:948–954.
8. Cho S, Kang H-C, Hahm J-H. Characteristics of vitiligo in Korean children. *Pediatr Dermatol*. 2000;17:189–193.
9. Howitz J, Brodthagen H, Schwartz M, Thomsen K. Prevalence of vitiligo. Epidemiological survey of the Isle of Bornholm, Denmark. *Arch Dermatol*. 1977;113:47–52.
10. Wang X, Du J, Wang T et al. Prevalence and clinical profile of vitiligo in China: A community-based study in six cities. *Acta Derm Venereol*. 2013;93:62–65.
11. Handa S, Dogra S. Epidemiology of childhood vitiligo: A study of 625 patients from North India. *Pediatr Dermatol*. 2003;20:207–210.
12. Hu Z, Liu J-B, Ma S-S, Yang S, Zhan XJ. Profile of childhood vitiligo in China: An analysis of 541 patients. *Pediatr Dermatol*. 2006;23:114–116.
13. Marinho Fde S, Cirino PV, Fernandes NC. Clinical epidemiological profile of vitiligo in children and adolescents. *An Bras Dermatol*. 2013;17:1096–1099.
14. Pajvani U, Ahmad N, Wiley A et al. The relationship between family medical history and childhood vitiligo. *J Am Acad Dermatol*. 2006;55:238–244.
15. Mu EW, Cohen BE, Orlow SJ. Early-onset childhood vitiligo is associated with a more extensive and progressive course. *J Am Acad Dermatol*. 2015;73:467–470.
16. A-Refu K. Vitiligo in children: A clinical-epidemiologic study in Jordan. *Pediatr Dermatol*. 2012;29:114–115.
17. Alikhan A, Felsten LM, Daly M et al. Vitiligo: A comprehensive overview Part I. Introduction, epidemiology, quality of life, diagnosis, differential diagnosis, associations, histopathology, etiology, and work-up. *J Am Acad Dermatol*. 2011;65:473–491.
18. Gan EY, Cario-André M, Pain C et al. Follicular vitiligo: A report of 8 cases. *J Am Acad Dermatol*. 2016;74:1178–1184.
19. Silverberg JI, Silverberg NB. Quality of life impairment in children and adolescents with vitiligo. *Pediatr Dermatol*. 2014;31:309–318.
20. Silverberg NB. Pediatric vitiligo. *Pediatr Clin North Am*. 2014;61:347–366.
21. van Geel N, Speeckaert M, Brochez L et al. Clinical profile of generalized vitiligo patients with associated autoimmune/autoinflammatory diseases. *J Eur Acad Dermatol Venereol*. 2014;28(6):741–746.
22. Iacovelli P, Sinagra JL, Vidolin AP et al. Relevance of thyroiditis and of other autoimmune diseases in children with vitiligo. *Dermatology*. 2005;210:26–30.
23. Kakourou T, Kanaka-Gantenbein C, Papadopoulou A et al. Increased prevalence of chronic auto-immune (Hashimoto's) thyroiditis in children and adolescents with vitiligo. *J Am Acad Dermatol*. 2005;53:220–223.
24. Kartal D, Borlu M, Çinar SL et al. Thyroid abnormalities in paediatric patients with vitiligo: Retrospective study. *Postepy Dermatol Alergol*. 2016;33(3):232–234.
25. Cho SB, Kim JH, Cho S et al. Vitiligo in children and adolescents: Association with thyroid dysfunction. *J Eur Acad Dermatol Venereol*. 2011;25:64–67.
26. Mazereeuw-Hautier J, Bezio S, Mahe E et al. Segmental and nonsegmental childhood vitiligo has distinct clinical characteristics: A prospective observational study. *J Am Acad Dermatol*. 2010;62:945–949.
27. Cohen BE, Mu EW, Orlow SJ. Comparison of childhood vitiligo presenting with or without associated halo nevi. *Pediatr Dermatol*. 2016;33:44–48.
28. Patrizi A, Bentivogli M, Raone B et al. Association of halo nevus/i and vitiligo in childhood: A retrospective observational study. *J Eur Acad Dermatol Venereol*. 2013;27(2):e148–e152.
29. Ezzedine K, Diallo A, Léauté-Labrèze C et al. Halo nevi association in nonsegmental vitiligo affects age at onset and depigmentation pattern. *Arch Dermatol*. 2012;148(4):497–502.
30. Bilgiç O, Bilgiç A, Akiş HK et al. Depression, anxiety and health-related quality of life in children and adolescents with vitiligo. *Clin Exp Dermatol*. 2011;36(4):360–365.
31. Krüger C, Panske A, Schallreuter KU. Disease-related behavioral patterns and experiences affect quality of life in children and adolescents with vitiligo. *Int J Dermatol*. 2014;53(1):43–50.

32. Catucci Boza J, Giongo N, Machado P et al. Quality of life impairment in children and adults with vitiligo: A cross-sectional study based on dermatology-specific and disease-specific quality of life instruments. *Dermatology*. 2016;232(5):619–625.

33. Amer AA, Mchepange UO, Gao XH et al. Hidden victims of childhood vitiligo: Impact on parents' mental health and quality of life. *Acta Derm Venereol*. 2015;95(3):322–325.

34. Manzoni AP, Weber MB, Nagatomi AR et al. Assessing depression and anxiety in the caregivers of pediatric patients with chronic skin disorders. *An Bras Dermatol*. 2013;88(6):894–899.

35. van Geel N, Speeckaert M, Chevolet I et al. Hypomelanoses in children. *J Cutan Aesthet Surg*. 2013;6(2):65–72.

36. Taieb A, Alomar A, Böhm M et al. Guidelines for the management of vitiligo: The European Dermatology Forum consensus. *Br J Dermatol*. 2013;168(1):5–19.

37. Kwinter J, Pelletier J, Khambalia A et al. High-potency steroid use in children with vitiligo: A retrospective study. *J Am Acad Dermatol*. 2007;56(2):236–241.

38. Ho N, Pope E, Weinstein M et al. A double-blind, randomized, placebo-controlled trial of topical tacrolimus 0.1% vs. clobetasol propionate 0.05% in childhood vitiligo. *Br J Dermatol*. 2011;165(3):626–632.

39. Köse O, Arca E, Kurumlu Z. Mometasone cream versus pimecrolimus cream for the treatment of childhood localized vitiligo. *J Dermatolog Treat*. 2010;21(3):133–139.

40. Rodrigues M, Ezzedine K, Hamzavi I et al. Current and emerging treatments for vitiligo. *J Am Acad Dermatol*. 2017;77(1):17–29.

41. Wu CS, Yu CL, Wu CS, Lan CCE, Yu HS. Narrow-band ultraviolet-B stimulates proliferation and migration of cultured melanocytes. *Exp Dermatol*. 2004;13:755–763.

42. Nicolaidou E, Antoniou C, Stratigos A et al. Narrowband ultraviolet B phototherapy and 308-nm excimer laser in the treatment of vitiligo: A review. *J Am Acad Dermatol*. 2009;60(3):470–477.

43. Njoo MD, Bos JD, Westerhof W. Treatment of generalized vitiligo in children with narrow-band (TL-01) UVB radiation therapy. *J Am Acad Dermatol*. 2000;42:245–253.

44. Koh MJ, Mok ZR, Chong WS. Phototherapy for the treatment of vitiligo in Asian children. *Pediatr Dermatol*. 2015;32(2):192–197.

45. Percivalle S, Piccinno R, Caccialanza M et al. Narrowband ultraviolet B phototherapy in childhood vitiligo: Evaluation of results in 28 patients. *Pediatr Dermatol*. 2012;29(2):160–165.

46. Nicolaidou E, Antoniou C, Stratigos AJ, Stefanaki C, Katsambas AD. Efficacy, predictors of response and long-term follow-up in vitiligo patients treated with narrow band UVB phototherapy. *J Am Acad Dermatol*. 2007;56:274–278.

47. Kanwar AJ, Dogra S. Narrow-band UVB for the treatment of generalized vitiligo in children. *Clin Exp Dermatol*. 2005;30(4):332–336.

48. Esfandiarpour I, Ekhlasi A, Farajzadeh S et al. The efficacy of pimecrolimus 1% cream plus narrow-band ultraviolet B in the treatment of vitiligo: A double-blind, placebo-controlled clinical trial. *J Dermatolog Treat*. 2009;20(1):14–18.

49. Majid I. Does topical tacrolimus ointment enhance the efficacy of narrowband ultraviolet B therapy in vitiligo? A left-right comparison study. *Photodermatol Photoimmunol Photomed*. 2010;26(5):230–234.

50. Dayal S, Sahu P, Gupta N. Treatment of childhood vitiligo using tacrolimus ointment with narrowband ultraviolet B phototherapy. *Pediatr Dermatol*. 2016;33(6):646–651.

51. Ezzedine K, Silverberg N. A practical approach to the diagnosis and treatment of vitiligo in children. *Pediatrics*. 2016;138(1):e20154126.

52. Cho S, Zheng Z, Park YK et al. The 308-nm excimer laser: A promising device for the treatment of childhood vitiligo. *Photodermatol Photoimmunol Photomed*. 2011;27(1):24–29.

53. Koh MJ, Mok ZR, Chong WS. Phototherapy for the treatment of vitiligo in Asian children. *Pediatr Dermatol*. 2015;32(2):192–197.

54. Hui-Lan Y, Xiao-Yan H, Jian-Yong F et al. Combination of 308-nm excimer laser with topical pimecrolimus for the treatment of childhood vitiligo. *Pediatr Dermatol*. 2009;26(3):354–356.

55. Hu JJ, Xu AE, Wu XG et al. Small-sized lesions of childhood vitiligo treated by autologous epidermal grafting. *J Dermatolog Treat*. 2012;23(3):219–223.

56. Sahni K, Parsad D, Kanwar AJ. Noncultured epidermal suspension transplantation for the treatment of stable vitiligo in children and adolescents. *Clin Exp Dermatol*. 2011;36(6):607–612.

57. Mulekar SV, Al Eisa A, Delvi MB et al. Childhood vitiligo: A long-term study of localized vitiligo treated by noncultured cellular grafting. *Pediatr Dermatol*. 2010;27(2):132–136.

58. Hong WS, Hu DN, Qian GP et al. Treatment of vitiligo in children and adolescents by autologous cultured pure melanocytes transplantation with comparison of efficacy to results in adults. *J Eur Acad Dermatol Venereol*. 2011;25(5):538–543.

59. Yao L, Li SS, Zhong SX et al. Successful treatment of vitiligo on the axilla in a 5-year-old child by cultured-melanocyte transplantation. *J Eur Acad Dermatol Venereol*. 2012;26(5):658–660.

Pharmacological therapy of vitiligo

8

IVANA BINIĆ and ANDRIJA STANIMIROVIĆ

CONTENTS

Topical therapy of vitiligo	49	Systemic therapy of vitiligo	60
Miscellaneous topical agents	52	References	64

TOPICAL THERAPY OF VITILIGO

Topical corticosteroids

Topical corticosteroids (TCSs) have been applied in vitiligo since the1950s for their anti-inflammatory and immunomodulating effects, and they still remain the first-line treatment option. Implication of both cellular and humoral immune responses in the pathogenesis of vitiligo provides a rationale for the use of corticosteroids.[1] Corticosteroids might decrease disease progression, but it should be clearly explained to the patient that the primary aim of TCS is to achieve disease stability. Advantages are a relative low cost, ease of application, and ability for home usage. Most repigmentation can be observed in the face and neck, while the trunk, extremities, and especially the hands/feet usually display only limited repigmentation.[2] Recent lesions have a higher tendency for repigmentation.[3] The efficacy rate between potent and ultrapotent corticosteroids seems to be similar. Topical steroids should be used only for a limited time and only in localized vitiligo (less than 10% total body surface).[4]

Since the 1970s, many studies have been conducted to test the efficacy of topical corticosteroids alone or in combination with phototherapy. Furthermore, many comparative studies with other topical preparations have also been performed. Most of these studies demonstrate good efficacy of topical corticosteroids, with varying percentages of repigmentation (Table 8.1). A recent meta-analysis has confirmed their effectiveness for localized vitiligo.[5] Steroid-induced repigmentation occurs within 1–4 months of treatment both in a perifollicular pattern and from the lesion margins (Figure 8.1).

In children and adults, once-daily application of potent TCS can be advised for patients with limited involvement for a period no longer than 3 months, according to a continuous treatment scheme or, better, a discontinuous scheme (15 days per month for 6 months with a strict assessment of response based on photographs).[6] Currently, there are still no studies on optimal duration of TCS therapy. Side effects include skin atrophy, telangiectasia, and striae, which are rare if a discontinuous treatment scheme is used (e.g., 15 days of application per month). In the case of the occurrence of acneiform eruptions (especially on the face), a switch to topical calcineurin inhibitors (TCIs) may be advisable. Also, the potential for systemic absorption should be kept in mind and regularly monitored, particularly in patients with head and/or neck locations of the disease.[7]

Calcineurin inhibitors

Topical tacrolimus and pimecrolimus belong to the drug group of calcineurin inhibitors, which affects T-cell activity, inhibits their activation and maturation, and decreases the production of proinflammatory cytokines. *In vitro* experiments showed their ability to enhance melanocyte migration and induce skin pigmentation.[18]

The use of tacrolimus for vitiligo was reported for the first time in 2002, particularly for skin areas where the use of potent TCS is contraindicated.[19] Further studies (Table 8.2) have shown efficacy and good tolerability of tacrolimus for children with vitiligo in Asia,[20] and very good response of segmental vitiligo of head and trunk lesions.[21] However, another study showed that treatment of lesions on the body (not the face) with pimecrolimus cream 1% was not effective in a group of adult patients.[22] So, as monotherapy, TCIs are used mainly for lesions on the head and neck both in adults and children (Figure 8.2).

In studies comparing tacrolimus and pimecrolimus, some authors have found equal efficacy,[23] but others have found slightly higher response rates in patients treated with tacrolimus (61%) than in those treated with pimecrolimus (54.6%).[24] Twice-daily application of tacrolimus has been shown to be more effective compared with once-daily application,[25] and occlusive treatment enhanced the efficacy of tacrolimus ointment 0.1% beyond the face and neck in a study that included 20 adult patients with vitiligo.[26] Ultraviolet radiation exposure during treatment with TCI may be favorable,[27] but long-term safety studies are not available. The most frequent side effect of topical calcineurin inhibitors is a burning sensation at the beginning of therapy, lasting for 10–14 days.[28] Data on the duration of therapy, as well as on the possibilities of intermittent therapy, are not yet available.[6]

TCI can be a safer alternative to topical corticosteroids, because of fewer side effects, but there is a need for longer follow-up studies.

Table 8.1 Topical corticosteroids alone or in combination in vitiligo treatment

Author/year	Type of study	Drug	Number of patients	Treatment duration	Results	Side effects	Observation
Kandil, 1974 (8)	Randomized controlled trial	0.1% betamethasone valerate in 50% isopropyl alcohol versus alcohol base	19	4 months	More lesions showed complete repigmentation with active product	Hypertrichosis (2 patients) Localised acneiform eruption (3 patients)	
Clayton, 1977 (9)	Randomized double-blind controlled trial	0.05% clobetasol propionate in a cream base versus cream base alone	23	4 months	Active product was significantly better, 50% of patients had partial repigmentation	All patients had skin atrophy	
Khalid et al., 1995 (10)	Randomized parallel group study	PUVAsol versus clobetasol propionate (0.05%) bd	50 (children)	6 months	Clobetasol showed favorable response	Mild atrophy (4 patients), telangiectasia, acneiform eruption (2 patients)	
Lepe et al., 2003 (11)	Randomized double-blind trial	0.1% tacrolimus versus 0.05% clobetasol propionate (CP)	20 (children)	2 months	The mean percentage of repigmentation for CP was 49.3%, and 41.3% for tacrolimus	Mild atrophy (3 patients), telangiectasia (2 patients) with CP	
Kumaran et al., 2006 (12)	Randomized trial	Betamethasone dipropionate (0.05%) versus calcipotriol 49 (0.005%) bd versus betamethasone dipropionate (0.05%) in the morning and calcipotriol (0.005%) in the evening		3 months	Combined therapy showed faster and more stable repigmentation	Atrophy and lesional burning sensation were more common in BD group	Combined therapy showed faster and stable repigmentation with lesser side effects
Sanclemente et al., 2008 (13)	Randomized, matched-paired, double-blind trial	0.05% betamethasone versus topical catalase/ dismutase superoxide	25	10 months	Percentage of skin repigmentation 18.5 ±93.14% with betamethasone and to 12.4 ± 59% with C/DSO, no statistical difference	Mild, not a reason for discontinuation of therapy	Used digital morphometry

(Continued)

Table 8.1 (Continued) Topical corticosteroids alone or in combination in vitiligo treatment

Author/year	Type of study	Drug	Number of patients	Treatment duration	Results	Side effects	Observation
Köse et al., 2010 (14)	Randomized parallel group study	0.1% mometasone (M-Furo) od versus 1% pimecrolimus (Elidel) bd	50 (children)	3 months	The mean repigmentation rate was 65% in the mometasone group and 42% in the pimecrolimus group	Some expected side effects were assessed such as atrophy, telangiectasia and erythema in the mometasone group and burning sensation and pruritus in the pimecrolimus group	
Yaghoobi et al., 2011 (15)	Randomized parallel group study	0.05% CP in isopropyl alcohol for body and 0.1% triamcinolone acetonide for the face and flexures, used twice daily for both groups Oral zinc was added in the combination group	35	4 months	The mean of responses in the corticosteroid group and the zinc sulfate-corticosteroid combination group were 21.43% and 24.7%, respectively, without statistical difference		
Kathuria et al., 2012 (16)	Randomized parallel group study	0.1% tacrolimus bd versus 0.05% fluticasone propionate od	60	6 months	Median repigmentation with tacrolimus was 15%, median repigmentation with fluticasone propionate was 5%	Side effects were minimal and did not warrant withdrawal from the study	
Iraji et al., 2017 (17)	Randomized, controlled study	Betamethasone valerate 0.1% cream bd versus betamethasone valerate 0.1% cream bd and oral simvastatin 80 mg	88	12 weeks	26.3% had more than 50% repigmentation in the betamethasone valerate group and 37% in the combination group, no statistical difference		

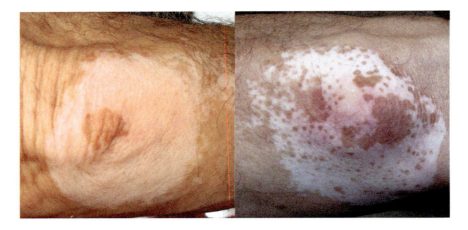

Figure 8.1 Vitiligo lesions on elbows before and after 8 weeks twice-daily topical treatment with 0.05% clobetasole propionate ointment.

Vitamin D analogues

Vitamin D3, or 1,25(OH)2D3, is a hormone responsible for regulating calcium homeostasis. It has already been proven that keratinocytes and melanocytes of vitiligo skin lesions show defective calcium uptake, which could inhibit melanogenesis through downregulation of tyrosinase activity. Two low calcemic synthetic analogs, with accentuated antiproliferative and cell-differentiating properties, calcipotriol and tacalcitol, have proven their efficacy in psoriasis, with the onset of perilesional hyperpigmentation during therapy. This feature has encouraged researchers to try to evaluate their efficacy in vitiligo,[32] used as monotherapy or in association with ultraviolet light or corticosteroids (Table 8.3). The exact mechanism of action is still unclear, but it is possible that they stimulate 1,25-dihydroxyvitamin D3 receptors, expressed on human melanocytes[33] and possibly adjusting calcium levels. The first results were encouraging,[34] with marked repigmentation in 55.6% of children treated; in this study, calcipotriol was used as once-daily application on all lesions for varying periods. Later studies used mostly combination therapy. Kumaran et al.[12] studied calcipotriol and betamethasone alone or in combination; repigmentation with the combined treatment was faster, stable, and with fewer side effects compared to either of the treatments used as monotherapy. Similar results were documented by Travis et al.,[35] where 83% of patients responded to combination therapy with an average of 95% repigmentation by body surface area and the best results achieved on eyelids and facial skin lesions. Some researchers have reported better results with calcipotriol ointment compared to cream.[36] The use of topical vitamin D analogues and sun exposure has been evaluated in several studies, but without good results,[37–39] so this combination is not recommended, due to its lack of significant efficacy and the possible carcinogenic risk associated with unregulated ultraviolet (UV) exposure.[38] The combination of calcipotriol and psoralen-ultraviolet A (PUVA) or narrowband ultraviolet B (NB-UVB) in vitiligo therapy has shown improvement in a few studies;[40–42] on the contrary, other investigators[43,44] could not find any such benefit when compared with phototherapy alone. The adverse effects due to calcipotriol are transient in the form of mild burning and irritation of the skin, and most of the investigators did not document them.

MISCELLANEOUS TOPICAL AGENTS
Pseudocatalase

The use of creams/ointments containing pseudocatalase may help in vitiligo repigmentation and in stabilizing the lesions (Table 8.4). Treatment is based on the evidence that the vitiligo epidermis shows oxidative stress, which is believed to have a important role in melanocyte degeneration. Pseudocatalase treatment aims to substitute low levels of catalase known to exist in vitiliginous skin and consequently aims to degrade excessive hydrogen peroxide.[45] Second, it aims to correct abnormalities in calcium homeostasis also known to exist in vitiligo. NB-UVB phototherapy is used to activate the pseudocatalase.

In the first study of pseudocatalase, 33 patients[46] were treated with pseudocatalase and calcium cream to the total body surface twice-daily, followed by suberythemogenic doses of UVB over 15 months. Results were encouraging; the first repigmentation was noted after 2–4 months and the best results were observed on the face and dorsa on the hands in 90% of cases. Also, disease activity was stopped in all cases. In an uncontrolled retrospective study of pseudocatalase cream plus NB-UVB in 71 children with generalized or segmental vitiligo, complete cessation of vitiligo progression was seen in 70 patients: more than 75% repigmentation was found in 66, with an observation that the response on the hands and feet was disappointing.[47] Later, several studies were conducted to confirm the usefulness of pseudocatalase as monotherapy or in combination with NB-UVB but failed to show any benefit.[48–50] One study compared topical catalase/dismutase superoxide (C/DSO) with topical corticosteroids and found

Table 8.2 Topical calcineurin inhibitors in vitiligo treatment

Author/year	Type of study	Drug/aim of study	Number of patients	Treatment duration	Results	Side effects	Observations
Silverberg et al., 2004 (21)	Randomized double-blind trial	Assess the efficacy of topical tacrolimus ointment in treatment of pediatric vitiligo	57 children	≥3 months	Partial response on head and neck (89%) and trunk and extremities (63%); segmental facial vitiligo had the best response rate	Two patients initially experienced burning on application	Topical tacrolimus ointment is effective alternative therapy for childhood vitiligo, particularly involving head and neck
Kanwar et al., 2004 (20)	Prospective pilot study	Topical 0.03% tacrolimus ointment twice daily	25 children	8 weeks	19 (86.4%) children showed some repigmentation at the end; another 3 had no response. Of 19 children, repigmentation was marked to complete in 11 (57.9%), moderate in 5 (26.3%), and mild in 3 (15.7%)	Side effects minimal, such as pruritus and burning in three patients	
Dawid et al., 2006 (22)	Double-blind, placebo controlled study	Pimecrolimus 1% cream vs vehicle cream, left–right comparison	20	6 months	Treatment with pimecrolimus cream 1% or vehicle resulted in no significant change in mean target lesion size. Modest repigmentation (1–25%). No side effects were noted with pimecrolimus at month 2 in 12 of 17 patients		In this group of adult patients with symmetrical vitiligo, treatment of body lesions (except face) with pimecrolimus cream 1% could not be shown to be effective
Radakovic et al., 2009 (25)	Controlled, prospective, randomized, observer-blinded trial	Assess the response of vitiligo to once- or twice-daily treatment with 0.1% tacrolimus	15 patients with 40 target lesions	6 months	Twice-daily treatment induced excellent (>75%) repigmentation in two lesions, moderate (>25–50%) and poor (1–25%) repigmentation in four lesions each, and no response in five lesions. Once-daily treatment resulted in moderate repigmentation in two lesions and poor repigmentation in five lesions, whereas no effect was observed in the remaining eight lesions. Facial lesions showed the best response		Tacrolimus ointment appears to be an effective treatment option for facial vitiligo

(Continued)

Table 8.2 (Continued)   Topical calcineurin inhibitors in vitiligo treatment

Author/year	Type of study	Drug/aim of study	Number of patients	Treatment duration	Results	Side effects	Observations
Xu et al., 2009 (29)	Prospective pilot study	Forty target lesions were selected to apply 0.1% tacrolimus ointment twice a day	30	4 months	25 (83.3%) patients showed some repigmentation at the end of 4 months. The mean percentage of repigmentation on the head and neck was greater than that on the trunk and extremities	Four patients initially experienced burning on application	Different sites of lesions
Lo et al., 2010 (30)	Multicenter, open-label, non-comparative study	To determine the efficacy and safety of topical tacrolimus as monotherapy for the treatment of face/neck vitiligo	61	12 weeks	At the end of treatment, all patients showed repigmentation and 45.9% of patients showed more than 25% repigmentation	15 adverse events related to the ointment were reported. All the reported adverse events were mild	
Shim et al., 2013 (31)	Prospective pilot study	Therapeutic efficacy and safety of 1% pimecrolimus cream for segmental childhood vitiligo			4 of 9 patients achieved mild to moderate responses after 3 months of treatment and continued with treatment; of these four patients, three achieved excellent response and one achieved moderate response, with a mean treatment duration of 7.3 months		Not double-blinded, treatment, duration not controlled, small number of patients

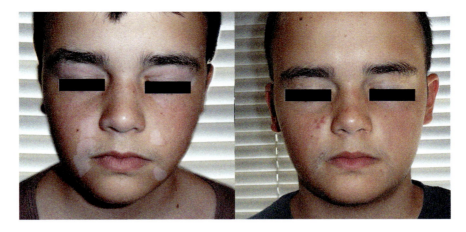

Figure 8.2 Vitiligo lesions on the face before and after 16 weeks twice-daily topical treatment with 0.1% tacrolimus ointment.

that objective vitiligo repigmentation with topical C/DSO at month 10 was similar to topical 0.05% betamethasone.[51] A very recent comparative, prospective, randomized study that included 30 patients demonstrated that the combination of excimer light and a topical antioxidant hydrogel was more effective compared to excimer light alone, especially on UV-sensitive areas.[52]

Prostaglandins

Prostaglandins (PGs) are biologically active derivatives of 20 carbon atom polyunsaturated essential fatty acids released from cell membrane phospholipids. Primary PGs are PGE2 and PGF2. PGE2 is synthesized in skin and affects keratinocytes, Langerhans cells, and melanocytes, causing proliferation of melanocytes and at the same time influencing the responsiveness of melanocytes to neuronal stimuli.[53]

The first study that used PGs in the treatment of vitiligo was reported in 2002 by Parsad et al.,[53] with encouraging results in patients with limited vitiligo with a body surface area involvement of less than 5% (Table 8.5). In this study, a translucent gel containing 0.5 mg/3 g (166.6 mg/g) PGE2 was used once daily on depigmented skin. Of the 24 patients included, marked to complete repigmentation was seen in 15, 3 patients showed moderate improvement, and 6 patients did not respond. In another study[54] that included 56 patients also with stable vitiligo and body surface area involvement less than 5%, repigmentation was seen in 40 of 56 patients (71%), with mean onset at 2 months. Patients with disease duration of 6 months or less repigmented best, with face and scalp responding earliest (1–1.5 months). In 8 of these 40 patients, 6 of whom had lesions on the face, complete repigmentation occurred. In a study by Anbar et al.,[55] latanoprost was found to be better than placebo and comparable with NB-UVB treatment. In the same study, the combination of latanoprost with NB-UVB produced significantly better results compared to NB-UVB monotherapy (Figure 8.3). Recently, a randomized, double-blind, controlled study that used another PGE, bimatoprost, for nonfacial vitiligo showed that bimatoprost alone or in combination with mometasone was more effective than mometasone monotherapy.[56]

Miscellaneous and new topical therapies for vitiligo

Melagenina is an alcohol extract of the human placenta, which has been considered for the topical treatment of vitiligo.[57] The exact mechanism of action is still unknown, but it seems to stimulate melanogenesis.[58] One pilot study evaluated the efficacy of topical melagenina, combined with 20 minutes of infrared exposure twice daily, for repigmentation in children with scalp vitiligo. The study concluded that the combination could be an efficient and safe treatment option for vitiligo, without side effects.[59] Recently, a new formulation has been created called Melagenina Plus, which consists of a placental extract with calcium; one study has shown efficacy in repigmentation of vitiligo lesions.[60]

In recent years, several studies have assessed some new drugs for the treatment of vitiligo. A very recent study showed that the use of a topical histamine for 5 weeks significantly reduced the size of vitiligo lesions and increased the melanin index by over 130%.[61] It is also important that the improvement of the melanin index did not correlate with disease duration. Another pilot study evaluated the efficacy of topical mycophenolate mofetil in the treatment of vitiligo.[62] The authors concluded that this drug can be effective in some cases of vitiligo, mostly on sun-exposed areas, but its use may not be warranted in cases resistant to topical steroids. The latest attempt for management of the disease is the use of topical Janus kinase (JAK) inhibitors. In the first study, the topical JAK inhibitor ruxolitinib was applied as a 1.5% cream in nine patients. A 23% improvement was reported in overall Vitiligo Area Scoring Index scores in all enrolled patients, with better results in facial vitiligo.[63] Some other studies underline the importance of the use of NB-UVB in combination with topical JAK inhibitors in order to achieve better results.[64,65] The above-mentioned studies are summarized in Table 8.6.

56 Pharmacological therapy of vitiligo

Table 8.3 Vitamin D3 analogues in vitiligo treatment

Author/year	Type of study	Drug/aim of study	Number of patients	Treatment duration	Results	Side effects	Observations
Parsad et al., 1999 (34)	Prospective pilot study	Topical calcipotriol–ultraviolet light (sunlight) therapy. Calcipotriol 50 lg/g+PUVA in the evening and exposure to sunlight the next day for 10–15 minutes	21 children	6–12 wks (3-week interval)	75%–100% repigmentation in 55.6% patients 50% repigmentation in 22.2% patients 0%–25% repigmentation in 22.2% patients	Three patients did not tolerate the drug and complained of mild irritation	Most of them were repigmented by 6–12 weeks of therapy
Yalçın et al., 2001 (42)	Prospective study	Patients received 60 sessions of PUVA 3 times a week and 0.005% topical calcipotriol twice daily	21	20 weeks	15 of 21 patients (71.5%) had some degree of pigmentation. Of these 15 patients, 6 (29%) had excellent or good response	Mild to moderate pruritus, irritation, and erythema on the regions in which calcipotriol had been applied were noted in 5 patients (24%)	
Gargoom et al., 2004 (36)	Randomized, Interventional study	Calcipotriol twice daily 50 lg/g cream or ointment for 2 wks then monthly for 4–6 mos	14 children	4–6 months	Of treated patients, 10 (77.8%) showed improvement; of responders, 3 (21.4%) showed complete resolution, 4 (28.6%) showed 50–80% improvement, and 3 (21.4%) showed 30%–50% improvement	One patient (5.5%) developed irritation	Better results obtained with ointment than with cream
Travis et al., 2004 (35)	Prospective study	Topical corticosteroid was applied in the morning and topical calcipotriene in the evening	12 patients, 10 children, 2 adults	3 months	83% responded to therapy, with an average of 95% repigmentation by body surface area	No adverse effects	This combination can repigment vitiligo even in those patients with topical corticosteroid failure
Sarma et al., 2004 (39)	Prospective, randomized and uncontrolled	Topical calcipotriol and sunlight for 15–20 min once daily	8 children	6 months	Mean repigmentation 41.5, range repigmentation 21%–100%		Earliest onset of pigmentation at the 4th week

(Continued)

Table 8.3 (Continued) Vitamin D3 analogues in vitiligo treatment

Author/year	Type of study	Drug/aim of study	Number of patients	Treatment duration	Results	Side effects	Observations
Kumaran et al., 2006 (12)	Randomized open-label	Group I patients were treated with betamethasone dipropionate (0.05%) cream twice daily. Group II patients were treated with calcipotriol ointment (0.005%) twice daily, and group III with betamethasone dipropionate (0.05%) in the morning and calcipotriol (0.005%) in the evening	45	3 months	No patient achieved excellent (>75%) pigmentation; Marked (50% to 75%) repigmentation was observed in 2 (13.3%), 1 (6.7%), and 4 (26.7%) patients in groups I, II, and III, respectively		Degree of repigmentation was greater in the combination group, but without statistical significance
Rodríguez-Martín et al., 2009 (37)	Rndomized double blind	30 min sunlight/day for 4 months+/–topical tacalcitol once daily	Tacalcitol 32 Control 32		Poor response: Tacalcitol 53% Control 31% >25% of lesional repigmentation Tacalcitol: none Control: 16%		No statistical difference found between the combination of tacalcitol and sunlight versus placebo and sunlight
Leone et al., 2006 (43)	Randomize open label	NB_UVB twice a week +/–topical tacalcitol ointment once daily	32 with paired lesions	6 months	Repigmentation score: Combination 2,4 NB-UVB: 1,2 Score 0: none, 1: <50%, 2: >50%		
Baysal et al., 2003 (44)	Randomized placebo-controlled	PUVA twice a week +/– topical calcipotriol twice a day	18 with paired lesions		Repigmentation rate on trunk: Combination 77% PUVA monoth: 78% Acral region: Combination 23% PUVA: 23% Extremities: Combination 78% PUVA: 77%		No statistical significance was found between combination calcipotriol and PUVA versus PUVA alone

Table 8.4 Topical pseudocatalase in vitiligo treatment

Author/year	Type of study	Drug	Number of patients	Treatment duration	Results	Side effects	Observation
Schallreuter et al., 2008 (47)	Retrospective study	Pseudocatalase PC-KUS twice daily to the entire body surface, followed by NB-UV-B irradiation	71 children	12 months	More than 75% repigmentation was achieved in 66 of 71 patients on the face/neck, 48 of 61 on the trunk, and 40 of 55 on the extremities	No adverse side effects	
Yuksel et al., 2009 (48)	Randomized placebo controlled	NB UVB + topical formulation including *Cucumis melo* superoxide dismutase and catalase (Vitix®) versus NB UVB alone	30	6 months	>75% repigmentation NB-UVB: 0% Combination: 2.8% >50% repigmentation NB-UVB 9.5% Combination: 19%	None	There was no statistically significant difference according to healing percentages between the two groups
Sanclemente et al., 2008 (51)	Randomized, matched paired study	Topical 0.05% betamethasone versus topical catalase/ dismutase superoxide twice a day	25 (paired lesions)	10 months	Catalase/dismutase superoxide 12% Betamethasone 19%, no statistical difference	Mild with corticosteroids	
Bakis-Petsoglou et al., 2009 (49)	Double-blind, placebo-controlled, randomized	Pseudocatalase cream/ placebo twice daily NB UVB three times a week	32	24 weeks	Pseudocatalase cream does not appear to add any incremental benefit to NB-UVB alone	No side effects	
Naini et al., 2012 (50)	Pilot randomized, double-blind, placebo-ontrolled	Pseudocatalase cream/ placebo twice daily 30 min sun exposure daily	23 (46 symmetrical lesions)	6 months	There were no significant changes in lesion area and no perifollicular pigmentation in each group		

Table 8.5 Prostaglandins in vitiligo treatment

Author/year	Type of study	Drug	Number of patients	Treatment duration	Results	Side effects	Observation
Parsad et al., 2002 (53)	Nonrandomized, uncontrolled	PGE2 Topicaly, 1×day	24	6 months	15 patients had moderate to marked repigmentation (50%–70%)	Not shown	
Kapoor et al., 2009 (54)	Nonrandomized, uncontrolled	Translucent PGE2 (0.25 mg g^{-1}) gel twice daily	56	6 months	Repigmentation in 40 (71%) patients, with mean onset at 2 months	In 18%, mainly a transient burning sensation especially on the lips	
Anbar et al., 2014 (55)	Randomized, controlled	Three groups of patients 1. Latanoprost (LP)/placebo 2. LP/NB-UVB 3. LP+NB-UVB/ NB-UVB	22	3 months	1. Better than placebo 2. Equal with NB-UVB 3. Better in combination	No observed side effects	Follow-up 6 months after termination of therapy
Grimes, 2016 (56)	Randomized, double-blind, controlled study	Three groups of patients: 1. Bimatoprost monotherapy 2. Bimatoprost+mometasone 3. Mometasone+placebo	32	20 weeks	Bimatoprost plus mometasone group had the maximum repigmentation	No side effects	

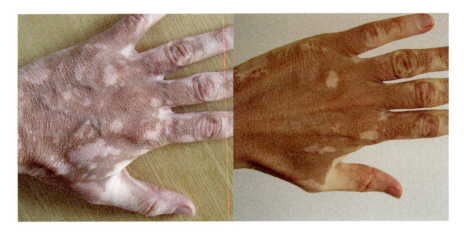

Figure 8.3 Vitiligo lesions on the dorsal side of the hands before and after 8 weeks topical treatment with 0.005% latanoprost solution twice-daily, combined with UVB 311-nm phototherapy three times weekly.

SYSTEMIC THERAPY OF VITILIGO
Systemic corticosteroids

Oral steroids are occasionally used in the treatment of fast-spreading adult vitiligo in an attempt to halt the spread of the disease (Table 8.7). Mostly, oral corticosteroids are administered as minipulse therapy. This mode of therapy refers to intermittent use of moderate or large doses of corticosteroids in order to enhance their therapeutic efficacy—and at the same time reduce their side effects. The first reported study was from India, with oral minipulse (OMP) of moderate doses of betamethasone/dexamethasone 5 mg on two consecutive days a week until adequate response was achieved.[66] Within 1–3 months, in 89% of patients with progressive vitiligo, spreading of the disease was stopped. The percentage of repigmentation varied a lot between patients, ranging from <10% to 90%. Another study used a daily dosing schedule of prednisolone for 4 months with an initial dose of 0.3 mg/kg body weight daily for the first 2 months, then halved in the third month, and again halved in the final, fourth month.[67] The results showed arrested progression of vitiligo and repigmentation in 87.7% and 70.4% of patients, respectively. Statistical significance was noted in patients under 15 years of age, male patients, and patients with a disease duration of less than 2 years. Side effects were minimal and did not affect the treatment. In another study, dexamethasone minipulses of 10 mg daily on two consecutive days per week up to 24 weeks were used. The authors concluded that this kind of treatment was effective in arresting progression of vitiligo, but failed to induce satisfactory repigmentation.[68] Side effects (weight gain, insomnia, agitation, acne, menstrual disturbances, and hypertrichosis) were observed in 69% of patients.

More recent studies have explored the efficacy of systemic steroids in combination with phototherapy, both the combination of intravenous prednisolone and psoralen ultraviolet A[69] and oral methylprednisolone (MPD) minipulse therapy combined with narrowband UVB.[70] The latter combination was effective in stopping the progression of the disease in 100% of patients, and it also induced rapid repigmentation. However, caution is warranted for long-term side effects when combining UVB with systemic immunosuppressants.[70] In a retrospective study by Kanwar et al., in 408 (91.8%) out of 444 patients, arrest of disease activity was achieved with low dose oral minipulse dexamethasone therapy, and the time needed for this varied from 12 to 24 weeks.[71] A randomized study comparing the effectiveness of dexamethasone oral minipulse therapy versus oral minocycline in patients with active vitiligo vulgaris showed that both drugs were effective in managing the arrest of disease activity.[72] A very recent randomized controlled trial aimed to evaluate the role of systemic steroid therapy and phototherapy in stable vitiligo; patients were divided into three groups: combined oral minipulses of prednisolone and NB-UVB, minipulses alone, and NB-UVB alone.[73] The authors concluded that both combination therapy and NB-UVB were superior to oral minipulses of steroids alone and suggested that adding steroid pulses to phototherapy can maintain success for a longer period.

Systemic immunosuppressive treatments

Systemic immunosuppressants are rarely used in vitiligo therapy and there are some anecdotal reports on a small number of patients or case reports (Table 8.8). Cyclophosphamide[74] and cyclosporine[75] have been studied, but there is not enough evidence of their effectiveness. Also, the potential side effects of these agents can be serious and do not justify their use in vitiligo.[6] Methotrexate has also been used in a number of small studies with limited success. The doses used ranged from 7.5 to 25 mg per week and the treatment was given for 3–16 months. It is important to note that no side effects were reported and the drug was well tolerated.[76–78] One study compared the efficacy of oral minipulses of dexamethasone (5 mg per week with 2.5 mg taken on two consecutive days) to that of methotrexate (10 mg per week); after 6 months of treatment, both group of patients had similar reduction in vitiligo disease activity score, and the investigators concluded that both drugs were equally effective in controlling the activity of the disease.[79]

Table 8.6 Miscellaneous and new topical therapies for vitiligo

Author/year	Type of study	Drug	Number of patients	Treatment duration	Results	Side effects	Observation
Xu et al., 2004 (59)	Nonrandomized, uncontrolled	Melagenina + 20 minutes Infrared exposure twice daily	22 (children)	2×3 months	18.2% full repigmenation, 8.2% no response	None	
Liu et al., 2017 (61)	Nonrandomized, uncontrolled	Topical histamine/placebo	23 (children and adults)	5 weeks	Melanin index increased by over 130%, histamin significantly reduced lesion size	Mild erythema and pruritus occurred in 8 patients	
Handjani et al., 2017 (62)	Nonrandomized uncontrolled	Topical 15% Mycophenolate mofetil	30	3 months	36.6% ($n=11$) of the patients showed 25% repigmentation	None	
Rothstein et al., 2017 (63)	Open-label, proof-of-concept trial	Topical ruxolitinib 1.5%	12	20 weeks	23% improvement in overall Vitiligo Area Scoring Index scores were observed in all enrolled patients	Minor, including erythema, hyperpigmentation, and transient acne	

62 Pharmacological therapy of vitiligo

Table 8.7 Systemic corticosteroid therapy for vitiligo

Author/year	Type of study	Drug	Number of patients	Treatment duration	Results	Side effects	Observation
Paricha et al., 1993 (66)	Prospective, open label trial	5 mg oral betamethasone/ dexamethasone /day 2d/week	40 (children and adults)	As long as the adequate response was achieved (>2 years)	Within 1–3 months, in 89% of patients with active disease, the progression was stopped. Rate of repigmentation varied from <10% to 90%	Weight gain, mild headache, general weakness, bad taste in the mouth	Extensive and/or rapidly spreading vitiligo
Kim et al., 1999 (67)	Prospective, open label trial	Oral prednisolone (0.3 mg/kg body weight) daily (2 months), halved (3rd month) halved (4th month)	81 (children and adults)	4 months	Arrested progression of vitiligo and repigmentation were noted in 87.7% and 70.4% of patients, respectively	Minimal, did not affect the course of treatment	
Radakovic-Fijan et al., 2001 (68)	Prospective, open label trial	10 mg oral dexamethasone/day 2d/week	29	24 weeks	Disease activity was arrested in 88% of patients. No effect on repigmentation	20 (69%) of patients: weight gain, insomnia, acne, agitation, menstrual disturbance, and hypertrichosis	
Kanwar et al., 2013 (71)	Retrospective	2.5 mg oral dexamethasone/day 2d/week	444	Until the arrest of disease activity (maximum 6 months)	In 408 (91.8%) of patients, arrest of disease activity was achieved	In 41(9.2%) of patients: weight gain, bloated appearance, gastric upset, lethargy acne, and joint pains	
El Mofty et al., 2016 (73)	Prospective, randomized, controlled	Group A: 30 mg prednisolone daily, 2d/week+ NB-UVB Group B: Prednisolone Group C: NB-UVB	45	3 months	Patients showing improvement Group A: 100% Group B: 33.33% Group C: 100%	None	Follow-up for 6 months

Table 8.8 Systemic immunosuppressive treatments for vitiligo

Author/year	Type of study	Drug	Number of patients	Treatment duration	Results	Side effects	Observation
Sandra et al., 1998 (76)	Case report	Methotrexate 7.5 mg/week	1	3 months	Stopping the appearance of new lesions	None	
Alghamdi et al., 2013 (77)	Pilot prospective	Methotrexate 25 mg/week	6	6 months	No change in vitiligo lesions	None	
Garza-Mayers et al., 2017 (78)	Case series	Methotrexate 12.5–25 mg/week	3	11–16 months	Clinically significant skin repigmentation	None	
Singh et al., 2015 (79)	Prospective randomized open label	Group 1: 10 mg methotrexate/week Group 2: OMP dexamethasone 2.5 mg on 2 consecutive days/week	52	24 weeks	Similar reduction in the vitiligo disease activity score	4% in I group (nausea) 5% in II group (weight gain, acne)	
Radmanesh et al., 2006 (80)	Prospective randomized	Group 1: azathioprine (0.6–0.75 mg/kg)+PUVA Group 2: PUVA	60	4 months	The mean total repigmentation rate was 58.4% for group 1 and 24.8% for group 2	None	

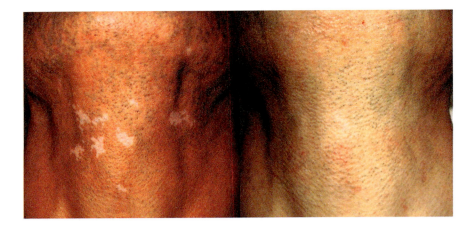

Figure 8.4 Vitiligo lesions on the neck before and after 8 weeks of therapy with perorally *Polypodium leucotomos* 240 mg per day combined with UVB 311-nm phototherapy twice weekly.

Azathioprine has also been used in combination with oral PUVA, in a study that compared this combination versus PUVA therapy alone.[80] The conclusion was that azathioprine may potentiate the repigmentary effects of PUVA therapy in vitiligo patients.

Systemic biologics and small molecules

In a few small case series, antitumor necrosis factor alpha biologic agents have been proposed for the treatment of vitiligo, with variable efficacy,[81,82] but also with no efficacy at all.[83,84] Moreover, there are reports of even initiation and worsening of the disease with their administration.[85,86] Recently, two very promising case reports with the oral JAK inhibitor tofacitinib citrate have been reported. In the first, nearly complete repigmentation after 5 months of treatment was achieved,[87] and in the other, there was only marginal improvement, also after 5 months of treatment.[88]

Systemic antioxidants

Therapy with oral antioxidants has its place in vitiligo therapy due to the etiopathogenetic role of cellular oxidative stress. Concerning the use of oral antioxidants, several clinical trials have been published; most of these studies are hampered by a limited patient number, and confirmatory results are mostly missing.[28] In a double-blind placebo-controlled trial, monotherapy with oral ginkgo biloba significantly reduced the progression of the disease compared to placebo.[89] Another study by Sczurko et al. showed that daily ingestion of 60 mg of ginkgo biloba extracts for 12 weeks was associated with a significant improvement of the spreading of vitiligo lesions.[90] Some studies have documented that the combination of oral antioxidants and NB-UVB therapy is useful. In a double-blind placebo-controlled trial, a mixture of alpha lipoic acid, vitamin C, vitamin E, and polyunsaturated fatty acids significantly improved the clinical efficacy of NB-UVB, with increased repigmentation rates and dose reduction of NB-UVB.[91] *Polypodium leucotomos*, an antioxidant immunomodulator and photosensitizing agent, significantly improved the repigmentation rates in the head and neck area when used in association with NB-UVB (Figure 8.4).[92]

REFERENCES

1. van den Wijngaard R, Wankowicz-Kalinska A, Pals S, Weening J, Das P. Autoimmune melanocyte destruction in vitiligo. *Lab Invest*. 2001;81:1061–1067.
2. Njoo MD, Spuls PI, Bos JD, Westerhof W, Bossuyt PM. Nonsurgical repigmentation therapies in vitiligo: Meta-analysis of the literature. *Arch Dermatol*. 1998;134:1532–1540.
3. Schaffer JV, Bolognia JL. The treatment of hypopigmentation in children. *Clin Dermatol*. 2003;21:296–310.
4. Lotti T, Berti S, Moretti S. Vitiligo therapy. *Expert Opin Pharmacother*. 2009;10:2779–2785.
5. Whitton M, Pinart M, Batchelor JM et al. Evidence-Based Management of vitiligo: Summary of a Cochrane systematic review. *Br J Dermatol*. 2015; 174:962–969.
6. Taieb A, Alomar A, Böhm M et al. Guidelines for the management of vitiligo: The European Dermatology Forum consensus. *Br J Dermatol*. 2013;168:5–19.
7. Kwinter J, Pelletier J, Khambalia A, Pope E. High-potency steroid use in children with vitiligo: A retrospective study. *J Am Acad Dermatol*. 2007;56:236–241.
8. Kandil E. Treatment of vitiligo with 0-1 per cent betamethasone 17-valerate in isopropyl alcohol – A double-blind trial. *Br J Dermatol*. 1974;91:457–460.
9. Clayton R. A double-blind trial of 0–05% clobetasol proprionate in the treatment of vitiligo. *Br J Dermatol*. 1977;96:71–73.
10. Khalid M, Mujtaba G, Haroon TS. Comparison of 0.05% clobetasol propionate cream and topical Puvasol in childhood vitiligo. *Int J Dermatol*. 1995;34:203–205.
11. Lepe V, Moncada B, Castanedo-Cazares JP, Torres-Alvarez MB, Ortiz CA, Torres-Rubalcava AB. A double-blind randomized trial of 0.1% tacrolimus

vs. 0.05% clobetasol for the treatment of childhood vitiligo. *Arch Dermatol.* 2003;139:581–585.

12. Kumaran MS, Kaur I, Kumar B. Effect of topical calcipotriol, betamethasone dipropionate and their combination in the treatment of localized vitiligo. *J Eur Acad Dermatol Venereol.* 2006;20:269–273.

13. Sanclemente G, Garcia JJ, Zuleta JJ, Diehl C, Correa C, Falabella R. A double-blind, randomized trial of 0.05% betamethasone vs. topical catalase/dismutase superoxide in vitiligo. *J Eur Acad Dermatol Venereol.* 2008;22:1359–1364.

14. Köse O, Arca E, Kurumlu Z. Mometasone cream versus pimecrolimus cream for the treatment of childhood localized vitiligo. *J Dermatolog Treat.* 2010;21:133–139.

15. Yaghoobi R, Omidian M, Bagherani N. Comparison of therapeutic efficacy of topical corticosteroid and oral zinc sulfate-topical corticosteroid combination in the treatment of vitiligo patients: A clinical trial. *BMC Dermatol.* 2011;11:7.

16. Kathuria S, Khaitan BK, Ramam M, Sharma VK. Segmental vitiligo: A randomized controlled trial to evaluate efficacy and safety of 0.1% tacrolimus ointment vs. 0.05% fluticasone propionate cream. *Indian J Dermatol Venereol Leprol.* 2012;78:68–73.

17. Iraji F, Banihashemi SH, Faghihi G, Shahmoradi Z, Tajmirriahi N, Jazi SB. A comparison of betamethasone valerate 0.1% cream twice daily plus oral simvastatin versus betamethasone valerate 0.1% cream alone in the treatment of Vitiligo patients. *Adv Biomed Res.* 2017;6:34.

18. Jung H, Chung H, Chang SE, Kang D-H, Oh E-S. FK506 regulates pigmentation by maturing the melanosome and facilitating their transfer to keratinocytes. *Pigment Cell Melanoma Res.* 2016;29:199–209.

19. Grimes PE, Soriano T, Dytoc MT. Topical tacrolimus for repigmentation of vitiligo. *J Am Acad Dermatol.* 2002;47:789–791.

20. Kanwar AJ, Dogra S, Parsad D. Topical tacrolimus for treatment of childhood vitiligo in Asians. *Clin Exp Dermatol.* 2004;29:589–592.

21. Silverberg NB, Lin P, Travis L et al. Tacrolimus ointment promotes repigmentation of vitiligo in children: A review of 57 cases. *J Am Acad Dermatol.* 2004;51:760–766.

22. Dawid M, Veensalu M, Grassberger M, Wolff K. Efficacy and safety of pimecrolimus cream 1% in adult patients with vitiligo: Results of a randomized, double-blind, vehicle-controlled study. *J Dtsch Dermatol Ges.* 2006;4:942–946.

23. Stinco G, Piccirillo F, Forcione M, Valent F, Patrone P. An open randomized study to compare narrow band UVB, topical pimecrolimus and topical tacrolimus in the treatment of vitiligo. *Eur J Dermatol.* 2009;19:588–593.

24. Lotti T, Buggiani G, Troiano M et al. Targeted and combination treatments for vitiligo. Comparative evaluation of different current modalities in 458 subjects. *Dermatol Ther.* 2008;21:S20–S26.

25. Radakovic S, Breier-Maly J, Konschitzky R et al. Response of vitiligo to once- vs. Twicedaily topical tacrolimus: A controlled prospective, randomized, observer-blinded trial. *J Eur Acad Dermatol Venereol.* 2009;23:951–953.

26. Hartmann A, Brocker EB, Hamm H. Occlusive treatment enhances the efficacy of tacrolimus 0.1% ointment in adult patients with vitiligo: Results of a placebo-controlled 12-month prospective study. *Acta Derm Venereol.* 2008;88:474–479.

27. Ostovari N, Passeron T, Lacour JP, Ortonne JP. Lack of efficacy of tacrolimus in the treatment of vitiligo in the absence of UV-B exposure. *Arch Dermatol.* 2006;142:252–253.

28. Speeckaert R, van Geel N. Vitiligo: An update on pathophysiology and treatment options. *Am J Clin Dermatol.* 2017;18:733–744.

29. Xu AE, Zhang DM, Wei XD, Huang B, Lu LJ. Efficacy and safety of tacrolimus cream 0.1% in the treatment of vitiligo. *Int J Dermatol.* 2009;48:86–90.

30. Lo YH, Cheng GS, Huang CC, Chang WY, Wu CS. Efficacy and safety of topical tacrolimus for the treatment of face and neck vitiligo. *J Dermatol.* 2010;37:125–129.

31. Shim WH, Suh SW, Jwa SW et al. A pilot study of 1% pimecrolimus cream for the treatment of childhood segmental vitiligo. *Ann Dermatol.* 2013;25:168–172.

32. Kanwar AJ, Kumaran MS. Childhood vitiligo: Treatment paradigms. *Indian J Dermatol.* 2012;57:466–474.

33. Leone G, Pacifico A. Profile of clinical efficacy and safety of topical tacalcitol. *Acta Biomed.* 2005;76:13–19.

34. Parsad D, Saini R, Nagpal R. Calcipotriol in vitiligo: Preliminary study. *Pediatr Dermatol.* 1999;16:317–320.

35. Travis LB, Silverberg NB. Calcipotriene and corticosteroid combination therapy for vitiligo. *Pediatr Dermatol.* 2004;21:495–498.

36. Gargoom AM, Duweb GA, Elzorghany AH, Benghazil M, Bugrein OO. Calcipotriol in the treatment of childhood citiligo. *Int J Clin Pharmacol Res.* 2004;24:11–14.

37. Rodríguez-Martín M, García Bustínduy M, Sáez Rodríguez M, Noda Cabrera A. Randomized, double-blind clinical trial to evaluate the efficacy of topical tacalcitol and sunlight exposure in the treatment of adult nonsegmental vitiligo. *Br J Dermatol.* 2009; 160:409–414.

38. Wat H, Dytoc M. Off-label uses of topical vitamin D in dermatology: A systematic review. *J Cutan Med Surg.* 2014;18:91–108.

39. Sarma N, Singh AK. Topical calcipotriol in childhood vitiligo: An Indian experience. *Int J Dermatol.* 2004;43:856–859.

40. Ermis O, Alpsoy E, Cetin L, Yilmaz E. Is the efficacy of psoralen plus ultraviolet a therapy for vitiligo

enhanced by concurrent topical calcipotriol? A placebo-controlled double-blind study. *Br J Dermatol.* 2001;145:472–475.

41. Leone G, Pacifico A, Iacovelli P, Paro Vidolin A, Picardo M. Tacalcitol and narrow-band phototherapy in patients with vitiligo. *Clin Exp Dermatol.* 2006;31:200–205.

42. Yalçin B, Sahin S, Bükülmez G et al. Experience with calcipotriol as adjunctive treatment for vitiligo in patients who do not respond to PUVA alone: A preliminary study. *J Am Acad Dermatol.* 2001;44:634–637.

43. Ada S, Sahin S, Boztepe G, Karaduman A, Kölemen F. No additional effect of topical calcipotriol on narrow-band UVB phototherapy in patients with generalized vitiligo. *Photodermatol Photoimmunol Photomed.* 2005;21:79–83.

44. Baysal V, Yildirim M, Erel A, Kesici D. Is the combination of calcipotriol and PUVA effective in vitiligo? *J Eur Acad Dermatol Venereol.* 2003;17:299–302.

45. Schallreuter KU, Wood JM, Berger J. Low catalase levels in the epidermis of patients with vitiligo. *J Invest Dermatol.* 1991;97:1081–1085.

46. Schallreuter KU, Wood JM, Lemke KR, Levenig C. Treatment of vitiligo with a topical application of pseudocatalase and calcium in combination with short-term UVB exposure: A case study on 33 patients. *Dermatology.* 1995;190:223–229.

47. Schallreuter KU, Krüger C, Würfel BA, Panske A, Wood JM. From basic research to the bedside: Efficacy of topical treatment with pseudocatalase PC-KUS in 71 children with vitiligo. *Int J Dermatol.* 2008;47:743–753.

48. Yuksel EP, Aydin F, Senturk N, Canturk T, Turanli AY. Comparison of the efficacy of narrow band ultraviolet B and narrow band ultraviolet B plus topical catalase-superoxide dismutase treatment in vitiligo patients. *Eur J Dermatol.* 2009;19:341–344.

49. Bakis-Petsoglou S, Le Guay JL, Wittal R. A randomized, double-blinded, placebo-controlled trial of pseudocatalase cream and narrowband ultraviolet B in the treatment of vitiligo. *Br J Dermatol.* 2009;161:910–917.

50. Naini FF, Shooshtari AV, Ebrahimi B, Molaei R. The effect of pseudocatalase/superoxide dismutase in the treatment of vitiligo: A pilot study. *J Res Pharm Pract.* 2012;1:77–80.

51. Sanclemente G, Garcia JJ, Zuleta JJ, Diehl C, Correa C, Falabella R. A double-blind, randomized trial of 0.05% betamethasone vs. topical catalase/dismutase superoxide in vitiligo. *J Eur Acad Dermatol Venereol.* 2008;22:1359–1364.

52. Soliman M, Samy NA, Abo Eittah M, Hegazy M. Comparative study between excimer light and topical antioxidant versus excimer light alone for treatment of vitiligo. *J Cosmet Laser Ther.* 2016;18:7–11.

53. Parsad D, Pandhi R, Dogra S, Kumar B. Topical prostaglandin analog (PGE2) in vitiligo--a preliminary study. *Int J Dermatol.* 2002;41:942–945.

54. Kapoor R, Phiske MM, Jerajani HR. Evaluation of safety and efficacy of topical prostaglandin E2 in treatment of vitiligo. *Br J Dermatol.* 2009;160:861–863.

55. Anbar TS, El-Ammawi TS, Abdel-Rahman AT, Hanna MR. The effect of latanoprost on vitiligo: A preliminary comparative study. *Int J Dermatol.* 2015;54:587–593.

56. Grimes PE. Bimatoprost 0.03% solution for the treatment of Nonfacial Vitiligo. *J Drugs Dermatol.* 2016;15:703–710.

57. Nordlund JJ, Halder R. Melagenina. An analysis of published and other available data. *Dermatologica.* 1990;181(1):1–4.

58. Zhao D, Li Y, Wang P et al. Melagenine modulates proliferation and differentiation of melanoblasts. *Int J Mol Med.* 2008;22:193–197.

59. Xu AE, Wei XD. Topical melagenine for repigmentation in twenty-two child patients with vitiligo on the scalp. *Chin Med J (Engl).* 2004;117:199–201.

60. Miyares CM, Hollands Barca I, Miyares Diaz E, Pernas González A. Effectiveness of human placental extract with calcium (Melagenina Plus) for the treatment of vitiligo. *Medicina cutánea ibero-latino-americana.* 2009;37:207–212.

61. Liu J, Xu Y, Lin TK, Lv C, Elias PM, Man MQ. Topical histamine stimulates repigmentation of nonsegmental vitiligo by a receptor-dependent mechanism. *Skin Pharmacol Physiol.* 2017;30:139–145.

62. Handjani F, Aghaei S, Moezzi I, Saki N. Topical mycophenolate mofetil in the treatment of vitiligo: A pilot study. *Dermatol Pract Concept.* 2017;7:31–33.

63. Rothstein B, Joshipura D, Saraiya A et al. Treatment of vitiligo with the topical Janus kinase inhibitor ruxolitinib. *J Am Acad Dermatol.* 2017;76: 1054–1060.e1.

64. Joshipura D, Alomran A, Zancanaro P, Rosmarin D. Treatment of vitiligo with the topical Janus kinase inhibitor ruxolitinib: A 32-week open-label extension study with optional narrow-band ultraviolet B. *J Am Acad Dermatol.* 2018;78:1205–1207.e1.

65. Joshipura D, Plotnikova N, Goldminz A et al. Importance of light in the treatment of vitiligo with JAK-inhibitors. *J Dermatolog Treat.* 2018;29:98–99.

66. Pasricha JS, Khaitan BK. Oral mini-pulse therapy with betamethasone in vitiligo patients having extensive or fast-spreading disease. *Int J Dermatol.* 1993;32:753–757.

67. Kim SM, Lee HS, Hann SK. The efficacy of low-dose oral corticosteroids in the treatment of vitiligo patients. *Int J Dermatol.* 1999;38:546–550.

68. Radakovic-Fijan S, Fürnsinn-Friedl AM, Hönigsmann H, Tanew A. Oral dexamethasone pulse treatment for vitiligo. *J Am Acad Dermatol.* 2001;44:814–817.

69. Lee Y, Seo YJ, Lee JH, Park JK. High-dose prednisolone and psoralen ultraviolet a combination therapy in 36 patients with vitiligo. *Clin Exp Dermatol.* 2007;32:499–501.

70. Lee J, Chu H, Lee H, Kim M, Kim DS, Oh SH. A retrospective study of methylprednisolone mini-pulse therapy combined with narrow-band UVB in non-segmental Vitiligo. *Dermatology.* 2016; 232(2):224–229.

71. Kanwar AJ, Mahajan R, Parsad D. Low-dose oral mini-pulse dexamethasone therapy in progressive unstable vitiligo. *J Cutan Med Surg.* 2013 Jul–Aug; 17(4):259–268.

72. Singh A, Kanwar AJ, Parsad D, Mahajan R. Randomized controlled study to evaluate the effectiveness of dexamethasone oral minipulse therapy versus oral minocycline in patients with active vitiligo vulgaris. *Indian J Dermatol Venereol Leprol.* 2014;80:29–35.

73. El Mofty M, Essmat S, Youssef R et al. The role of systemic steroids and phototherapy in the treatment of stable vitiligo: A randomized controlled trial. *Dermatol Ther.* 2016;29:406–412.

74. Dogra S, Kumar B. Repigmentation in vitiligo universalis: Role of melanocyte density, disease duration, and melanocytic reservoir. *Dermatol Online J.* 2005;11(3):30.

75. Pardue SL, Fite KV, Bengston L, Lamont SJ, Boyle ML 3rd, Smyth JR Jr. Enhanced integumental and ocular amelanosis following the termination of cyclosporine administration. *J Invest Dermatol.* 1987;88:758–761.

76. Sandra A, Pai S, Shenoi SD. Unstable vitiligo responding to methotrexate. *Indian J Dermatol Venereol Leprol.* 1998;64:309.

77. Alghamdi K, Khurrum H. Methotrexate for the treatment of generalized vitiligo. *Saudi Pharm J.* 2013;21:423–424.

78. Garza-Mayers AC, Kroshinsky D. Low-dose methotrexate for vitiligo. *J Drugs Dermatol.* 2017; 16:705–706.

79. Singh H, Kumaran MS, Bains A, Parsad D. A randomized comparative study of oral corticosteroid minipulse and low-dose oral methotrexate in the treatment of unstable vitiligo. *Dermatology.* 2015; 231:286–290.

80. Radmanesh M, Saedi K. The efficacy of combined PUVA and low-dose azathioprine for early and enhanced repigmentation in vitiligo patients. *J Dermatolog Treat.* 2006;17(3):151–153.

81. Kim NH, Torchia D, Rouhani P, Roberts B, Romanelli P. Tumor necrosis factor-α in vitiligo: Direct correlation between tissue levels and clinical parameters. *Cutan Ocul Toxicol.* 2011;30:225–227.

82. Webb KC, Tung R, Winterfield LS et al. Tumour necrosis factor-α inhibition can stabilize disease in progressive vitiligo. *Br J Dermatol.* 2015;173:641–650.

83. Rigopoulos D, Gregoriou S, Larios G, Moustou E, Belayeva-Karatza E, Kalogeromitros D. Etanercept in the treatment of vitiligo. *Dermatology.* 2007;215:84–85.

84. Alghamdi KM, Khurrum H, Taieb A, Ezzedine K. Treatment of generalized vitiligo with anti-TNF-α Agents. *J Drugs Dermatol.* 2012;11:534–539.

85. Maruthappu T, Leandro M, Morris SD. Deterioration of vitiligo and new onset of halo naevi observed in two patients receiving adalimumab. *Dermatol Ther.* 2013;26:370–372.

86. Alghamdi KM, Khurrum H, Rikabi A. Worsening of vitiligo and onset of new psoriasiform dermatitis following treatment with infliximab. *J Cutan Med Surg.* 2011;15:280–284.

87. Craiglow BG, King BA. Tofacitinib citrate for the treatment of Vitiligo: A pathogenesis-directed therapy. *JAMA Dermatol.* 2015;151:1110–1112.

88. Vu M, Heyes C, Robertson SJ, Varigos GA, Ross G. Oral tofacitinib: A promising treatment in atopic dermatitis, alopecia areata and vitiligo. *Clin Exp Dermatol.* 2017;42:942–944.

89. Parsad D, Pandhi R, Juneja A. Effectiveness of oral Ginkgo biloba in treating limited, slowly spreading vitiligo. *Clin Exp Dermatol.* 2003;28:285–287.

90. Szczurko O, Shear N, Taddio A, Boon H. Ginkgo biloba for the treatment of vitilgo vulgaris: An open label pilot clinical trial. *BMC Complement Altern Med.* 2011;11:21.

91. Dell'Anna ML, Mastrofrancesco A, Sala R et al. Antioxidants and narrow band-UVB in the treatment of vitiligo: A double-blind placebo controlled trial. *Clin Exp Dermatol.* 2007;32:631–636.

92. Middelkamp-Hup MA, Bos JD, Rius-Diaz F, Gonzalez S, Westerhof W. Treatment of vitiligo vulgaris with narrow-band UVB and oral Polypodium leucotomos extract: A randomized double-blind placebo-controlled study. *J Eur Acad Dermatol Venereol.* 2007;21:942–950.

Surgical treatment of vitiligo

9

MUHAMMED RAZMI T., T. P. AFRA, and DAVINDER PARSAD

CONTENTS

Introduction	69	Conclusion	76
Patient selection	69	Acknowledgments	76
Recipient area preparation	69	References	76
Types of vitiligo surgery	69		

INTRODUCTION

Vitiligo is the most common acquired depigmentation disorder, with a reported worldwide prevalence of around 2%. Cosmetically disfiguring depigmented patches due to the loss of melanocytes cause great concern and psychological distress to affected patients.[1] While medical modalities address the stabilization of the patches followed by repigmentation, surgical modalities may need to be employed to those patches that do not repigment with medical modalities. Inadequate residual melanocytes or inducible stem cells may be the reasons for lack of repigmentation even after attaining stability. In vitiligo surgery, such resistant achromic patches are supplied with melanocytes or, recently, with additional melanocyte precursors. Here, we highlight the different aspects of vitiligo surgery, including patient selection, recipient area preparation, and methodology of various types of vitiligo surgery.

PATIENT SELECTION

Patient selection is an important aspect of successful vitiligo surgery. Currently, a patch with at least 1 year lesional stability is best suited for a surgical intervention.[2] A minigraft test prior to the proposed surgery will help to rule out microscopic lesional activity of the disease. Amelanotic lesions with sharp borders are best suited for surgery compared to hypopigmented lesions with poorly defined borders. Regarding the type of vitiligo, segmental vitiligo yields better repigmentation, followed by focal and common vitiligo, with acrofacial types giving a poorer repigmentation outcome. Repigmentation of lesions over hairy regions is better compared to lesions on nonhairy regions. Koebner sites like bony areas, flexures, and eyelids also respond poorly. With the advent of cellular transplantation and combination therapies, the definition of acral sites is being shifted more distally, with acceptable repigmentation outcome achieved nowadays proximal to the proximal phalanges. Even though the repigmentation outcome is good even in children, it's prudent to wait until they become mature enough to endure the pain of the procedure and follow the postprocedure instructions. Patients with smaller

lesions are preferred for tissue grafts, and those with larger lesions are preferred for cellular grafts. Patients with unrealistic expectations should be properly counseled regarding surgical outcomes, including the possibility of a failed surgery.

RECIPIENT AREA PREPARATION

Various methods of recipient area preparation have been described in the literature. These include the use of liquid nitrogen, mechanical dermabrasion, diathermy or chemical peeling–assisted dermabrasion, suction blisters, psoralen plus ultraviolet A (PUVA), and CO_2 and Er:YAG lasers. Lasers are very versatile and offer a precise depth of recipient bed at the cost of increase in expense. Mechanical dermabrasion devices are less costly and simpler to use, but may result in scarring with inexperienced hands. PUVA, suction blister, and liquid nitrogen–based recipient area preparation increase the procedural time for the surgery since it takes some time to prepare the recipient bed.

Laser devices are largely used in resource-rich settings, and manual dermabrasion methods are commonly used in resource-poor settings. Acral skin and the skin previously exposed to phototherapy are difficult to dermabrade. Local infiltrative anesthesia is commonly used for the procedure. General or regional anesthesia can be used for the surgery of large extensive patches or in the pediatric population.

TYPES OF VITILIGO SURGERY

Different types of vitiligo surgery have been tabulated in Table 9.1. Tissue-based methods were the initial choices of surgery. Nowadays, cellular methods, especially noncultured epidermal cell suspensions, are increasingly used for the surgery.

Tissue grafts

The source of melanocytes here is epidermal-dermal punches, ultrathin skin sheets, the epidermal roof of a blister, and hair follicles. There will not be much augmentation of donor-to-recipient area factor, but the expected repigmentation is denser and diffuse compared to cellular transplantation methods. Postoperative

Table 9.1　Vitiligo surgery techniques

Method			Efficacy[a]	Advantages	Disadvantages
Tissue Grafts	Full-Thickness Punch Grafts, 1983[27] (mini-punch grafts)		Varies from 50%–100% RP in 38%–74.5% of patients in various studies[28,29]	Inexpensive. Easy to perform. Minimal equipment. Suitable for difficult locations such as the lips, palms, soles, and fingers.[30,31]	Cannot be expanded. Limited use in the treatment of large areas. Cosmetic complications like color mismatch, cobblestoning, speckled appearance, and donor site scarring.[29,31,32]
	Split-Thickness Skin Grafts Theirsch-Ollier (0.125–0.275 mm thick), 1973[3] or Ultrathin (0.08–0.15 mm thick), 1993[4]	Flip-Top Grafts, 1999[5] Seed/Smash Grafts, 2012[6]	Rate of RP is 78%–91%[6,33–35]	High rate of RP. Suitable for multiple or large areas and difficult areas, such as the eyelid, inner canthus of the eyes, areola, nipples, and genitals. The donor site can be reused for subsequent grafts.[36]	Requires a high degree of skill and dexterity. Cosmetic damage to the recipient and donor areas in case of thick grafts. Temporary milia-like cysts, partial loss of graft, and thick margins at the recipient site.[33] Donor site scarring and hypopigmentation (less with ultrathin grafts). Not suitable for palms, soles, body folds, and nonkeratinized mucosa.
	Suction Blister Grafts, 1971,[37] 1988[38]		50%–100% RP[9]	Safe, effective, easy, and inexpensive technique. Fast and uniform repigmentation. No risk of scarring at the donor site, and donor sites can be used more than once. Suitable for difficult areas such as the eyelids, lips, and bony prominences.	Time-consuming and painful procedure. Cannot be expanded. Limited use in the treatment of large areas and areas such as the palms, soles, and body folds. Repigmentation results are inferior to split-thickness grafts and noncultured epidermal cell suspensions.[39] Cosmetic complications are temporary hyperpigmentation of the donor site and perigraft halo.[40]
	Hair Follicle Tissue Grafts, 1998[41]		RP in 70% of grafts with a mean diameter of repigmentation of 5 mm[42]	Suitable in hair-bearing areas and patches with leukotrichia.	Cannot be expanded. Limited use in the treatment of large areas and non-hair-bearing areas. Scarring of the donor site is common.
Cellular Grafts	Cultured Grafts	Cultured Epidermal Cellular Suspensions, 1989[43,44]	RP rate similar to noncultured epidermal Transplantation (more than 70%)[10]	Cover 100- to 500-fold the surface area of the original donor site.	Requires significantly greater resources in terms of procedure cost, equipment, and skilled personnel hours. Failure of the culture procedure.
		Cultured Melanocyte Cellular Suspensions, 1987[45]	50%–90% RP[46]	Requires significantly less culture medium and flasks, so less expense. Being a cellular suspension, can be used in the treatment of difficult areas, such as irregularly shaped surfaces.	

Table 9.1 (Continued) Vitiligo surgery techniques

Method			Efficacy[a]	Advantages	Disadvantages
	Noncultured Grafts	Noncultured, Epidermal Cellular Suspensions (NCES), 1992[47]	RP rates varies from 69%[48] to more than 95%[49]	Five- to 10-fold greater surface area than the donor site can be treated. Can be used on difficult-to-treat areas including the hands, feet, extensor surfaces, eyelids, and genitalia with good results and color matching.[50] Risk of scarring at the donor site is low.	Taking an ideal graft from donor site requires skill and dexterity. Specialized laboratory equipment and trained personnel are needed. Not suitable for the palms and soles.
		Noncultured Outer Root Sheath Hair Follicle Suspensions (NCORSHFS or FCS), 2009[15]	RP outcomes inferior to noncultured epidermal suspension grafts[17]	Hair follicle–derived melanocytes are more resistant to future depigmentation and are more numerous compared to epidermal-derived melanocytes.	Though theoretically superior to noncultured epidermal grafts, studies have not shown similar results.
Nongrafting Surgical Techniques	Therapeutic Wounding		RP rate is inferior to grafting techniques[51]	No specialized training or supplies needed. Improved efficacy with concomitant photo/chemotherapy, use of 5-fluorouracil with an erbium YAG-laser.[52]	Limited efficacy, with similar or greater risks of scarring in comparison to other techniques.
	Local Excision			A quick technique for correcting a small area of depigmentation if located in a cosmetically acceptable location.	Suboptimal cosmetic outcome such as anatomic deformation, persistent nerve injury, koebnerization, keloid formation, dehiscence, or infection.
	Micropigmentation			A rapid method for providing persistent camouflage that is recalcitrant to future depigmentation by underlying vitiligo.	Risk of vitiligo reactivation, infection, the pigment can occasionally induce phototoxic reactions, granuloma formation, loss of hair, and keloid formation.

[a] The reported efficacy is not directly comparable owing to differences in outcome measures and study design. RP, repigmentation.

immobilization plays an important role in the success of surgery, which limits patient convenience.

a. *Split-thickness skin grafts*: Here, a thin skin graft is harvested using a skin-harvesting knife and transplanted over denuded recipient skin (Figure 9.1). If meshing is not done, the donor skin should be 10%–25% larger than the recipient area owing to the dermal elastin contracture. A rapid and uniform repigmentation can be achieved with this method, but temporary milia-like cysts, a partial loss of graft, and thick graft margins or scarring at the donor area are a possibility as well as a lack of donor-to-recipient ratio augmentation. Behl[3] has demonstrated repigmentation of vitiligo patches with autologous thin Thiersch's grafts of 0.1–0.2 mm thickness. Ultrathin skin grafts[4] of 0.08–0.15 mm thickness have now become the preferred tissue source for melanocytes. For a successful outcome, Thiersch's grafts of 0.1–0.2 mm thickness should be engrafted to the recipient area, unlike ultrathin grafts, which are detached from the recipient bed by 1–2 weeks after transferring melanocytes. Plucking or chemical epilation before surgery avoids graft lift-off after split-thickness grafting on hair-bearing vitiligo patches.

Various modifications of split-thickness grafts have been proposed. In flip top grafting,[5] small pieces of split-thickness grafts are placed under a hinge of raised epidermal flaps, which act as a natural dressing. The borders of the hinge are secured with cyanoacrylate glue, and a transparent dressing is placed that is removed after 1 week. The success of the graft can be ascertained by observing the pigmentation through the depigmented epidermal hinge. Smash grafting,[6] a modification of split-thickness grafting, cuts down split-thickness grafts into tiny pieces using scissors and transplants these pieces admixed with normal saline as a semisolid preparation over the recipient dermal bed. Even though it is simple to perform and can cover a larger area than ultrathin grafts, evidence for its efficacy is poor.

b. *Mini-punch graft*: Grafts are harvested from the donor area (gluteal region) with the help of biopsy punches and transplanted to the pits created in the recipient depigmented patches (Figure 9.2). Punches measuring 1–3 mm in diameter can be placed at 5–10 mm gaps (dark skin) or 3–5 mm gaps (light skin) because of the differential melanosome properties.[7] The punches are secured with tape dressing and removed after 1–2 weeks. The melanocytes in the donor punches start migrating horizontally to the surrounding depigmented skin with the resultant production and transfer of melanin to the keratinocytes.[8] Repigmentation starts by 3 weeks and an adequate outcome can be expected by 4–6 months.

Cobblestoning is a common adverse effect that can be prevented by adjusting the donor-to-recipient punch height-to-depth ratio by trimming excess fat in the donor punch or creating deeper punches in the recipient area. This is the simplest and cheapest method of vitiligo surgery and can be done under any setting.

c. *Suction blister epidermal grafting*: Epidermal roofs raised by applying negative pressure (300–500 mmHg) on the pigmented donor skin are transected and transplanted to the recipient de-epithelialized skin (Figure 9.3). Since the blisters are raised above the lamina lucida level, scarring at the recipient site is not a possibility. Dressings are removed on day 7. Grafts may detach by this time or some days later; however, the melanocytes will be transferred from the donor epidermis to the recipient bed. The patient should be well informed prior to surgery to avoid erroneous interpretation of this as a graft failure by the patient.

Suction can be applied using a syringe attached to a 50-cc syringe through a three-way rubber tubing system, an oil rotary vacuum connected to a manometer, or a manual suction unit with transparent plastic cups. A modified suction-blister device has recently been introduced to raise multiple blisters simultaneously.[9] It takes at least 3 hours to form a suction blister, or longer during the winter. Injecting warm saline to the donor bed, use of a heat lamp or hair dryer, or placing blisters over bony prominences may hasten blister formation. Too much negative pressure that results in hemorrhagic blistering should be avoided to get "nonstressed" melanocytes. It is a simple office-based procedure with minimal adverse effects and rapid repigmentation outcome. However, increased procedural time for the initial blister raising, learning curve for final placement of thin epidermal grafts, and a lower donor-to-recipient augmentation are the limitations.

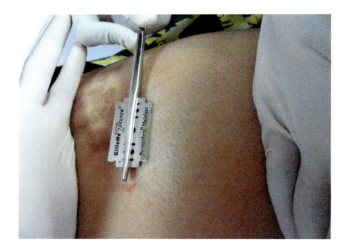

Figure 9.1 Method of skin harvesting using straight artery forceps and disposable shaving blade. It is a common step in split-thickness skin grafting as well as cultured and noncultured cellular transplantation. Applying petroleum jelly, using field block anesthesia, and stretching the skin away and laterally from the donor area will help to get a uniform ultrathin graft. Thinness of the graft can be ascertained by its ability to float in normal saline, ability to read the letters on the blade due to its translucency, and absence of shrinking of the tissue (dermal elastin contraction). (Courtesy of Dr Rajsmita Bhattacharjee, MD, DNB.)

Types of vitiligo surgery 73

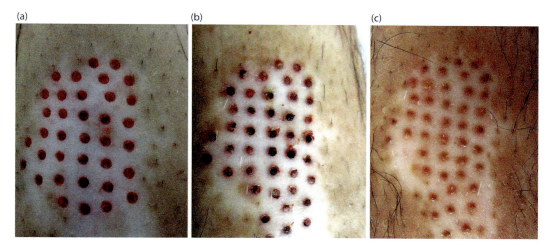

Figure 9.2 Method of mini-punch grafting and repigmentation outcome. (a) Recipient area being punched to receive the donor tissue. (b) Engrafted tissue punches at day 8. (c) Completely depigmented recipient area has now become partially pigmented at third month due to melanocyte-melanin transfer from the grafted tissues. (Courtesy of Dr Amit Dalla, MBBS.)

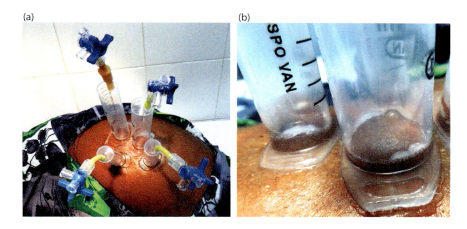

Figure 9.3 Method of suction blister epidermal grafting. (a) Syringe with tubing and three-way cannula system to create a negative suction pressure using 50-cc syringe. (b) Development of minute vesicles (after 2 hours) that later coalesce to form a single large blister. Blister roofs will be detached at their peripherally attached borders using corneal scissors and placed on a glass slide with their dermal side facing upward. Attached minimal dermal fibers will be scored and removed. The blister roof will now be placed carefully on the dermabraded recipient bed by sandwiching the epidermal graft between the recipient bed and glass slide.

d. *Hair follicle transplantation*: Here, hair follicles including the hair bulb are harvested either using the strip or follicular unit extraction method, then punched into the recipient dermal bed. Since hair follicles contain various immature melanocytes, stem cells, and melanocytes with superior melanogenic properties and different antigen expression (compared to epidermal melanocytes), it appears to be a good option for refractory vitiligo. A mean diameter of repigmentation up to 5 mm has been achieved with this method. This method is especially useful for patches with leukotrichia.

Cellular transplantation

Individual cells from a tissue are transplanted to the recipient depigmented patch in this method. It may be either a cultured or noncultured process. Both processes involve harvesting of skin, similar to ultrathin grafting, which is later trypsinized using 0.25% trypsin-EDTA solution.

1. Cultured cellular grafts
   a. *Autologous, cultured epidermal cellular grafts*: Keratinocytes and melanocytes obtained after trypsinization of tissue grafts are later cultured *in vitro* for 15–30 days to produce large epidermal sheets expanding more than 100–500 times that of donor tissue. Once adequate cell lines have been achieved, the epidermal sheets are detached from the culture plates using dispase and shrunk to half to two-thirds of their original culture size. This shrinkage increases the concentration of melanocytes per area of cultured sheets to 1000–2000 cells/mm^2. Since the culture sheets are often fragile, these are made into cell suspensions before transplanting into the

recipient site. A recent study comparing cultured vs. noncultured melanocyte transfer has documented a similar repigmentation outcome.[10]

b. *Autologous, cultured melanocyte grafts*: Unlike cultured epidermal cellular grafts, a pure isolate of melanocyte population will be cultured to yield cultured melanocyte grafts. During the culturing process as described above, calcium is added to remove keratinocytes and genticin is added to remove fibroblasts.

Cultured cellular grafting requires a sophisticated laboratory setup, skilled personnel, and a 3-week period for cell expansion. Even though the use of 12-tetradecanoylphorbol 13 acetate (TPA), a tumor promoter, has been discarded nowadays, the use of xenobiotics and growth factors still poses a concern regarding its safety. However, no serious adverse effects have been reported with the use of cultured cellular grafts since their inception 25 years ago.

2. Noncultured cellular grafts

a. *Autologous noncultured epidermal cell suspension (NCES)*: In the noncultured epidermal cell suspension method, individual melanocytes and keratinocytes are transplanted to the recipient de-epithelized area concurrently, thus circumventing the costly and time-consuming step of culturing the cells. It has similar repigmentation outcome to that of tissue grafts, with a donor-to-recipient augmentation factor of 10.

Ultrathin grafts are immersed in trypsin-ethylenediaminetetraacetic acid (EDTA) solution for 1 hour under 37°C (hot trypsinization) or for 18 hours under 4°C (cold trypsinization). Proteolytic dissociation of the tissue aided by mechanical dissociation with forceps leaves individual cells in the solution (Figure 9.4). The resultant solution is centrifuged to get a cell pellet, which is resuspended in phosphate buffer saline (PBS) and mixed to get a thick cell suspension. The cell suspension is either injected into a blister raised on the recipient area or spread on the de-epithelized recipient surface. After that, dressings are applied with collagen sheets, paraffin embedded mesh, absorbable gauze, transparent polyurethane dressing, and elastic adhesive bandage, inside to outside in that order. Dressings are removed after 1 week. Various modifications of noncultured epidermal cell suspension have been described (Table 9.2).

Nowadays, vitiligo surgeons prefer this method owing to its acceptable repigmentation outcome, better donor-recipient area augmentation and procedural simplicity (Figure 9.5). PBS has now replaced melanocyte culture medium and trypsin inhibitors, which were previously employed for NCES preparation.[11] Optimal repigmentation (>75%) can be attained in more than two-thirds of patients as per a number of clinical trials.[12] However, color mismatch

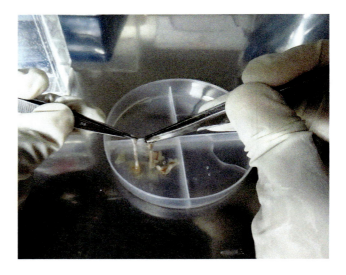

Figure 9.4 Method of noncultured epidermal cell suspension preparation using a four-compartment technique. Harvested ultrathin graft will be placed on the first chamber containing trypsin-EDTA solution for 90 minutes under 37°C. Excess trypsin is washed off using phosphate-buffered saline (PBS) in second and third chamber. An adequate amount of PBS (based on recipient area size) is added to the fourth chamber and dermal (left-hand side in the image) and epidermal (right-hand side in the image) sides of the graft will be separated using forceps. Attached melanocytes from the dermal side will be separated and the remaining whitish dermal tissue will be discarded. Pipetting the cell containing the PBS solution using a 2-mL syringe yields a uniform epidermal cell suspension.

was noted in more than half of the study population as per the studies.[13,14] At present, in the absence of a better alternative, such color mismatch is acceptable to the patient, provided there is a uniform coverage of the repigmentation. Moreover, such a conclusion cannot be made in the real-world scenario, as most clinical trials are limited by a short trial period of 4–6 months, and we often observe improvement of color match as time progresses.

b. *Autologous noncultured hair follicular cell suspension (FCS)*: Hair follicles as a source of better melanocytes and various melanocyte precursors for vitiligo surgery were first reported by Vanscheidt et al. through the plucked hair follicle method of cell harvesting.[15] Poor cell yield of this method was rectified by Mohanty et al. by employing follicular unit extraction followed by sequential trypsinization.[16] It is estimated that one hair follicle is enough to provide melanocytes for a 1-cm² area of depigmented skin. Melanocytes from the outer root sheath of hair follicles are extracted through a three-step trypsinization-neutralization process, each having a duration of 20–30 minutes. This is to avoid prolonged unopposed action of trypsin to individual melanocytes shedding into the solution owing to the columnar shape of hair follicles.

Table 9.2 Modifications of noncultured epidermal cell suspension transplantation

Study	Modification
Gauthier et al.[47]	Pioneered the NCES method. Cold trypsinization (under 4°C for 18 hours).
Olsson and Juhlin[53]	Hot trypsinization (60 minutes under 37°C). Cell suspension in melanocyte culture media.
van Geel et al.[54]	Addition of hyaluronic acid to the cell suspension to increase viscosity and adherence to the recipient site.
Mulekar et al.[55]	Demonstrated repigmentation outcome with the ReCell-kit.
Gho et al.[56]	Proposed the "six-well plate" technique for the preparation of epidermal cell suspension.
Holla et al.[11]	Modifications addressing the cost reduction. Proposed the use of PBS in place of melanocyte culture medium and trypsin inhibitor.
Sahni et al.[57]	Better repigmentation outcome by suspending the melanocytes in the patients' own serum.
Kumar et al.[58]	Proposed four-compartment method, a simple and clinic-based method of NCES preparation.
Benzekri et al.[59]	Transepidermal transplantation of melanocytes using a 0.2-mm dermaroller system.
Razmi et al.[20]	Addition of noncultured hair follicular cell suspension into the NCES to improve its repigmentation outcome.

However, this complexity of the procedure was not translated to better repigmentation outcomes, especially in acral areas. Even though there are better melanocytes and stem cells with melanogenic properties, the repigmentation outcome of this method is comparable or inferior to NCES.[17,18]

c. *Combined epidermal and follicular cell suspension*: In this method, NCES and FCS are mixed in equal proportion of cell numbers before transplanting into the depigmented skin. Such a combined cell suspension was found to have better repigmentation at acral areas compared to NCES or FCS alone.[19] In a randomized clinical trial, this method was found to give quicker and optimal repigmentation even in difficult-to-treat vitiligo. This response was superior to that obtained through NCES, the active control.[20] Authors proposed that better keratinocyte-derived growth factors and OCT4+ stem cells found in NCES+FCS vs. NCES alone might be the reason for the superior outcome with the combined cell suspension.

3. Other methods

Excision and primary closure can be employed for small lesions. This method results in rapid correction of the depigmented patch, but at the cost of possible scarring.[21] In micropigmentation, inert exogenous pigments are inserted into the papillary dermis, similar to tattooing, to impart a permanent camouflage. Even though it is rapid in concealing depigmentation, there is a risk of infection and various tattoo reactions like granuloma formation and phototoxic reactions. After years, the pigment starts to fade and sometimes is deposited into the dermis to give a bluish discoloration due to the Tyndall effect. In therapeutic wounding, trauma is inflicted to the vitiligo patch so

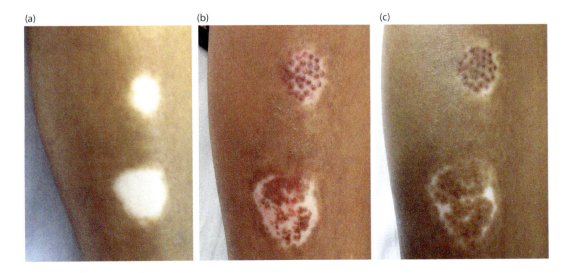

Figure 9.5 Comparison of repigmentation outcome with mini-punch graft and noncultured epidermal cell suspension. (a) Baseline image showing depigmented patches on the legs. (b) Repigmentation outcome after 1 month; mini-punch graft—upper patch, and noncultured epidermal cell suspension—lower patch. (c) Repigmentation outcome at third month. In our experience, the peri-graft halo on both the sites at this early follow-up usually repigments at a longer (1–2 year) follow-up. However, the speckled appearance of mini-punch graft site persists for a long time. (Courtesy of Dr Amit Dalla, MBBS.)

that various pro-pigmentary inflammatory cascade ensures repigmentation. Various tools like ablative and non-ablative lasers (fractional and nonfractional), microneedling, cryotherapy, chemical wounding (e.g., trichloroacetic acid, phenol), and dermabrasion have been used to induce trauma. However, the repigmentation outcome is not at all comparable to that of tissue or cellular grafts.

4. Future trends and authors' hypotheses

Multilineage differentiating stress enduring (Muse) cells, naturally present within mesenchymal tissues, including the dermis, are a possible source of pluripotent cells. Muse cells efficiently hone in on damaged tissues, as in melanocyte-keratinocyte-fibroblast damaged vitiligo tissue, and help in tissue regeneration and functional recovery.[22] In the late quiescent stages of vitiligo, when the inducible stem cells are exhausted due to the incessant contribution to melanocyte revival, we believe stem cell replenishment may help in repigmentation. In fact, using a 3D skin equivalent, Li et al. have shown that OCT4+ dermal stem cells could differentiate into HMB45-positive melanocytes and migrate to the epidermis.[23]

Dermal mesenchymal stem cells have various immunomodulatory properties. Zhou et al. have demonstrated in an *in vitro* co-culture that human dermal stem cells were able to deplete CD8+ T cells, the presence of which was found to be a marker of poor repigmentation outcome after surgery.[24] In a pilot clinical study,[25] we could demonstrate the superior repigmentation outcome of NCES combined with dermal cell suspension over NCES alone only in patches with lesional stability between 3 and 6 months (cf. patches with more than 1 year stability).

Immune regulatory cells like T-regulatory cells (T-regs) can halt immune attack by cytotoxic T cells against melanocytes. Replenishment of T-regs resulted in halting the depigmentation in a mouse model.[26] Tyrosinase-specific T-reg replenishment can be employed to halt melanocyte destruction in active vitiligo.

CONCLUSION

Surgical options in vitiligo can be employed in carefully selected patches of stable vitiligo that do not respond to medical modalities. To begin with, suction blister epidermal grafts or mini-punch grafts can be tried in small patches of vitiligo involving non-acral areas. With experts and laboratory support, noncultured epidermal cell suspension can be tried in larger lesions. Even though there is considerable development in the field of surgical management of vitiligo, the repigmentation of extreme acral (periungual) vitiligo is still an enigma.

ACKNOWLEDGMENTS

The authors thank Drs. Rajsmita Bhattacharjee, MD, DNB, and Amit Dalla, MBBS, for their kind permission to use the clinical and procedural images.

REFERENCES

1. Silverberg JI, Silverberg NB. Association between vitiligo extent and distribution and quality-of-life impairment. *JAMA Dermatol.* 2013;149:159–164.
2. Ezzedine K, Lim HW, Suzuki T et al. Revised classification/nomenclature of vitiligo and related issues: The Vitiligo Global Issues Consensus Conference. *Pigment Cell Melanoma Res.* 2012;25:E1–13.
3. Behl PN, Bhatia RK. Treatment of vitiligo with autologous thin Thiersch's grafts. *Int J Dermatol.* 1973;12:329–331.
4. Kahn AM, Cohen MJ, Kaplan L, Highton A. Vitiligo: Treatment by dermabrasion and epithelial sheet grafting—A preliminary report. *J Am Acad Dermatol.* 1993;28:773–774.
5. McGovern TW, Bolognia J, Leffell DJ. Flip-top pigment transplantation: A novel transplantation procedure for the treatment of depigmentation. *Arch Dermatol.* 1999;135:1305–1307.
6. Krishnan A, Kar S. Smashed skin grafting or smash grafting—A novel method of vitiligo surgery. *Int J Dermatol.* 2012;51:1242–1247.
7. Mutalik S, Ginzburg A. Surgical management of stable vitiligo: A review with personal experience. *Dermatol Surg.* 2000;26:248–254.
8. Kovacs D, Abdel-Raouf H, Al-Khayyat M et al. Vitiligo: Characterization of melanocytes in repigmented skin after punch grafting. *J Eur Acad Dermatol Venereol.* 2015;29:581–590.
9. Li J, Fu WW, Zheng ZZ, Zhang QQ, Xu Y, Fang L. Suction blister epidermal grafting using a modified suction method in the treatment of stable vitiligo: A retrospective study. *Dermatol Surg.* 2011;37:999–1006.
10. Verma R, Grewal RS, Chatterjee M, Pragasam V, Vasudevan B, Mitra D. A comparative study of efficacy of cultured versus non cultured melanocyte transfer in the management of stable vitiligo. *Med J Armed Forces India.* 2014;70:26–31.
11. Holla AP, Kumar R, Parsad D, Kanwar A. Modified procedure of noncultured epidermal suspension transplantation: Changes are the core of vitiligo surgery. *J Cutan Aesthet Surg.* 2011;4:44–45.
12. Razmi TM, Parsad D. Cellular transplantation procedures in vitiligo: What is in a name? *Int J Dermatol.* 2018;57:e36–e7.
13. Silpa-Archa N, Griffith JL, Huggins RH et al. Long-term follow-up of patients undergoing autologous noncultured melanocyte-keratinocyte transplantation for vitiligo and other leukodermas. *J Am Acad Dermatol.* 2017;77:318–327.
14. van Geel N, Ongenae K, De Mil M, Haeghen YV, Vervaet C, Naeyaert JM. Double-blind placebo-controlled study of autologous transplanted epidermal cell suspensions for repigmenting vitiligo. *Arch Dermatol.* 2004;140:1203–1208.

15. Vanscheidt W, Hunziker T. Repigmentation by outer-root-sheath-derived melanocytes: Proof of concept in vitiligo and leucoderma. *Dermatology.* 2009;218:342–343.

16. Mohanty S, Kumar A, Dhawan J, Sreenivas V, Gupta S. Noncultured extracted hair follicle outer root sheath cell suspension for transplantation in vitiligo. *Br J Dermatol.* 2011;164:1241–1246.

17. Singh C, Parsad D, Kanwar AJ, Dogra S, Kumar R. Comparison between autologous noncultured extracted hair follicle outer root sheath cell suspension and autologous noncultured epidermal cell suspension in the treatment of stable vitiligo: A randomized study. *Br J Dermatol.* 2013;169:287–293.

18. Donaparthi N, Chopra A. Comparative study of efficacy of epidermal melanocyte transfer versus hair follicular melanocyte transfer in stable vitiligo. *Indian J Dermatol.* 2016;61:640–644.

19. Razmi TM, Parsad D, Kumaran SM. Combined epidermal and follicular cell suspension as a novel surgical approach for acral vitiligo. *J Am Acad Dermatol.* 2017;76:564–567.

20. Razmi TM, Kumar R, Rani S, Kumaran SM, Tanwar S, Parsad D. Combination of follicular and epidermal cell suspension as a novel surgical approach in difficult-to-treat vitiligo: A randomized clinical trial. *JAMA Dermatol.* 2018;154:301–308.

21. Shilpa K, Sacchidanand S, Savitha S, Ranjitha R, Lakshmi DV, Divya G. A study of the outcome of primary excision and closure technique in the management of lip leukoderma in 30 patients. *J Cutan Aesthet Surg.* 2016;9:20–26.

22. Tsuchiyama K, Wakao S, Kuroda Y et al. Functional melanocytes are readily reprogrammable from multilineage-differentiating stress-enduring (Muse) cells, distinct stem cells in human fibroblasts. *J Invest Dermatol.* 2013;133:2425–2435.

23. Li L, Fukunaga-Kalabis M, Yu H et al. Human dermal stem cells differentiate into functional epidermal melanocytes. *J Cell Sci.* 2010;123:853–860.

24. Zhou MN, Zhang ZQ, Wu JL et al. Dermal mesenchymal stem cells (DMSCs) inhibit skin-homing CD8+ T cell activity, a determining factor of vitiligo patients' autologous melanocytes transplantation efficiency. *PLOS ONE.* 2013;8:e60254.

25. Thakur V, Parsad D. Clinical Trial: A Novel Surgical Method in the Treatment of Unstable Vitiligo. Clinical Trial Identifier:NCT03013049. Available at https://clinicaltrials.gov/ct2/show/NCT03013049?cond=Vitiligo&cntry=IN&rank=1. Last accessed on April 25, 2018

26. Le Poole IC, Mehrotra S. Replenishing regulatory T cells to halt depigmentation in vitiligo. *J Investig Dermatol Symp Proc.* 2017;18:S38–S45.

27. Falabella R. Repigmentation of segmental vitiligo by autologous minigrafting. *J Am Acad Dermatol.* 1983;9:514–521.

28. Feetham HJ, Chan JL, Pandya AG. Characterization of clinical response in patients with vitiligo undergoing autologous epidermal punch grafting. *Dermatol Surg.* 2012;38:14–19.

29. Malakar S, Dhar S. Treatment of stable and recalcitrant vitiligo by autologous miniature punch grafting: A prospective study of 1,000 patients. *Dermatology.* 1999;198:133–139.

30. Babu A, Thappa DM, Jaisankar TJ. Punch grafting versus suction blister epidermal grafting in the treatment of stable lip vitiligo. *Dermatol Surg.* 2008;34:166–178; discussion 78.

31. Khandpur S, Sharma VK, Manchanda Y. Comparison of minipunch grafting versus split-skin grafting in chronic stable vitiligo. *Dermatol Surg.* 2005;31:436–441.

32. Gupta S, Jain VK, Saraswat PK. Suction blister epidermal grafting versus punch skin grafting in recalcitrant and stable vitiligo. *Dermatol Surg.* 1999;25:955–958.

33. Njoo MD, Westerhof W, Bos JD, Bossuyt PM. A systematic review of autologous transplantation methods in vitiligo. *Arch Dermatol.* 1998;134:1543–1549.

34. Olsson MJ, Juhlin L. Epidermal sheet grafts for repigmentation of vitiligo and piebaldism, with a review of surgical techniques. *Acta Derm Venereol.* 1997;77:463–466.

35. Lu N, Xu A, Wu X. Follow-up study of vitiligo patients treated with autologous epidermal sheet transplants. *J Dermatolog Treat.* 2014;25:200–204.

36. Majid I, Imran S. Ultrathin split-thickness skin grafting followed by narrowband UVB therapy for stable vitiligo: An effective and cosmetically satisfying treatment option. *Indian J Dermatol Venereol Leprol.* 2012;78:159–164.

37. Falabella R. Epidermal grafting. An original technique and its application in achromic and granulating areas. *Arch Dermatol.* 1971;104:592–600.

38. Koga M. Epidermal grafting using the tops of suction blisters in the treatment of vitiligo. *Arch Dermatol.* 1988;124:1656–1658.

39. Budania A, Parsad D, Kanwar AJ, Dogra S. Comparison between autologous noncultured epidermal cell suspension and suction blister epidermal grafting in stable vitiligo: A randomized study. *Br J Dermatol.* 2012;167:1295–1301.

40. Gou D, Currimbhoy S, Pandya AG. Suction blister grafting for vitiligo: Efficacy and clinical predictive factors. *Dermatol Surg.* 2015;41:633–639.

41. Na GY, Seo SK, Choi SK. Single hair grafting for the treatment of vitiligo. *J Am Acad Dermatol.* 1998;38:580–584.

42. Mapar MA, Safarpour M, Mapar M, Haghighizadeh MH. A comparative study of the mini-punch grafting and hair follicle transplantation in the treatment of refractory and stable vitiligo. *J Am Acad Dermatol.* 2014;70:743–747.

43. Brysk MM, Newton RC, Rajaraman S et al. Repigmentation of vitiliginous skin by cultured cells. *Pigment Cell Res.* 1989;2:202–207.

44. Falabella R, Escobar C, Borrero I. Transplantation of *in vitro*-cultured epidermis bearing melanocytes for repigmenting vitiligo. *J Am Acad Dermatol.* 1989;21:257–264.

45. Lerner AB, Halaban R, Klaus SN, Moellmann GE. Transplantation of human melanocytes. *J Invest Dermatol.* 1987;89:219–224.

46. Chen YF, Yang PY, Hu DN, Kuo FS, Hung CS, Hung CM. Treatment of vitiligo by transplantation of cultured pure melanocyte suspension: Analysis of 120 cases. *J Am Acad Dermatol.* 2004;51:68–74.

47. Gauthier Y, Surleve-Bazeille JE. Autologous grafting with noncultured melanocytes: A simplified method for treatment of depigmented lesions. *J Am Acad Dermatol.* 1992;26:191–194.

48. van Geel N, Goh BK, Wallaeys E, De Keyser S, Lambert J. A review of non-cultured epidermal cellular grafting in vitiligo. *J Cutan Aesthet Surg.* 2011;4:17–22.

49. Mulekar SV. Long-term follow-up study of 142 patients with vitiligo vulgaris treated by autologous, non-cultured melanocyte-keratinocyte cell transplantation. *Int J Dermatol.* 2005;44:841–845.

50. Mulekar SV, Al Issa A, Al Eisa A. Treatment of vitiligo on difficult-to-treat sites using autologous noncultured cellular grafting. *Dermatol Surg.* 2009;35:66–71.

51. Toossi P, Shahidi-Dadras M, Mahmoudi Rad M, Fesharaki RJ. Non-cultured melanocyte-keratinocyte transplantation for the treatment of vitiligo: A clinical trial in an Iranian population. *J Eur Acad Dermatol Venereol.* 2011;25:1182–1186.

52. Anbar T, Westerhof W, Abdel-Rahman A, El-Khayyat M, El-Metwally Y. Treatment of periungual vitiligo with erbium-YAG-laser plus 5-flurouracil: A left to right comparative study. *J Cosmet Dermatol.* 2006;5:135–139.

53. Olsson MJ, Juhlin L. Leucoderma treated by transplantation of a basal cell layer enriched suspension. *Br J Dermatol.* 1998;138:644–648.

54. van Geel N, Ongenae K, De Mil M, Naeyaert JM. Modified technique of autologous noncultured epidermal cell transplantation for repigmenting vitiligo: A pilot study. *Dermatol Surg.* 2001;27:873–876.

55. Mulekar SV, Ghwish B, Al Issa A, Al Eisa A. Treatment of vitiligo lesions by ReCell vs. conventional melanocyte-keratinocyte transplantation: A pilot study. *Br J Dermatol.* 2008;158:45–49.

56. Goh BK, Chua XM, Chong KL, de Mil M, van Geel NA. Simplified cellular grafting for treatment of vitiligo and piebaldism: The "6-well plate" technique. *Dermatol Surg.* 2010;36:203–207.

57. Sahni K, Parsad D, Kanwar AJ, Mehta SD. Autologous noncultured melanocyte transplantation for stable vitiligo: Can suspending autologous melanocytes in the patients' own serum improve repigmentation and patient satisfaction? *Dermatol Surg.* 2011;37:176–182.

58. Kumar R, Parsad D, Singh C, Yadav S. Four compartment method: A simplified and cost-effective method of noncultured epidermal cell suspension for the treatment of vitiligo. *Br J Dermatol.* 2014;170:581–585.

59. Benzekri L, Gauthier Y. The first transepidermal transplantation of non-cultured epidermal suspension using a dermarolling system in vitiligo: A sequential histological and clinical study. *Pigment Cell Melanoma Res.* 2017;30:493–497.

Phototherapy and lasers in the treatment of vitiligo

10

VIKTORIA ELEFTHERIADOU

CONTENTS

Introduction	79
Mechanism of action of phototherapy	79
Hospital and home phototherapy	79
Narrowband ultraviolet B and psoralen and ultraviolet A phototherapy for vitiligo	80
Narrowband ultraviolet B phototherapy side effects and contraindications	80
Narrowband ultraviolet B phototherapy and carcinogenicity	80
Targeted phototherapy devices	80
Monochromatic excimer light	81
Combination treatments with phototherapy	81
References	81

INTRODUCTION

Phototherapy is one of the well-known therapeutic modalities for the treatment of various skin diseases. The use of ultraviolet light dates back to the early 1900s. Extensive research has expanded our understanding of various skin disease pathophysiology. Advancements in technology have led to the development of UV devices that are more precise, safer, and more effective for the treatment of a wide variety of dermatologic conditions, including vitiligo.

In Egypt around 2000 BC, topical psoralens and sun exposure were used for treatment of vitiligo. Since then, PUVA (topical or oral psoralen and UVA) and PUVAsol (topical or oral psoralen and ultraviolet A [UVA] sun exposure) have been widely used to treat various skin conditions, including vitiligo and psoriasis. Although PUVA phototherapy proved effective, it has several limitations, including phototoxic effects, nausea and vomiting due to psoralens, and the potential risk for skin cancer. In addition, systemic PUVA phototherapy is contraindicated for children or pregnant women because of the systemic use of psoralen.[1] Since narrow-band ultraviolet B (NB-UVB) phototherapy was first reported to be effective for treatment of vitiligo in 1997, it has gradually taken the place of PUVA phototherapy.[2] NB-UVB phototherapy is also associated with adverse events such as erythema, itching, and mild burning or pain, which are usually better tolerated and spontaneously disappear a few hours after treatment in most cases.[3]

In summary, the lack of a photosensitizer, the lower cumulative dose, and fewer adverse effects are considered major advantages of NB-UVB over PUVA.[2,3]

MECHANISM OF ACTION OF PHOTOTHERAPY

The mechanism of action of NB-UVB is the inhibition of cytokines and stimulation of melanocyte-stimulating hormone. The latter enhances the proliferation and migration of melanocytes in the outer root sheath of hair follicles into depigmented lesions. In addition, NB-UVB induces tyrosinase enzyme activity and T-cell apoptosis.

The above supports the fact that repigmentation usually begins around the hair follicle, that is, perifollicularly, in vitiliginous lesions. Lack of hair follicles in areas such as hands and feet might explain poorer response to phototherapy.[4,5]

HOSPITAL AND HOME PHOTOTHERAPY

Hospital UVB usually involves whole-body cabinets suitable for extensive cutaneous involvement, such as large or multiple lesions. During the session, the patient goes into a specially designed cabinet containing fluorescent light tubes (whole-body units). Usually the whole body is exposed to the UVB for a short time (seconds to minutes). Hand and feet units for UVB are also available in some hospitals.[6]

In recent years, targeted phototherapy has been developed to overcome many of the limitations of full-body cabinets. Terms such as microphototherapy, concentrated phototherapy, and focused phototherapy have been used for targeted phototherapy.[6,7] There are several benefits of using targeted phototherapy devices, such as sparing of uninvolved skin and treating areas not easily reached by light, such as scalp and skin folds.

In addition, home phototherapy has gained popularity recently. Home phototherapy using whole-body units is available for the treatment of various dermatological conditions. A study comparing home versus hospital whole-body phototherapy (NB-UVB) for psoriasis concluded that home phototherapy is equally effective and implies no additional safety hazards compared to hospital phototherapy. Most of the participants said they would prefer future phototherapy at home over the hospital.[8] Other benefits of home phototherapy include:

- Reduction in attendance at the hospital. Traditionally, patients receiving NB-UVB treatment would be required to attend the hospital 2–3 times per week.
- Cheaper cost and less opportunity cost for patients, such as traveling costs.
- Treatment can be provided at an early stage of their disease, when the intervention might be more effective.[6]

NARROWBAND ULTRAVIOLET B AND PSORALEN AND ULTRAVIOLET A PHOTOTHERAPY FOR VITILIGO

Although several interventions are available to treat patients with vitiligo, there is no cure nor firm clinical recommendations.[3] Phototherapy, including psoralen–UV-A (PUVA) and narrowband UV-B therapy, has been historically used for the management of generalized or extensive vitiligo, whereas targeted phototherapy, including lasers and various topical agents, are used to treat localized disease. Management of vitiligo requires a long-term time commitment and can be challenging.

Currently there is no agreed protocol for NB-UVB in vitiligo and therefore a variety of treatment regimens are used in different institutions and countries. Usually, NB-UVB is administered twice or thrice a week. Patients with vitiligo have traditionally been regarded as skin type 1 and consequently were treated with doses between 150 and 250 mj/cm^2 with increments of 10%–15% at each visit.[9] However, minimal erythema dose (MED) values in vitiligo skin are on average only 35% (95% confidence interval 31%–39%) lower than in normal skin, suggesting photoadaptation.[2,10–13] Total-body NB-UVB is suggested for vitiligo covering over 15%–20% of the body surface area or for actively spreading vitiligo.[9]

A recently conducted meta-analysis of studies on phototherapy for vitiligo included 35 studies (1428 patients). Randomized, nonrandomized, and open trials were included. Single-arm meta-analyses were performed for the NB-UVB and PUVA groups. The primary outcomes were mild (≥25%), moderate (≥50%), and marked (≥75%) responses on a quartile scale. This meta-analysis was conducted with the aim to provide references to the expected treatment response to phototherapy in the management of vitiligo. Mild response to narrowband UV-B phototherapy occurred in 74% at 6 months and 75% at 12 months, and a marked response was achieved in 19% at 6 months and 36% at 12 months. The face and neck achieved better repigmentation compared to the trunk and extremities.[14] The authors concluded that phototherapy requires at least 1 year to achieve a maximal treatment response and suggested that at least 6 months of treatment are required to determine the responsiveness to NB-UVB phototherapy. Moreover, overall treatment response to PUVA phototherapy was inferior to that to NB-UVB, although statistical comparisons were not conducted in this study. Long-duration phototherapy should be encouraged to enhance the treatment response, with the greatest response anticipated on the face and neck.[14]

In addition, Yones et al. demonstrated the superiority of NB-UVB phototherapy to oral PUVA therapy. In their study, the rate of more than 50% repigmentation was significantly higher in the NB-UVB group (64%) than in the PUVA group (36%) after 6 months of treatment. In addition, repigmented skin showed excellent color match in all patients in the NB-UVB group but only 44% of those in the PUVA group.[14,15]

Recurrence of vitiligo after discontinuation of NB-UVB can occur. Relapses of previously repigmented lesions have been reported in approximately 50% of patients (44%–55%).[16,17]

NARROWBAND ULTRAVIOLET B PHOTOTHERAPY SIDE EFFECTS AND CONTRAINDICATIONS

Whole-body NB-UVB as well as targeted NB-UVB are well tolerated. The most common adverse events are dose- and skin type–dependent erythema occurring 12–24 hours post treatment. Mild erythematous reaction in vitiliginous skin is generally considered a desirable outcome and indicates adequate dosimetry.[9]

NB-UVB is absolutely contraindicated in patients with xeroderma pigmentosum and lupus erythematosus. Relative contraindications include photodermatoses, immunosuppression, and inability to stand still in a whole-body cubicle, among others. NB-UVB can be administered to children, pregnant and lactating women, and patients with renal or hepatic diseases.[9]

NARROWBAND ULTRAVIOLET B PHOTOTHERAPY AND CARCINOGENICITY

The issue of how great the risk of carcinogenicity is for NB-UVB is unclear, as there is no good evidence to date.

Several studies were unable to detect any definite increased risk of skin cancer following NB-UVB phototherapy.[18–21] A larger study on 1380 participants also showed that UVB remains a relatively low-risk treatment for psoriasis.[22]

A study performed on 1514 participants with vitiligo and 2813 participants with no vitiligo, showed that there is a mutually exclusive relationship between susceptibility to vitiligo and susceptibility to melanoma, that is, vitiligo patients may have protection against melanoma.[23] However, there have been no trials performed on the risk of carcinogenicity of NB-UVB phototherapy on vitiligo patients and the consensus is made mainly on data from psoriasis patients.

TARGETED PHOTOTHERAPY DEVICES

For localized vitiligo and in particular for small lesions of recent onset and childhood vitiligo, targeted phototherapies are indicated. In the management of vitiligo, several different types of targeted phototherapy have been reported: excimer laser, monochromatic excimer lamp, hand-held multichromatic incoherent UV sources, and low-level laser therapy.

NB-UVB devices have a peak emission spectrum between 311–313 nm. The first targeted NB-UVB device was described by Lotti et al. in 1999 (Bioskin).[24] Other devices have been reported since with similar efficacy results.[25–27]

MONOCHROMATIC EXCIMER LIGHT

Monochromatic excimer light (MEL) is a xenon chloride (XeCl) device, which emits a single 308-nm wavelength either as a lamp or laser. MEL has shown therapeutic success in the treatment of various skin conditions such as vitiligo, psoriasis, and mycosis fungoides. Various excimer lamp and laser devices are commercially available. The photobiologic effects of MEL are similar to those of 311–313 nm. They include greater T-cell apoptosis and melanin production from perifollicular dihydroxyphenylalanine (DOPA)-depleted amelanotic melanocytes than traditional NB-UVB.[28,29] Treatment regimens studied included excimer laser two to three times weekly for up to 36 weeks. Patients commonly achieved >75% repigmentation.[30] Differences between excimer lamp and laser include lower cost of excimer lamp, different hand pieces with various spot sizes for excimer lamp compared to a fixed spot size of excimer laser, and more expensive maintenance costs for excimer laser. No significant difference in the effectiveness of excimer laser and lamp have been found.[29,31]

The optimal frequency and duration of treatment of excimer light are unclear. However, the success of the excimer laser appears to vary by anatomical site similar to other sources of NB-UVB.[32]

Other targeted phototherapy devices include:

- UVA device, Dualite (Theralight, Inc., USA), which emits at 330–380 nm. No trials with this device's UVA spectrum have been reported in the treatment of vitiligo.
- Low-level laser devices, which emit at 600–1100 nm. These include ruby, gallium-aluminum-arsenide, and helium-neon lasers. Some evidence exists to support the effectiveness of HeNe lasers.[33,34]

In summary, targeted phototherapy is an emerging form of phototherapy with advantages and limitations compared to whole-body phototherapy as described above. Targeted phototherapy is a safer option for both children and adults with limited vitiligo covering up to 10% of the total body surface.

COMBINATION TREATMENTS WITH PHOTOTHERAPY

Several combination treatments have been proposed with the aim to enhance the effectiveness of phototherapy for the treatment of vitiligo.

Topical steroids and phototherapy

European guidelines for the management of vitiligo recommend that the combination of topical steroids and phototherapy (NB-UVB, excimer light or laser) may be promising, especially for difficult-to-treat areas such as bony prominences. Potent topical steroids applied once a day can be used on vitiligo lesions for the first three months of phototherapy.[9] One study compared 308-nm excimer laser in combination with topical hydrocortisone 17-butyrate cream and as monotherapy. Combination therapy showed significantly higher repigmentation that the laser alone for resistant head and neck lesions.[35]

Topical cancineurin inhibitors and phototherapy

Good evidence exists that combination of topical calcineurin inhibitors (TCIs) (tacrolimus, pimecrolimus) with light therapy is more effective than monotherapy. TCIs showed encouraging results when combined with UVB phototherapy and laser.[3,14] Concerns were expressed regarding possible increased risk of carcinogenicity; a long-term follow-up of 9813 tacrolimus-treated eczema patients showed no evidence of an increased risk of nonmelanoma skin cancer.[36] However, long-term data on vitiligo patients are still missing.

Vitamin D analogues and phototherapy

A combination of vitamin D analogues and phototherapy is not recommended due to contradictory results in trials.[3,9]

Oral corticosteroids and narrowband ultraviolet B

One study comparing the combination of oral minipulse of prednisolone (OMP) and NB-UVB versus OMP alone showed that combination therapy was better.[37] Expert consensus recommends that the benefit of adding OMP for repigmentation of stable vitiligo is not considered useful. Weekend OMP starting with a low dose (2.5 mg daily of dexamethasone) for fast-spreading vitiligo could be considered.[9]

In summary, light and laser therapies in combination treatments with topical agents were shown to be statistically significantly better at achieving over 75% repigmentation compared with monotherapies.[3,9,14]

In conclusion, targeted phototherapy (including lasers) is an emerging, effective form of phototherapy with advantages and limitations compared to conventional phototherapy. A recent shift toward using phototherapy earlier in the course of disease seems to be promising. However, further trials are needed to definitively demonstrate the effectiveness of various phototherapy treatment modalities both as monotherapies and in combination with topical treatments for vitiligo.

REFERENCES

1. Ling TC, Clayton TH, Crawley J et al. British Association of Dermatologists and British Photodermatology Group guidelines for the safe and effective use of psoralen-ultraviolet A therapy 2015. *Br J Dermatol.* January 2016;174(1):24–55.
2. Westerhof W, Nieuweboer-Krobotova L. Treatment of vitiligo with UV-B radiation vs topical psoralen plus UV-A. *Arch Dermatol.* December 1997;133(12):1525–1528.
3. Whitton ME, Pinart M, Batchelor J, Leonardi-Bee J, González U, Jiyad Z, Eleftheriadou V, Ezzedine K. Interventions for vitiligo. *Cochrane Database Syst Rev.* February 2015;24(2):CD003263.
4. Weichenthal M, Schwarz T. Phototherapy: How does UV work? *Photodermatol Photoimmunol Photomed.* October 2005;21:260–266.

5. De Francesco V, Stinco G, Laspina S, Parlangeli ME, Mariuzzi L, Patrone P. Immunohistochemical study before and after narrow band (311 nm) UVB treatment in vitiligo. *Eur J Dermatol.* May 2008–June;18(3):292–296.

6. Eleftheriadou V. Setting priorities and reducing uncertainties for the treatment of vitiligo. *PhD thesis.* The University of Nottingham; 2013.

7. Mysore V. Targeted phototherapy. *Indian J Dermatol Venereol Leprol.* 2009;75:119–125.

8. Koek M, Buskens E, van Weelden H, et al. Home versus outpatient ultraviolet B phototherapy for mild to severe psoriasis: Pragmatic multicentre randomised controlled non-inferiority trial (PLUTO study). *Br Med J.* 2009; 338:b1542.

9. Taieb A, Alomar A, Böhm M et al. Vitiligo European Task Force. Guidelines for the management of vitiligo: The European Dermatology Forum consensus. *Br J Dermatol.* January 2013;168:5–b1519.

10. Anbar TS, Westerhof W, Abdel-Rahman AT, El-Khayyat MA. Evaluation of the effects of NB-UVB in both segmental and non-segmental vitiligo affecting different body sites. *Photodermatol Photoimmunol Photomed.* June 2006;22:157–163.

11. Diffey BL, Farr PM. The challenge of follow-up in narrowband ultraviolet B phototherapy. *Br J Dermatol.* August 2007;157:344–349.

12. Njoo MD, Bos JD, Westerhof W. Treatment of generalized vitiligo in children with narrow-band (TL-01) UVB radiation therapy. *J Am Acad Dermatol.* February 2000;42:245–255.

13. Parsad D, Kanwar AJ, Kumar B. Psoralen–ultraviolet A vs. narrow-band ultraviolet B phototherapy for the treatment of vitiligo. *J Eur Acad Dermatol Venereol.* February 2006; 20:175–177.

14. Yones SS, Palmer RA, Garibaldinos TM, Hawk JLM. Randomized double-blind trial of treatment of vitiligo efficacy of psoralen–UV-A therapy vs narrowband–UV-B therapy. *Arch Dermatol.* May 2007;143(5):578–584.

15. Bae JM, Jung HM, Hong BY, Lee JH, Choi WJ, Lee JH, Kim GM. Phototherapy for vitiligo: A systematic review and meta-analysis. *J Am Acad Dermatol.* July 2017; 153(7):666–674.

16. Nicolaidou E, Antoniou C, Stratigos AJ, Stefanaki C, Katsambas AD. Efficacy, predictors of response, and long-term follow-up in patients with vitiligo treated with narrowband UVB phototherapy. *J Am Acad Dermatol.* February 2007;56(2):274–278.

17. Sitek JC, Loeb M, Ronnevig JR. Narrowband UVB therapy for vitiligo: does the repigmentation last? *J Eur Acad Dermatol Venereol.* August 2007;21(7):891–896.

18. Studniberg HM, Weller P. PUVA, UVB, psoriasis, and non-melanoma skin cancer. *J Am Acad Dermatol.* December 1993;29(6):1013–1022.

19. Weischer M, Blum A, Eberhard F et al. No evidence for increased skin cancer risk in psoriasis patients treated with broadband or narrowband UVB phototherapy: a first retrospective study. *Acta Derm Venereol.* 2004;84(5):370–374.

20. Man I, Crombie I, Dawe R, Ibbotson S, Ferguson J. The photocarcinogenic risk of narrowband UVB (TL-01) phototherapy: Early follow-up data. *Br J Dermatol.* April 2005;152(4):755–757.

21. Hearn R, Kerr A, Rahim K, Ferguson J, Dawe R. Incidence of skin cancers in 3867 patients treated with narrow-band ultraviolet B phototherapy. *Br J Dermatol.* September 2008; 159(4):931–935.

22. Lim JL, Stern RS. High levels of ultraviolet B exposure increase the risk of non-melanoma skin cancer in psoralen and ultraviolet A-treated patients. *J Invest Dermatol.* March 2005;124(3): 505–513.

23. Jin Y, Birlea SA, Fain PR et al. Common variants in FOXP1 are associated with generalized vitiligo. *Nat Genet.* July 2010;42(7):576–578.

24. Lotti TM, Menchini G, Andreassi L. UV-B radiation microphototherapy. An elective treatment for segmental vitiligo. *J Eur Acad Dermatol Venereol.* September 1999; 13(2):102–108.

25. Menchini G, Tsoureli-Nikita E, Hercogova J. Narrow-band UV-B micro-phototherapy: A new treatment for vitiligo. *J Eur Acad Dermatol Venereol.* March 2003;17(2):171–177.

26. Majid I. Efficacy of targeted narrowband ultraviolet B therapy in vitiligo. *Indian J Dermatol.* September 2014; 59(5):485–489.

27. Shanmuga SC, Srinivas CR. Fractional-targeted phototherapy. *Indian Dermatol Online J.* December 2014; 5(Suppl 2):S104–S105.

28. Yang Y, Cho H, Ryou J, Lee M. Clinical study of repigmentation patterns with either narrow-band ultraviolet B (NBUVB) or 308 nm excimer laser treatment in Korean vitiligo patients. *Intern J Dermatol.* February 2010; 49:317–323.

29. Chimento SM, Newland M, Ricotti C, Nistico S, Romanelli P. A pilot study to determine the safety and efficacy of monochromatic excimer light in the treatment of vitiligo. *J Drugs Dermatol.* March 2008; 7(3):258–263.

30. Park K, Liao W, Murase J. A review of monochromatic excimer light in vitiligo. *British Journal of Dermatology.* 2012;167:468–478.

31. Leone G, Iacovelli P, Paro Vidolin A, Picardo M. Monochromatic excimer light 308 nm in the treatment of vitiligo: A pilot study. *J Eur Acad Dermatol Venereol.* August 2003;17:531–537.

32. Hofer A, Hassan A, Legat F, Kerl H, Wolf P. The efficacy of excimer laser (308 nm) for vitiligo at different body sites. *J Eur Acad Dermatol Venereol.* August 2006;20:558–564.

33. AlGhamdi KM, Kumar A, Moussa NA. Low-level laser therapy: A useful technique for enhancing the proliferation of various cultured cells. *Lasers Med Sci.* January 2012;27:237–249.

34. Yu HS, Wu CS, Yu CL, Kao YH, Chiou MH. Helium–neon laser irradiation stimulates migration and proliferation in melanocytes and induces repigmentation in segmental-type vitiligo. *J Investig Dermatol.* January 2003;120(1):56–264.

35. Sassi F, Cazzaniga S, Tessari G, Chatenoud L, Reseghetti A, Marchesi L, Girolomoni G, Naldi L. Randomized controlled trial comparing the effectiveness of 308-nm excimer laser alone or in combination with topical hydrocortisone 17-butyrate cream in the treatment of vitiligo of the face and neck. *Br J Dermatol.* October 2008;159:1186–1191.

36. Naylor M, Elmets C, Jaracz E, Rico JM. Non-melanoma skin cancer in patients with atopic dermatitis treated with topical tacrolimus. *J Dermatol Treatm.* July 2009; 16(3):149–153.

37. Rath N, Kar HK, Sabhnani S. An open labeled, comparative clinical study on efficacy and tolerability of oral minipulse of steroid (OMP) alone, OMP with PUVA and broad/narrow band UVB phototherapy in progressive vitiligo. *Indian J Dermatol Venereol Leprol.* August 2008;74(4):357–360.

Emerging treatments for vitiligo

11

ANGELO MASSIMILIANO D'ERME and GIOVANNI BAGNONI

CONTENTS

Introduction	85	Emerging surgical treatments	87
Topical emerging treatments	85	Concluding remarks	87
Emerging phototherapies and lasers	85	References	87
Emerging systemic treatments	86		

INTRODUCTION

There are several safe and effective treatments that are available for vitiligo. Existing treatments include topical and systemic immunosuppresants, phototherapy, and surgical techniques that, alone or together, may halt disease progression, stabilize lesions, and lead to repigmentation. The choice of the treatment depends on the type of the disease, the percent of body area surface affected, the effect on the quality of life, the compliance of the patient, and the patient's perception with regards to the risk-benefit ratio.[1–8] Currently, no treatment has been approved by the U.S. Food and Drug Administration (FDA) for vitiligo. Topical treatments may be applied alone when a small area is involved, or together with phototherapy or systemic treatments when the area affected is more than 5%–10% or there is a progression of the disease. Based on our current understanding of vitiligo pathogenesis, a successful strategy to treat vitiligo should incorporate three distinct approaches: reducing melanocyte stress, regulating autoimmune response, and stimulating melanocyte regeneration. Existing treatments partially address these needs; however, emerging therapies may do this in a more targeted way, and combination therapies may synergize to produce a better overall response.[1–8]

TOPICAL EMERGING TREATMENTS

Topical corticosteroids and calcineurin inhibitors are common and effective first-line therapies. They can be used as monotherapy or combined with phototherapy.

An emerging topical treatment is a liposomal cream that contains in high concentration a natural phytocomplex obtained from black pepper fruit (piper nigrum phytocomplex) (Pigmerise Fagron) (Figure 11.1). Piperine, the major alkaloid of black pepper, and its synthetic derivatives can stimulate pigmentation in the skin by inducing melanocyte proliferation and dendrite formation *in vitro*.[9] In a sparsely pigmented mouse model, piperine and its analogues induced greater pigmentation than vehicle, with additional exposure to ultraviolet radiation (UVR) leading to darker pigmentation than did the compound or UVR alone, together with greater numbers of dihydroxy-phenylalanine (DOPA) + melanocytes in skin histology.[9]

Clinical studies on Pigmerise are ongoing and recent results also seem to underline its efficacy in humans. Recently, an evaluation of the efficacy of topical piperine in combination with narrowband ultraviolet B (NB-UVB) in patients with facial vitiligo was published. The authors reported that the combination therapy with NB-UVB/topical piperine had more influence on facial vitiligo than that of NB-UVB alone.[10]

Piperine cream has the advantage of having fewer adverse side effects than topical corticosteroids. The most common side effect reported in daily practice and in the literature is a burning sensation and redness when applied on the skin. However, further studies on its clinical efficacy and pathogenic mechanisms are needed.

EMERGING PHOTOTHERAPIES AND LASERS

The efficacy of UVR in the treatment of vitiligo has long been a well-known therapy. Even today, phototherapies are considered the first-line therapy, especially for extensive vitiligo, because of their good efficacy and tolerance. Phototherapy should be reserved for patients who have vitiligo covering more than 5%–10% of body surface area (BSA) or patients who fail to respond to topical therapy. Narrowband UVB light phototherapy is superior to UVA light phototherapy for the treatment of vitiligo.

The monochromatic excimer laser is indicated as targeted treatment of specific lesions and yields better results than conventional light therapy. Helium neon laser therapy is effective for segmental vitiligo.

Within this context, some lasers have recently been studied for the treatment of vitiligo, such as fractional erbium-YAG laser,[11] fractional CO_2 laser,[12] and UVA1 laser,[13] with good results. However, more studies are needed before these lasers are recommended for vitiligo treatment.

Despite being the most effective current treatment, patient access to phototherapy is often difficult, and patients have to attend a specialized clinic two to three times weekly for months. Sun exposure, on the other hand, is an inexpensive alternative to phototherapy, but nontherapeutic wavelengths of sunlight produce erythema and sunburn. To overcome this limitation of sun exposure, a topical formulation of

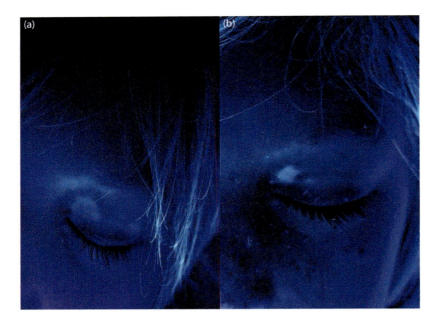

Figure 11.1 (a) Vitiligo lesions in an 8-year-old child; (b) rapid improvement in under 3 months of treatment of Pigmerise cream in combination with tacrolimus ointment.

dimethicone 1% was recently produced with the ability to permit therapeutic wavelengths in the NB-UVB range (~311 nm) to reach the skin and contemporaneously to block nontherapeutic wavelengths of sunlight below 300 nm. A first study found that sun exposure with application of this cream was safe and effective at inducing repigmentation.[14] These promising results have to be confirmed in larger clinical trials, opening new, easy, and more accessible methods of vitiligo treatment. However, UVA light is not blocked by this cream, and thus this approach may not be as safe as NB-UVB phototherapy.

EMERGING SYSTEMIC TREATMENTS
Antioxidants/hormones

Oxidative stress, including reduction of catalase enzyme, as well as elevated levels of reactive oxygen species (ROS) in lesional skin, has been implicated in the pathogenesis of vitiligo. These data prompted the hypothesis that treating patients with antioxidants or otherwise controlling ROS might be an effective treatment strategy.

For example, methionine sulfoxide reductase (MSR), an important reducing agent, is less active and present in lower amounts in patients with vitiligo, leading to an increase of melanocyte sensitivity to oxidative stress and cell death.

Oral or topical natural health products, vitamins, and supplements have been suggested as possible therapies based on their elevated catalase activity, antioxidant, and anti-inflammatory properties.[1–8,15]

The herbal supplement gingko biloba has been tested in two trials and reported to decrease disease progression of vitiligo compared to placebo.[16–18]

Polypodium leucotomos (PL) is a fern found in the American subtropics. The extract has antioxidant, immunomodulating, and photoprotective qualities and is used to treat a variety of inflammatory and degenerative diseases.[19]

The plant extract *Polypodium leucotomos* improved repigmentation responses to NB-UVB. Furthermore, in subjects with or without vitiligo, it reduced the cutaneous phototoxicity of PUVA and UVB phototherapies.[19]

Other studies revealed that the supplementation of an *antioxidant pool* of alpha lipoic acid, vitamin C, vitamin E, and polyunsaturated fatty acids improved repigmentation rates in combination with NB-UVB phototherapy but not with PUVA.[16]

In conclusion, there is good evidence to support oral antioxidant supplementation, specifically together with NB-UVB phototherapy. It is also likely a safe, widely available, and inexpensive adjunct. However, defining dosing parameters, efficacy, and side effect profiles requires further research.

Hormones

Afamelanotide, a synthetic analogue of alpha-melanocyte-stimulating hormone (α-MSH), has recently been approved by the European Medicines Agency to mitigate photosensitivity in erythropoietic protoporphyria. Afamelanotide also seems to improve the efficacy of NB-UVB in vitiligo. A randomized trial with afamelanotide in combination with NB-UVB was carried out in adults with generalized vitiligo. The addition of afamelanotide resulted in faster and increased total repigmentation compared to NB-UVB monotherapy, especially in patients with darker skin. The combination therapy was somewhat well tolerated, although side effects including nausea and skin hyperpigmentation were reported.[20]

Immunosuppressants

Over the past decade, significant progress has been made in the development of immunomodulators for inflammatory skin disease, such as psoriasis and atopic dermatitis. The identification of novel immune targets and pathways will also help the development of new vitiligo treatments.[1-8]

The IFN-γ/CXCL10 axis is emerging as a critical signaling pathway required for both the progression and maintenance of vitiligo. Interfering with the IFN-γ/CXCL10 chemokine axis may be an effective strategy to develop novel, targeted immunotherapies.[21,22]

A variety of antibodies and small-molecule inhibitors have already been found to be efficacious and safe in targeting components of this pathway in early-phase clinical trials for treatment of other autoimmune diseases. Recent findings in patients and a mouse model suggest that vitiligo patients may benefit in the future from these new drugs.[23,24]

Janus kinase (JAK)-signal transduction and transcription (STAT) signaling, essential to transmitting extracellular signals of many cytokines, including IFN-γ, to the nucleus, has been studied in the last years.[25] There are four members of the JAK family: JAK1, JAK2, JAK3, and tyrosine kinase 2 (TYK2), that are directly involved in IFN-γ signaling, which activates STAT1 and thus induces the transcription of IFN-γ-induced genes, including CXCL10.

Several small-molecule JAK inhibitors with distinct selectivity have been tested in patients or are under development for several autoimmune or autoinflammatory diseases. Interestingly, significant repigmentation in one patient with generalized vitiligo after the oral administration of tofacitinib (a Janus kinase inhibitor [JAK 1/3])[26] and in another patient with facial and trunk vitiligo at the beginning of treatment with oral ruxolitinib [JAK 1/2 inhibitor])[27] have been reported, opening new scenarios in the pathogenesis and treatment of vitiligo. However, the treatment response from these inhibitors did not appear to be durable, as patients lost the repigmentation after discontinuing treatment. Similar to all other immunosuppressive drugs, adverse events may limit their daily use. Topical formulations of these drugs, however, may provide therapeutic benefit without increasing the risk of adverse events. Topical ruxolitinib for 20 weeks resulted in 76% repigmentation of facial lesions in four patients and 23% improvement of all lesions in nine patients in a recent small study.[28] Clinical trials testing the efficacy of topical ruxolitinib 1.5% in the treatment of vitiligo are ongoing.[29]

Last, successful use of immunotherapy to treat metastatic melanoma by the modulation of T-cell responses to inflammation, including cytotoxic T-lymphocyte-associated protein 4 (CTLA-4) and programmed cell death protein 1 (PD-1), has gained recent attention.[30,31] Interestingly, the treatment response of melanoma patients to immunotherapy correlates with the development of vitiligo, opening new insights into the pathogenesis of the disease.

Some have hypothesized that activating these surface receptors could restore tolerance in vitiligo patients.

CTLA-4 agonists, such as abatacept (recently approved by the FDA for rheumatoid arthritis) or PD-1 ligand (PD-L1, a PD-1 agonist), are under development or in testing in trials for inflammatory diseases and may be effective, especially for vitiligo patients.[32]

EMERGING SURGICAL TREATMENTS

Surgical treatment for vitiligo is invasive and not without risks; however, it can be an excellent option for patients who fail nonsurgical therapy. There are several melanocyte transplant techniques available, including suction blister grafting, split-thickness grafting, punch grafting, and melanocyte suspension. Surgical techniques are most successful in late-stage segmental vitiligo, and they may be considered in those with nonresponsive, stable vitiligo.

Noncultured epidermal melanocyte cell grafting demonstrates superior extent and quality of pigmentation compared with other surgical techniques

Adverse outcomes include scarring, graft failure, koebnerization, infection, cobblestoning, and variegated pigmentation.

Not so many surgical treatments have emerged for vitiligo in recent years.

Noncultured, extracted follicular outer root sheath suspension (NC-EHF-ORS-CS) is a recently introduced technique for the treatment of stable vitiligo. Melanocytes are extracted from follicles from the occipital scalp and incubated with trypsin-ethylenediaminetetraacetic acid to separate outer root sheath cells, then reintroduced. This technique is minimally invasive and promising for vitiligo.[33]

CONCLUDING REMARKS

At all stages of therapy, we should always keep in mind that vitiligo can be a lifelong disease that may extensively damage one's psychosocial sense of well-being. Thus, treatment in the future should also stress the use of nonmedical treatment in helping patients to deal with the psychological disease burden.

The correct use of proper camouflage, tattoos, cosmetic agents, and psychological support will help patients to face the psychosocial effects of vitiligo and also positively affect disease progression.

Personalized nonmedical support is fundamental and will be always more important in vitiligo treatment.

REFERENCES

1. Cohen BE, Elbuluk N, Mu EW, Orlow SJ. Alternative systemic treatments for vitiligo: A review. *Am J Clin Dermatol.* 2015;16(6):463–474.
2. Dell'Anna MLEK, Hamzavi I, Harris J, Parsad D, Taieb A, Picardo M. Vitiligo. *Nature Reviews Disease Primers.* 2015;1(1):1–16.
3. Frisoli ML, Harris JE. Vitiligo: Mechanistic insights lead to novel treatments. *J Allergy Clin Immunol.* September 2017;140(3):654–662.
4. Harris JE. Cellular stress and innate inflammation in organ-specific autoimmunity: Lessons learned from vitiligo. *Immunol Rev.* 2016;269(1):11–25.

5. Lotti T, Gianfaldoni S, Valle Y, Rovesti M, Feliciano C, Satolli F. Controversial issues in vitiligo patients: A review of old and recent treatments. *Dermatol Ther.* 2019;32(1):e12745.

6. Rashighi M, Harris JE. Vitiligo pathogenesis and emerging treatments. *Dermatol Clin.* April 2017;35(2):257–e12265.

7. Rodrigues M, Ezzedine K, Hamzavi I, Pandya AG, Harris JE; Vitiligo Working Group. Current and emerging treatments for vitiligo. *J Am Acad Dermatol.* July 2017;77(1):17–29.

8. Spritz RA. Six decades of vitiligo genetics: Genome-wide studies provide insights into autoimmune pathogenesis. *J Invest Dermatol.* 2012;132(2):268–273.

9. Faas L, Venkatasamy R, Hider RC, Young AR, Soumyanath A. *In vivo* evaluation of piperine and synthetic analogues as potential treatments for vitiligo using a sparsely pigmented mouse model. *Br J Dermatol.* May 2008;158(5):941–950.

10. Shafiee A, Hoormand M, Shahidi-Dadras M, Abadi A. The effect of topical piperine combined with narrowband UVB on vitiligo treatment: A clinical trial study. *Phytother Res.* September 2018;32(9):1812–1817.

11. Yan R, Yuan J, Chen H et al. Fractional Er:YAG laser assisting topical betamethasone solution in combination with NB-UVB for resistant non-segmental vitiligo. *Lasers Med Sci.* 2017;32:1571–1577.

12. Kim HJ, Hong ES, Cho SH et al. Fractional Carbon Dioxide Laser as an "Add-on" treatment for vitiligo: A meta-analysis with systematic review. *Acta Derm Venereol.* 2018;98:180–184.

13. Lotti T, Tchernev G, Wollina U et al. Successful treatment with UVA 1 laser of non-responder vitiligo patients. *Open Access Maced J Med Sci* 2018;6:43–45.

14. Goren A, Salafia A, McCoy J, Keene S, Lotti T. Novel topical cream delivers safe and effective sunlight therapy for vitiligo by selectively filtering damaging ultraviolet radiation. *Dermatol Ther.* 2014;27(4):195–197.

15. Shalbaf M, Gibbons NC, Wood JM et al. Presence of epidermal allantoin further supports oxidative stress in vitiligo. *Exp Dermatol.* 2008;17(9):761–770.

16. Dell'Anna ML, Mastrofrancesco A, Sala R et al. Antioxidants and narrow band-UVB in the treatment of vitiligo: A double-blind placebo controlled trial. *Clin Exp Dermatol.* 2007;32(6):631–636.

17. Parsad D, Pandhi R, Juneja A. Effectiveness of oral ginkgo biloba in treating limited, slowly spreading vitiligo. *Clin Exp Dermatol.* 2003;28(3):285–287.

18. Szczurko O, Shear N, Taddio A, Boon H. Ginkgo biloba for the treatment of vitiligo vulgaris: An open label pilot clinical trial. *BMC Complement Altern Med.* 2011;11:21.

19. Middelkamp-Hup MA, Bos JD, Rius-Diaz F, Gonzalez S, Westerhof W. Treatment of vitiligo vulgaris with narrow-band UVB and oral *Polypodium leucotomos* extract: A randomized double-blind placebo-controlled study. *J Eur Acad Dermatol Venereol.* 2007;21(7):942–950.

20. Grimes PE, Hamzavi I, Lebwohl M, Ortonne JP, Lim HW. The efficacy of afamelanotide and narrowband UV-B phototherapy for repigmentation of vitiligo. *JAMA Dermatol.* 2013;149(1):68–73.

21. Rashighi M, Harris JE. Interfering with the IFN-gamma/CXCL10 pathway to develop new targeted treatments for vitiligo. *Ann Transl Med.* 2015;3(21):343.

22. Macdonald JB, Macdonald B, Golitz LE, LoRusso P, Sekulic A. Cutaneous adverse effects of targeted therapies: Part II: Inhibitors of intracellular molecular signaling pathways. *J Am Acad Dermatol.* 2015;72(2):221–236. quiz 37-8.

23. Rashighi M, Agarwal P, Richmond JM et al. CXCL10 is critical for the progression and maintenance of depigmentation in a mouse model of vitiligo. *Sci Transl Med.* 2014;6(223):223ra23.

24. Wang XX, Wang QQ, Wu JQ, Jiang M, Chen L, Zhang CF, Xiang LH. Increased expression of CXCR3 and its ligands in vitiligo patients and CXCL10 as a potential clinical marker for vitiligo. *Br J Dermatol.* 2016;174(6):1318–1326.

25. Villarino AV, Kanno Y, Ferdinand JR, O'Shea JJ. Mechanisms of JAK/STAT signaling in immunity and disease. *J Immunol.* 2015;194(1):21–27.

26. Craiglow BG, King BA. Tofacitinib citrate for the treatment of vitiligo: A pathogenesis-directed therapy. *JAMA Dermatol.* 2015;151(10):1110–1112.

27. Harris JE, Rashighi M, Nguyen N et al. Rapid skin repigmentation on oral ruxolitinib in a patient with coexistent vitiligo and alopecia areata (AA). *J Am Acad Dermatol.* 2016;74(2):370–371.

28. Rothstein B, Joshipura D, Sarayia A et al. Treatment of vitiligo with the topical Janus kinase inhibitor ruxolitinib. *J Am Acad Dermatol.* 2017;76:1054–1060.

29. Tufts Medical Center. *ClinicalTrials.gov [Internet].* Bethesda (MD): National Library of Medicine (US); Topical Ruxolitinib for the Treatment of Vitiligo. Available from https://clinicaltrials.gov/ct2/show/NCT02809976 NLM Identifier: NCT02809976 [2000-[cited June 29, 2016]

30. Moreland L, Bate G, Kirkpatrick P. Abatacept. *Nat Rev Drug Discov.* 2006;5(3):185–186.

31. Weber J. Immune checkpoint proteins: A new therapeutic paradigm for cancer—Preclinical background: CTLA-4 and PD-1 blockade. *Semin Oncol.* 2010;37(5):430–439.

32. Speerchaert R, van Geel N. Targeting CTLA-4, PD-L1 and IDO to modulate immune responses in vitiligo. *Exp Dermatol.* 2017;26:630–636.

33. Kumar P, Bhari N, Tembhre MK, Mohanty S, Arava S, Sharma VK, Gupta S. Study of efficacy and safety of noncultured, extracted follicular outer root sheath cell suspension transplantation in the management of stable vitiligo. *Int J Dermatol.* February 2018;57(2):245–249.

Tuberous sclerosis complex

12

VESNA PLJAKOSKA, KATERINA DAMEVSKA, and NATASA TEOVSKA MITREVSKA

CONTENTS

Introduction	89	Angiofibromas	91
Clinical features	89	Shagreen patches	91
Cutaneous manifestations of tuberous		Fibrous cephalic plaques	91
sclerosis complex	90	Ungual fibromas (Koenen tumors)	91
Hypopigmented macules	90	Treatment of cutaneous lesions	92
"Confetti"-like hypopigmentation	91	References	92

INTRODUCTION

Tuberous sclerosis complex (TSC) is a genetically determined autosomal disorder that causes substantial complications in multiple organ systems.[1] Benign tumor growth represents the hallmark of the disease, with the central nervous system (CNS), the kidneys, and the skin being the most commonly affected organs.[1]

The incidence of TSC may be as high as 1:5800 live births.[2] Population-based studies of TSC are rare. Studies in the United Kingdom reported a frequency of 1 in 12,000 to 1 in 14,000 in children under 10 years of age.[3]

Tuberous sclerosis is caused by mutations in one of two tumor suppressor genes: TSC1 (9q34) and TSC2 (16p13.3), which encode the proteins hamartin (TSC1) and tuberin (TSC2). The hamartin-tuberin complex inhibits the mammalian target of rapamycin pathway, which controls cell growth and proliferation.[4]

TSC can be diagnosed by the presence of clinical criteria and by genetic testing. The identification of either a TSC1 or TSC2 pathogenic mutation in DNA from normal tissue is sufficient to make a definite diagnosis of TSC.[5-7] Disease-causing mutations can be detected in 75%–90% of patients who meet the diagnostic criteria.[6] Therefore, negative genetic testing does not exclude the diagnosis of TSC.[5] International TSC guidelines recommend obtaining a three-generation family history to assess for additional family members at risk for TSC.[7] However, clinical features continue to be the principal means of diagnosis.[7,8]

Updated clinical diagnostic criteria for TSC include 11 major and six minor features (Table 12.1).[7] A definite TSC diagnosis requires identifying either two major symptoms or one major and two or more minor symptoms.[7] However, a combination of lymphangioleiomyomatosis (LAM) and angiomyolipomas without other features does not meet criteria for a definite diagnosis. The classic TSC diagnostic triad of seizures, intellectual disability, and facial angiofibromas (Vogt triad) occurs in less than one-third of patients with TSC.[8]

Table 12.1 Clinical criteria for the diagnosis of tuberous sclerosis complex

Major criteria	Minor criteria
Hypomelanotic macules (≥3, at least 5 mm diameter)	"Confetti" skin lesions
Angiofibromas (≥3) or fibrous cephalic plaque	Dental enamel pits (≥3)
Ungual fibromas (≥2)	Intraoral fibromas (≥2)
Shagreen patch	Retinal achromic patch
Multiple retinal hamartomas	Multiple renal cysts
Cortical dysplasia	Nonrenal hamartomas
Subependymal nodules	
Subependymal giant cell astrocytoma	
Cardiac rhabdomyoma	
Lymphangioleiomyomatosis (LAM)	
Angiomyolipomas (≥2)	

Source: Adapted from Northrup H, Krueger DA; International Tuberous Sclerosis Complex Consensus Group. *Pediatr Neurol.* October 2013;49(4):243–54, with permission.

Definite diagnosis: Two major features or one major feature with two minor features.

Possible diagnosis: Either one major feature or two minor features.

CLINICAL FEATURES

TSC is characterized by the development of a variety of benign, noninvasive tumors in multiple organs, most commonly in the brain, heart, skin, eyes, kidneys, and lungs, but also in the gastrointestinal tract, liver, and reproductive organs.[4]

According to a recent national surveillance study in Germany conducted using the current revised criteria for TSC, the three most common clinical features identified with TSC patients were central nervous system involvement in 73.3% of patients (of these, 95.2% experienced seizures), cutaneous involvement in 58.1% of patients, and cardiac rhabdomyoma. The annual incidence rate of TSC is estimated at a minimum of 1:17,785 live births.[9]

Central nervous system tumors are the leading cause of morbidity and mortality. They exhibit various neurological symptoms, including epilepsy, seizures, developmental delay, intellectual disability, and autism, which are referred to as TSC-associated neuropsychiatric disorders.[10]

Other possible TSC symptoms include vascular anomalies, cardiovascular and pulmonary issues, ophthalmologic problems such as multiple retinal hamartomas, and retinal achromic patches. Dental enamel pits and intraoral fibromas can occur in about 20%–50% of individuals with TSC, appearing on the buccal or labial mucosa and even the tongue.[7]

The management of TSC patients is very oppressive in terms of time, and might increase healthcare costs and the cost for the healthcare system. Management options include conservative approaches, surgery, pharmacotherapy with mammalian target of rapamycin inhibitors, and recently proposed options such as therapy with anti-EGFR antibodies and ultrasound-guided percutaneous microwaves. However, no systematically accepted strategy has been found that is both clinically and economically efficient. Thus, decisions are tailored to patients' characteristics, resource availability, and the clinical and technical expertise of each single center.[8,11]

CUTANEOUS MANIFESTATIONS OF TUBEROUS SCLEROSIS COMPLEX

Cutaneous findings are the most common and readily visible manifestation of TSC. More than 90% of patients with TSC have one or more skin lesions early in life, although none are pathognomonic.[4,12] It is important for the pediatrician to be able to identify TSC-associated skin manifestations to ensure prompt diagnosis, early treatment initiation, and appropriate referral for follow-up of other TSC-related sequelae.

The spectrum of cutaneous manifestation is wide and includes:[1,4,12,13]

- Ash leaf macules, 90%
- Confetti macules, 67%
- Café au lait spots, 90%
- Angiofibromas, 73%
- Shagreen patch, 67%
- Fibrous plaque, 86%
- Periungual fibromas, 100%
- Poliosis, 100%
- Molluscum fibrosum pendulum, 100%

Ash leaf macules are the first to appear, usually at birth or during infancy, and are present in more than 90% of patients; shagreen patches and facial angiofibromas also usually develop during childhood; angiofibromas typically appear from 3–4 years of age and progressively worsen as a patient gets older; ungual fibromas may develop during adolescence or early adulthood. Skin lesions can negatively impact a patient's quality of life, confidence, and psychological well-being. On occasion, the lesions may bleed and become infected.[13]

HYPOPIGMENTED MACULES

One of the terms used in the past to describe hypopigmented macules in tuberous sclerosis is white ash leaf spots; the term is now discouraged from use since the macules can be any shape or size (Figures 12.1 and 12.2). Hypopigmented macules of a certain size and shape are not indicative of a definite TSC diagnosis.[14]

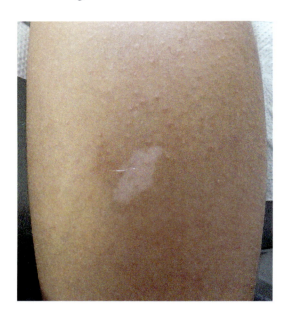

Figure 12.1 Ash leaf spot.

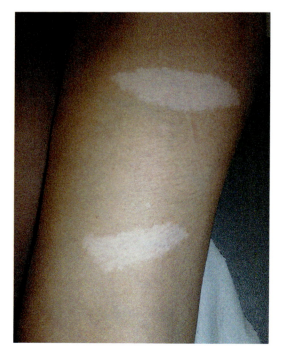

Figure 12.2 Large hypopigmented macules with serrated margins.

Hypopigmented macules are observed in about 90% of patients with TSC and are usually elliptic in shape.[13–15] In the updated criteria,[7] it was recommended that hypomelanotic macules meet a size requirement of at least 5 mm in diameter to distinguish hypomelanotic macules from smaller and more numerous "confetti" lesions. Furthermore, it is suggested to include polioses (circumscribed areas of hypomelanosis of hair) in the hypomelanotic macule count. While hypomelanotic macules are the more frequent cutaneous presentation of TSC in children, they fade with age and are detected less frequently in older patients.[16] Minimally visible hypopigmented spots are more easily visualized with a Wood's lamp.

Congenital onset may help distinguish TSC-related hypomelanotic macules from acquired causes of hypopigmentation, such as vitiligo, idiopathic guttate hypomelanosis, post-inflammatory hypopigmentation, and hypopigmented scars.[13,16,17]

Treatment usually is not necessary, but is considered for the cosmetically sensitive area of the face. An option for this treatment can be topical mTOR inhibitors, but long-term treatment may be necessary and the cost can be substantial.[16,17]

"CONFETTI"-LIKE HYPOPIGMENTATION

"Confetti" skin lesions, another typical TSC symptom, are numerous 1-mm to 3-mm hypopigmented macules scattered over regions of the body, such as the arms and legs.[7] This symptom is less common in children with TSC but has over 50% overall prevalence. Confetti skin lesions can appear any time from childhood to adulthood.[17–19]

ANGIOFIBROMAS

Moreover, about 75% of TSC patients between ages 2 and 5 years develop angiofibromas on the malar regions of the face.[8] Facial angiofibromas, sometimes erroneously referred to as adenoma sebaceum, are the most visually apparent TSC-associated symptom. They are usually pink to red-brown papulonodules with a smooth, glistening surface and are typically distributed symmetrically on the face, at times mistaken for acne. Angiofibromas start small and gradually increase in size, with their growth being augmented by puberty.[17,20]

To be regarded as a symptom of TSC, patients must exhibit at least three facial angiofibroma lesions, since one or two isolated sporadic lesions are often found among the general population. When there are only several angiofibromas, or if they are developed at a later age, a skin biopsy may be required. It is important to note that multiple facial angiofibromas have also been observed in Birt-Hogg-Dubé (BHD) syndrome and multiple endocrine neoplasia type 1 (MEN1).[20]

Treatment options for facial angiofibroma could be topical mTOR inhibitors, and there are benefits from various laser surgeries (vascular and ablative), using sedation with minimum surgical risks. Continual therapy is necessary, because improvements are temporary.[17]

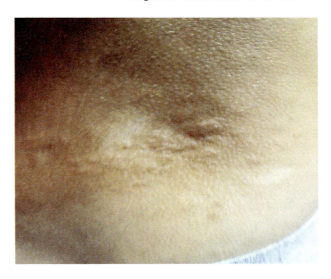

Figure 12.3 Shagreen patch.

SHAGREEN PATCHES

Shagreen patches are usually apparent before 10 years of age and increase in number as a patient ages. Shagreen patches are also a major symptom of TSC, seen most commonly over the lower back (Figure 12.3), in the form of large plaques that have a bumpy or orange-peel surface. Smaller collagenomas on the trunk exhibit the same histologic changes as shagreen patches but are less specific for TSC, since they may also occur as an isolated finding or in other genetic syndromes, including MEN1, BHD, and Cowden syndrome.[21]

FIBROUS CEPHALIC PLAQUES

Histologically similar to angiofibromas, fibrous cephalic plaques are regarded as the most specific skin finding for TSC, present in about 25% of TSC patients.[20] Initially referred to as forehead plaque, this symptom was renamed to fibrous cephalic plaque in order to increase awareness that fibrous plaques, although often located unilaterally on the forehead, may occur on other parts of the face or scalp. If there is rapid progression of fibrous cephalic plaques, treatment options include surgical intervention and sedation if necessary.[15,20]

UNGUAL FIBROMAS (KOENEN TUMORS)

Ungual fibromas are smooth, firm, flesh-colored lumps that emerge from the nail folds. Ungual fibromas are less common compared to other TSC-related skin findings, appearing with a frequency of about 20% overall, but as high as 80% in older adults with TSC.[15,20] They often develop during adolescence or adulthood and are more commonly found on toenails. Longitudinal nail grooves without visible fibromas are also commonly seen. Less frequent acral lesions include subungual red comets, splinter hemorrhages, and longitudinal leukonychia.[20]

If lesions are symptomatic or larger than 3 mm, the treatment options include ablative laser or surgical excision, and this treatment can be repeated if necessary.

TREATMENT OF CUTANEOUS LESIONS

All individuals with TSC are at risk for life-threatening conditions related to brain tumors, kidney lesions, or LAM. Treatment options are aimed at managing the symptoms of the disorder and often require input from a multidisciplinary team. Continued monitoring by physicians experienced with TSC is crucial.

Skin features are among the most prominent features of TSC. Individuals diagnosed with TSC should undertake a detailed dermatologic exam annually. Rapidly changing, disfiguring, or symptomatic TSC-associated skin lesions should be treated as appropriate for the lesion and clinical context, using approaches such as surgical excision, lasers, or possibly topical mTOR inhibitors. Sun protection is highly recommended, since hypopigmented macules are susceptible to sunburn, and ultraviolet-induced DNA damage may play a role in the development of facial angiofibromas. Disfiguring lesions may improve with laser therapy and dermabrasion. Symptomatic or deforming dental lesions and oral fibromas should be treated with surgical excision or curettage.

Limited data suggest that topical mTOR inhibitors such as sirolimus are effective for the treatment of facial angiofibromas, ungual fibromas, and hypomelanotic macules.[21,22] Long-term and comparative studies between topical rapamycin and ablative techniques are required to establish which treatment has a better outcome and a lower recurrence rate.[23]

Complication risks, adverse effects, cost, length of treatment, and potential impact on TSC-associated comorbidities should be considered when determining the best treatment option. Management strategies should be based on the clinical profile of each patient and on evidence-based good practice guidelines.

REFERENCES

1. Sparagana SP, Roach ES. Tuberous sclerosis complex. *CurrOpin Neurol.* April 2000;13(2):115–119.
2. Osborne JP, Fryer A, Webb D. Epidemiology of tuberous sclerosis. *Ann NY Acad Sci.* 1991;615:125–127.
3. O'Callaghan FJ, Shiell AW, Osborne JP, Martyn CN. Prevalence of tuberous sclerosis estimated by capture-recapture analysis. *Lancet.* 1998;351:1490.
4. Curatolo P, Bombardieri R, Jozwiak S. Tuberous sclerosis. *Lancet.* 2008;23:372(9639):657–1468.
5. Rosset C, Netto CBO, Ashton-Prolla P. TSC1 and TSC2 gene mutations and their implications for treatment in tuberous sclerosis complex: A review. *Genet Mol Biol.* 2017;40(1):69–79.
6. Caban C, Khan N, Hasbani DM, Crino PB. Genetics of tuberous sclerosis complex: Implications for clinical practice. *Appl Clin Genet.* 2016;10:1–8. doi:10.2147/TACG.S90262
7. Northrup H, Krueger DA; International Tuberous Sclerosis Complex Consensus Group. Tuberous sclerosis complex diagnostic criteria update: Recommendations of the 2012 International Tuberous Sclerosis Complex Consensus Conference. *Pediatr Neurol.* October 2013;49(4):243–254.
8. Schwartz RA, Fernández G, Kotulska K, Jóźwiak S. Tuberous sclerosis complex: Advances in diagnosis, genetics and management. *J Am Acad Dermatol.* 2007;57:189–202.
9. Ebrahimi-Fakhari D, Mann LL, Poryo M et al. Incidence of tuberous sclerosis and age at first diagnosis: New data and emerging trends from a national, prospective surveillance study. *Orphanet J Rare Dis.* July 17, 2018;13(1):117.
10. de Vries PJ, Whittemore VH, Leclezio L et al. Tuberous sclerosis associated neuropsychiatric disorders (TAND) and the TAND checklist. *Pediatr Neurol.* 2014;52(1):25–135.
11. Kohrman MH. Emerging treatments in the management of tuberous sclerosis complex. *Pediatr Neurol.* May 2012;46(5):267–275.
12. Roach ES, Gomez MR, Northrup H. Tuberous sclerosis complex consensus conference: Revised clinical diagnostic criteria. *J Child Neurol.* 1998;13:624–628.
13. Webb DW, Clarke A, Fryer A, Osborne JP. The cutaneous features of tuberous sclerosis: A population study. *Br J Dermatol.* 1996;135(1):1–5.
14. Northrup H, Koenig MK, Pearson DA et al. Tuberous Sclerosis Complex. July 13, 1999 [Updated July 12, 2018]. In: Adam MP, Ardinger HH, Pagon RA et al. eds. *GeneReviews.* Seattle (WA): University of Washington, Seattle; 1993–2018. Available from: https://www.ncbi.nlm.nih.gov/books/NBK1220/
15. Wataya-Kaneda M, Tanaka M, Hamasaki T, Katayama I. Trends in the prevalence of tuberous sclerosis complex manifestations: An epidemiological study of 166 Japanese patients. *PLOS ONE.* 2013;8:e63910.
16. Seibert D, Hong CH, Takeuchi F et al. Recognition of tuberous sclerosis in adult women: Delayed presentation with life-threatening consequences. *Ann Intern Med.* 2011;154:806–e63813.
17. Cardis MA, DeKlotz CMC. Cutaneous manifestations of tuberous sclerosis complex and the paediatrician's role. *Arch Dis Child.* September 2017;102(9):858–863.
18. Sehgal VN, Srivastava G. Hereditary hypo/de-pigmented dermatoses: An overview. *Int J Dermatol.* 2008;47:1041–1050.
19. Jimbow K. Tuberous sclerosis and guttate leukodermas. *SeminCutan Med Surg.* 1997;16:30–35.
20. Jozwiak S, Schwarz RA, Janniger CK et al. Skin lesions in children with tuberous sclerosis complex: Their prevalence, natural course, and diagnostic significance. *Int J Dermatol.* 1998;37:911–917.
21. Wataya-Kaneda M, Ohno Y, Fujita Y et al. Sirolimus gel treatment vs placebo for facial angiofibromas in patients with tuberous sclerosis complex: A randomized clinical trial. *JAMA Dermatol.* July 1, 2018;154(7):781–788.
22. Sasongko TH, Ismail NF, Zabidi-Hussin Z. Rapamycin and rapalogs for tuberous sclerosis complex. *Cochrane Database Syst Rev.* July 13, 2016;7:CD011272.
23. Balestri R, Neri I, Patrizi A, Angileri L, Ricci L, Magnano M. Analysis of current data on the use of topical rapamycin in the treatment of facial angiofibromas in tuberous sclerosis complex. *J Eur Acad Dermatol Venereol.* January 2015;29(1):14–20.

Oculocutaneous albinism

13

MIRA KADURINA, ANASTASIYA A. CHOKOEVA, and TORELLO LOTTI

CONTENTS

Introduction	93	Diagnosis	94
Epidemiology	93	Treatment	95
Etiology and pathogenesis	93	Prognosis	95
Clinical manifestations	93	References	95
Histology	94		

INTRODUCTION

Albinism represents a large family of inherited disorders, characterized by enzyme defects, leading to impaired melanin production with decreased or absent melanin in the skin, hair, and eyes, resulting in hypo- or depigmentation, depending on the degree of lack of tyrosinase.[1,2] The name of the disease comes from the Latin "albus," meaning "white," to emphasize the hallmark of its clinical manifestation. In contrast to vitiligo, the number of melanocytes in the skin is normal. This rare genetic condition can clinically present affecting the pigmentation of the eyes only or the eyes as well as the skin and hair, resulting in ocular (OA) or oculocutaneous albinism (OCA), respectively.[3] To date, seven types of nonsyndromic albinism have been described, and oculocutaneous albinism is the most commonly presented form.[1] Oculocutaneous albinism is caused by a mutation in specific genes that inhibit melanin biosynthesis within melanocytes. The deficiency of melanin pigment causes the clinical presentations of albinism.

Albinism may be a clinical symptom in a variety of other syndromes, classified as "albinoid disorders." Fifteen genes are currently associated with different types of albinism, although new genes have recently been described in association with autosomal recessive oculocutaneous albinism, which is phenotypically similar, but with diverse molecular origin.[1,2,4] Clinical manifestation depends on the residual activity of tyrosinase, as well as on the underlying genetic mutation, impairing different levels of melanin production, accumulation, or melanosome function.[1] Mild, moderate, or severe visual problems are associated with almost all of the clinical types of OCA.[5] Other associated symptoms, such as mental retardation, anemia or bleeding, deafness, recurrent infections, and so on, should direct the clinician's differential diagnostic plan toward the diagnosis of other syndromes. Hermansky-Pudlak syndrome, Chediak-Higasi syndrome, and Griscelli syndrome are thought to represent OCA with systemic manifestations and will be described in detail in separate chapters.[6]

EPIDEMIOLOGY

The condition was first described in detail by Pearson et al. in 1911, but the earliest description of this disorder was made by the Greek Ctesis in 400 BC and the Roman Plini, four centuries later.[7]

Nowadays, the incidence varies between racial groups, as the highest morbidity has been found in Nigeria (1:1000), and Cuna Indians in Panama (7:1000).[7] Worldwide incidence has been estimated around 1:20,000, but still varies for the different phenotypes of the disease (Table 13.1). Males and females are equally affected by this condition, although ocular albinism occurs primarily in males.[2,3]

ETIOLOGY AND PATHOGENESIS

The variety of forms of this rare genetic condition is a result of lack or reduction of melanin in skin and eyes, caused by mutations in genes involved in the biosynthesis of melanin pigment. Almost all of the forms are inherited in an autosomal recessive pattern, and they are classified based on the identified gene defect. Mutations in genes responsible for different types of oculocutaneous and ocular albinism include the tyrosinase gene (TYR) in OCA1. TYR hydroxylates L-tyrosine to L-DOPA and oxidates L-DOPA to DOPA quinone, while loss of this function leads to an inability to synthesize melanin.[1,2] The product of the OCA2 gene in OCA2 is melanosome transmembrane protein P, while the OCA3 gene in OCA3 produces the tyrosinase-related protein-1 gene (TYRP1), responsible for the stabilization and modulation of the activity of tyrosinase and contributing to melanosome integrity. The SLC45A2 gene in OCA4 codes for a solute carrier family 45, member 2 membrane-associated transport protein (MATP), associated with the transport substances required for melanin biosynthesis into the melanosome.[1,4] The former separation between tyrosinase-positive and tyrosinase-negative types of albinism has been replaced by a gene defect–based classification (Table 13.1).

CLINICAL MANIFESTATIONS

The two main affected organs in albinism are the skin and eyes. However, patients with ocular albinism may also have skin problems, while patients with cutaneous albinism show ocular findings quite often.[7] The degree of hypo- and depigmentation varies widely between the different types of albinism based on the activity of tyrosinase. Patients with

94 Oculocutaneous albinism

Table 13.1 Prevalence and genetics of albinism

Type of albinism	Worldwide prevalence	Most commonly seen in	Pattern of inheritance	Gene defect
OCA1	1:40,000	America, China	AR	The TYR gene; product: tyrosinase
OCA2	1:39,000	African Americans, Sub-Saharan Africa	AR	OCA2 gene; product: OCA2 melanosome transmembrane protein P
OCA3	1:8500	Southern Africa, Pakistan, Germany, India, Japan	AR	The TYRP1 gene; product: tyrosinase-related protein 1
OCA4	1:100,000	Japan, Turkey, Korea, Morocco	AR	SLC45A2 gene codes for a solute carrier family 45, member 2 membrane-associated transport protein (MATP)
OCA5	Very rare	Pakistan	AR	Not identified
OCA6	Very rare	China, India		SLC24A5 gene (solute carrier family 24, member 5) codes for a Na/K/Ca cation exchange protein
OCA7	Very rare		AR	LRMDA gene (leucine-rich melanocyte differentiation–associated protein)
Ocular albinism	1:50,000		X-linked	GPR143 gene

Source: Federico JR, Krishnamurthy K. *Albinism. StatPearls [Internet].* Treasure Island, FL: StatPearls Publishing; January 2018–July 28, 2018.

completely inactive tyrosinase are totally depigmented at birth with no melanin in irises and retina, leading to red reflex and severe ocular defects. Their hair is totally white, and they never get darker or tanned. If there is some degree of functional tyrosinase, it may lead to some hair color, seen in patients with the so-called OCA1-b form of albinism, where a mild degree of skin pigmentation may develop later in life. One extremely rare form of OCA1-B is the so-called "temperature-sensitive OCA1-b," where tyrosinase is only active when the temperature is lower than the body temperature, resulting in some degree of peripheral pigmentation of the extremities.[1,3,7]

OCA2 is the most common form among the tyrosinase-positive types of albinism. Although totally depigmented at birth, patients develop some degree of pigmentation later in life. The clinical findings in MATP-related albinism (OCA4) are almost similar.

In so-called "red albinism" (OCA3), patients have tan skin and red-brown hair. The irises are pigmented. The condition most commonly affects dark-skinned individuals (Africans and African Americans), and it is caused by defects in the P gene. The condition is known as "brown" or "rufous" OCA and it is often diagnosed because of the associated ocular problems.[1,7,8]

Ocular albinism is associated with mutations in the GPR143 gene, resulting in dysfunctional melanosome biogenesis with "macromelanosomes." The pigment dysfunction is limited to the eyes, and the ocular problems are severe, including nystagmus, foveal hypoplasia, and photophobia with impaired visual acuity. Pale skin may be seen in addition. Almost all of the female carriers show X-inactivation with pigmentary mosaicism in the retina, which is an important diagnostic clue for affected male children.[5,8,9]

Importantly, ocular problems in all forms of albinism are the most concerning clinical findings. They may be divided into refractive and nonrefractive errors, including photophobia, foveal hypoplasia with lack of foveal reflex, nystagmus, strabismus with binocular vision, reduced fine depth perception, and iris pigmentation and refractive disorders such as astigmatism, myopia, pyperopia, and so on. Pigmented disorders can also be presented as iris transillumination, yellow or orange retina due to hypomelanosis of retinal epithelium with prominent choroidal vessels.[2,10]

HISTOLOGY

The histopathologic examination is not helpful. In contrast to vitiligo, normal melanocytes are present and skin defects are not observed in hematoxylin and eosin staining. Special melanin staining such as dopa oxidase or HMB45 could be moderately positive. Specific histologic features could be seen only in some of the albinoid disorders.[7,11]

DIAGNOSIS

The diagnosis of albinism is basically clinical. Skin depigmentation at birth as a clinical finding should always include albinism in a differential diagnostic plan. Evaluation should focus on hair and skin color, presence of freckles and ability to tan, evaluation of pigmented and nonpigmented melanocytic nevi, and ophthalmologic evaluation for eye visual acuity.[1,2] The diagnosis is often made at birth as the skin and hair color of the baby will be much lighter or paler than the rest of the family. The presence of light patches on the skin is a clue to the presence of albinism. The diagnostic approach will include a physical examination, including comparison of the pigmentation of the child with that of the parents and other members of the family.

Further follow-up is also mandatory in order to assess the potential residual pigmentation that can increase with time, mostly through pheomelanin.[5] Comparison with other family members may be also a helpful diagnostic tool. Ophthalmologic examination is also essential for the correct diagnosis.[12] As a number of vision-related problems are often associated with albinism, a detailed eye examination may be needed. The ophthalmologist will assess the baby for nystagmus, strabismus, and photophobia. Electrodiagnostic testing in which small electrodes are placed on the scalp to test the connection of the brain and eyes is also sometimes conducted.[12]

Detailed directed evaluation for other associated symptoms is essential, in order to exclude some of the albinoid disorders. Recurrent infections, mental retardation, anemia, or bleeding episodes should be a diagnostic sign for an underlying syndromic albinism.

Molecular genetic testing with multigene or comprehensive genome sequencing provide the highest sensitivity for correct diagnosis and differentiation between the types of albinism.[1,13] This method is expensive and not routinely applied worldwide. Prenatal diagnosis can be also helpful, if the genetic mutation is already identified among family members.[1]

TREATMENT

There is no curative treatment for albinism and associated conditions. The most essential part of the patients' education is to maximize light (ultraviolet radiation A and B) protection with high sun protection factors, protective clothing, and sunglasses. Collaboration with an experienced ophthalmologist is needed for optimal management of the visual problems.[12] Dermatologic follow-up is crucial for the timely diagnosis and management of cutaneous malignancies. Patients should be educated in self-skin examination with the melanoma ABCDE rules.[1] Recent clinical trials established that nitisinone (an inhibitor of 4-hydroxyphenylpyruvate dioxygenase) can trigger tyrosine accumulation in blood, suggesting that it could improve pigmentation in OCA1B patients.[14] Potential gene therapy includes adeno-associated viruses' vectors, introducing a functional copy of the tyrosinase gene in OCA1 and OA1 patients, but clinical trials are still missing.[1]

PROGNOSIS

The overall lifetime prognosis is not affected in OCA. The mortality rate is due to a higher incidence of cutaneous malignancies. Although rare, albinism patients could be also affected by melanoma, because of the preserved melanocyte number and distribution.[15] Squamous cell carcinoma is the most commonly seen cutaneous malignancy among albinism patients (75%), with increased relative risk up to 1000 times, followed by basal cell carcinoma (23.4%) and melanoma (1.6%).[16]

REFERENCES

1. Federico JR, Krishnamurthy K. *Albinism. StatPearls [Internet]*. Treasure Island, FL: StatPearls Publishing; January 2018 – July 28, 2018.
2. Orlow SJ. Albinism: An update. *Semin Cutan Med Surg*. 1997;16(1):24–29.
3. Oetting WS. Albinism. *Curr Opin Pediatr*. 1999;11(6):565–571.
4. Suzuki T, Tomita Y. Recent advances in genetic analyses of oculocutaneous albinism types 2 and 4. *J Dermatol Sci*. 2008;51(1):1–9.
5. Kubasch AS, Meurer M. Oculocutaneous and ocular albinism. *Hautarzt*. 2017;68(11):867–875.
6. Toro C, Nicoli ER, Malicdan MC, Adams DR, Introne WJ. Chediak-Higashi syndrome. In: Adam MP, Ardinger HH, Pagon RA, Wallace SE, Bean LJH, Stephens K, Amemiya A, ed. *GeneReviews [Internet]*. Seattle (WA): University of Washington, Seattle; 1993–2018. March 3, 2009 [updated July 5, 2018].
7. Ramrath K, Stolz W. Disorders of melanin pigmentation/amelanosis and hypomelanosis/albinism, Chapter 65. In: Burgdorf WHC, Plewig G, Wolf HH, Landthaler M. ed. *Braun-Falco's Dermatology*. 3rd ed. Springer Verlag, Munchen, Germany; 2009, pp. 969–971.
8. Kamaraj B, Purohit R. Mutational analysis of oculocutaneous albinism: A compact review. *Biomed Res Int*. 2014;2014:905472.
9. Mártinez-García M, Montoliu L. Albinism in Europe. *J Dermatol*. 2013;40(5):319–24.
10. Khordadpoor-Deilamani F, Akbari MT, Karimipoor M, Javadi G. Sequence analysis of tyrosinase gene in ocular and oculocutaneous albinism patients: introducing three novel mutations. *Mol Vis*. 2015;21:730–735. eCollection 2015.
11. Dotta L, Parolini S, Prandini A, Tabellini G, Antolini M, Kingsmore SF, Badolato R. Clinical, laboratory and molecular signs of immunodeficiency in patients with partial oculo-cutaneous albinism. *Orphanet J Rare Dis*. October 17, 2013;8:168.
12. Kirkwood BJ. Albinism and its implications with vision. *Insight*. 2009;34(2):13–166.
13. Montoliu L, Grønskov K, Wei AH, Martínez-García M, Fernández A, Arveiler B, Morice-Picard F, Riazuddin S, Suzuki T, Ahmed ZM, Rosenberg T, Li W. Increasing the complexity: New genes and new types of albinism. *Pigment Cell Melanoma Res*. 2014;27(1):11–18.
14. Onojafe IF, Adams DR, Simeonov DR, Zhang J, Chan CC, Bernardini IM, Sergeev YV, Dolinska MB, Alur RP, Brilliant MH, Gahl WA, Brooks BP. Nitisinone improves eye and skin pigmentation defects in a mouse model of oculocutaneous albinism. *J. Clin. Invest*. 2011;121(10):3914–3923.
15. Emadi SE, Juma Suleh A, Babamahmoodi F, Ahangarkani F, Betty Chelimo V, Mutai B, Raeeskarami SR, Ghanadan A, Emadi SN. Common malignant cutaneous conditions among albinos in Kenya. *Med J Islam Repub Iran*. 2017;31:3.
16. Mabula JB, Chalya PL, Mchembe MD, Jaka H, Giiti G, Rambau P, Masalu N, Kamugisha E, Robert S, Gilyoma JM. Skin cancers among albinos at a university teaching hospital in Northwestern Tanzania: A retrospective review of 64 cases. *BMC Dermatol*. 2012;12:5.

Hermansky-Pudlak syndrome, Chediak-Chigasi syndrome, and Griscelli syndrome

14

VESNA PLJAKOSKA, SILVIJA DUMA, and ANDREJ PETROV

CONTENTS

Hermansky-Pudlak syndrome	97	Griscelli syndrome	99
Chediak-Higashi syndrome	98	References	99

HERMANSKY-PUDLAK SYNDROME

Introduction

Hermansky-Pudlak syndrome (HPS) is an autosomal recessive and a rare genetic group of disorders associated with oculocutaneous albinism, bleeding diathesis, granulomatous colitis, and highly penetrant pulmonary fibrosis in some subtypes.[1-3] The disorder was initially identified in 1959 and was named after the two Czechoslovakian pathologists, Hermansky and Pudlak, who were the first to identify patients with a unique combination of oculocutaneous albinism and bleeding diathesis.

Prevalence and prognosis

Hermansky-Pudlak syndrome is a rare hereditary disorder, with a worldwide prevalence of 1–9 in 1,000,000 individuals,[4] though prevalence differs per subtype and region. The disorder is more commonly found in certain populations of the world. For example, the prevalence of certain subtypes of HPS is significantly higher in Puerto Rico.[5] Individuals with HPS have also been identified in other regions, including China, India, South America, and Western Europe. Although initial symptoms usually appear in infancy or early childhood, they may develop at an older age as well. The prognosis for patients with HPS varies depending on the subtype. The course of subtypes 3, 5, and 6, or HPS without pulmonary fibrosis as a complication, is mild with no pulmonary involvement. Prognosis of subtypes 1, 2, and 4 is poor, as pulmonary fibrosis is fatal.[4]

Clinical features

Depending on the genetic mutation that causes the disorder, there are 10 subtypes of human HPS identified to date. These mutations, observed in HPS patients, are known to cause impairment of the specialized secretory cells, including melanocytes, platelets, and lung alveolar type II epithelial cells.[6] Different symptoms are associated with the different subtypes of HSP.

Initial clinical symptoms of HPS often include bleeding diathesis (bleeding from the nose, gums, or surgical wounds, especially in women during menstruation). Bleeding may become life-threatening, and aspirin may deteriorate the bleeding.

In addition to prolonged bleeding, classic symptoms of Hermansky-Pudlak syndrome include a lack of color (pigmentation) in the skin, hair, and eyes, known as oculocutaneous albinism, and the color may vary from very pale to almost normal coloring. Retinal hypopigmentation is characterized by reduced iris and retinal pigment associated with a severe decline in visual acuity and horizontal nystagmus. Tyrosinase-positive oculocutaneous albinism implies that the eumelanin, that is, the brown/black pigment, is absent from hair, eyes, and skin, while pheomelanin or the yellow/orange pigment is present and builds up with age.[7] It is important to note that the degree of albinism varies and can be subtle in HPS patients, potentially masked by use of hair-coloring products.

Pulmonary fibrosis occurs in HPS patients with subtypes 1, 2, or 4, which may prove fatal in their 30s, 40s, or 50s.[8]

The differential diagnosis of HPS includes Chediak-Higashi syndrome, a recessive disorder that shares the features of mild albinism and bleeding.[9]

Diagnosis

The diagnosis of HPS is established by clinical findings of hypopigmentation of the skin and hair, characteristic eye findings, and demonstration of absent delta granules (dense bodies) on whole-mount electron microscopy of platelets.[10] Furthermore, high-resolution computed tomography of the chest (HRCT) is used for diagnosing interstitial lung disease.

Should clinical features prove inconclusive, the diagnosis is confirmed via identification of biallelic pathogenic variants in the protein coding genes associated with the disorder.[11] Genetic testing is recommended to determine the specific disease subtype in individuals with

HPS[10] (multigene panel containing the 10 genes associated with HPS). However, platelet transmission electron microscopy (PTEM), used to determine hereditary platelet disorders, is currently available only in a limited number of laboratories.

Management

HPS patients with oculocutaneous albinism are at an increased risk of skin cancers, such as squamous and basal cell carcinomas, as well as melanoma. Recommendations toward the prevention of complications include protection from the sun starting from a young age, as well as yearly screening examinations by a dermatologist.

Furthermore, HPS patients with bleeding diathesis should be evaluated and managed by a hematologist, and female patients should be also evaluated by gynecologists if abnormally abundant menstrual bleeding is present. If present, gastrointestinal complications associated with ceroid deposition, such as gastroduodenitis, proctocolitis, or a granulomatous colitis, should be addressed by gastroenterologists. In addition, patients with subtypes 1, 2, or 4 should be diagnosed and managed by a pneumologist, due to the risk of developing severe pulmonary fibrosis.

CHEDIAK-HIGASHI SYNDROME

Introduction

Chediak-Higashi syndrome (CHS) is a rare autosomal recessive disorder, characterized by partial oculocutaneous albinism, immunodeficiency, recurring infections, mild bleeding tendency, and various neurological issues.[12–14] This disorder was first reported by Beguez Cesar, a Cuban pediatrician, in 1943.[15]

Prevalence and prognosis

With fewer than 500 cases reported worldwide, the exact prevalence of CHS is unknown.[16] The disorder can appear in individuals of all age groups. There are two types of CHS: classic and late onset. Predominantly, the classical accelerated CHS phase affects newborns and children under the age of 5. Generally, a mutation resulting in a loss of neurological function leads to a severe childhood onset of the disease. Milder than the classic form, the late-onset form occurs later in childhood or adulthood, and individuals experience minor pigmentation changes and are less likely to develop severe infections, but are at risk of developing neurological problems.

It has been observed that the severity of the disease correlates with the molecular phenotype, as well as the cellular phenotype. In terms of race or ethnicity, no predilection is determined.

CHS patients have poor prognosis if the disorder is left untreated. Most children with the classic form die within the first 10 years of their lives as a result of chronic infections or organ failure. Patients with late-onset CHS may live with the disorder into early adulthood, but typically have shorter lifespans due to complications.[17]

Clinical features

Eight known gene allele defects are associated with the Chediak-Higashi disorder.[18] Patients with CHS exhibit hypopigmentation, immunodeficiency and recurring infections, mild coagulation defects, and different levels of neurological dysfunction.[19]

The classical, early-onset CHS phase is known as the accelerated phase, with a mortality rate of 90% in the first decade of life. While this phase was initially thought to be caused by a malignancy, such as lymphoma, it is now known to be hemophagocytic lymphohistiocytosis, associated with multiorgan inflammation. In addition to this classical, early-onset CHS phase, patients might also have a later-onset form, known as atypical CHS phenotype. They exhibit abnormal granules within leukocytes, with neurodegeneration as the predominant symptom with only mild alterations in pigmentation, immune function, and reduced platelet-dense bodies with subtle bleeding manifestations.[16] These patients have subtle or absent oculocutaneous albinism, as well as insignificant infections or infections that become less frequent with age. Patients with this phenotype may be diagnosed after the third decade of life.

CHS patients often exhibit various neurological issues. Neurological manifestations include strokes, coma, ataxia, tremor, motor and sensory neuropathies, and absent deep-tendon reflexes.

In terms of partial oculocutaneous albinism, the quantity of pigment dilution can vary from normal, partial, or totally absent on skin, hair, and eyes. The classical form of the disease is characterized by a metallic or "silvery" appearance of the hair, observable under a light microscope. A decrease in pigmentation of the iris leads to a decrease in pigmentation of the retina. The visual acuity may be affected, and patients can either have normal acuity or exhibit some moderate impairment. Other ophthalmologic symptoms include photophobia, increasing red reflex, and a horizontal or rotating nystagmus.

Skin infections and upper respiratory tract infections are some of the most common infections associated with CHS. Affected individuals often have recurring bacterial and fungal infections with staphylococcal, streptococcal, pneumococcal, and beta-hemolytic species. Periodontitis has been identified as an important indicator of immune dysfunction and can help in establishing the correct diagnosis.

When it comes to bleeding tendency among individuals with CHS, epistaxis, mucosal, or gum bleeding are usually mild symptoms and generally do not require any medical intervention.

The differential diagnosis for CHS should include other genetic conditions with oculocutaneous albinism, such as Hermansky-Pudlak syndrome and Griscelli syndrome.

Diagnosis

Clinical diagnosis can be given to patients with immunodeficiency; pigment dilution of the skin, hair, or eyes; congenital or transient neutropenia; and signs of unexplained neurologic symptoms or neurodegeneration. Light microscopy and polarized microscopy of hair shafts aids in the differential diagnosis of CHS.[20]

Specific molecular genetic testing, which can include single-gene testing or multigene panel testing, can be conducted in order to detect the biallelic variants in the LYST gene.[17] Molecular genetic testing is necessary for detecting the carrier status of the parents, since CHS follows an autosomal recessive pattern of inheritance. The best time for determining genetic risk is before pregnancy.

Management

CHS patients have poor prognosis if the disorder is left untreated. The hematological and immune deficiency associated with the accelerated phase, which usually develops in the first 10 years of life, can only be cured with an allogeneic hematopoietic stem cell transplantation (HSCT), which should be performed as soon as the diagnosis is established.[21] Nevertheless, neurological problems may occur despite the bone marrow transplantation.

Since individuals with CHS exhibit varying degrees of hypopigmentation, CHS patients should apply sunscreen with a high protection factor to prevent skin cancers and skin damage. The SPF is in direct correlation to the severity of the hypopigmentation. Furthermore, sunglasses should be worn for protecting sensitive eyes against UV rays.[22]

GRISCELLI SYNDROME

Introduction

Initially identified by Griscelli and Prunieras in 1978, Griscelli syndrome (GS) is a rare autosomal recessive disorder characterized by unusual hypopigmentation of skin and hair, as well as immunodeficiency.[23]

Prevalence and prognosis

The exact prevalence of GS is unknown. There are around 100 cases reported worldwide, mostly from Turkish and Mediterranean populations.[24] The age and onset of the disorder range between 4 months to 7 years, and there is no sex predilection. In most patients, GS usually manifests between the ages of 4 months to 7 years, with the youngest occurring at 1 month. type II appears to be the most common of the three known types of GS.

The prognosis for patients with type I depends on the severity of their neurological impairment, and there is no cure. Bone marrow transplant extend survival for patients with type II.

Clinical features

Griscelli syndrome is classified into three types, depending on the gene mutation.[25] Type I[26] is due to MYO5A gene mutations and is manifested by hypomelanosis, associated with primary dysfunction of central nervous system. Patients with this type of GS exhibit silvery-gray sheen of their hair and light-colored skin, as well as early and severe psychomotor retardation. They typically have delayed development, intellectual disability, seizures, weak muscle tone (hypotonia), and eye and vision abnormalities. Type II[27] is caused by a mutation in the RAB27A gene, and presents with hypopigmentation, combined with variable cellular immunodeficiency. Prone to recurring infections, affected individuals may develop hemophagocytic lymphohistiocytosis, which manifests by overproduction and infiltration of activated histiocytes (T lymphocytes and macrophages), which may damage various organs and tissues, occasionally with a fatal outcome. Type III[28] is also characterized by hypomelanosis, but without neurological or immunological manifestations. This type may result from a mutation in melanophilin (MLPH) or the MIO5A gene.

GS differs from Chediak-Higashi syndrome by the evident lack of observable giant granules in GS granulocytes.

Diagnosis

Clinical diagnosis can be made in individuals who exhibit symptoms caused by the mutations in the MYO5A or RAB27A gene. These include pigmentary dilution, such as granulomatous skin lesions, partial albinism, and generalized lymphadenopathy. The hair appears silvery gray, silvery, grayish golden, or dusty, and the skin is pale. Similar to Chediak-Higashi syndrome, light microscopy and polarized microscopy of hair shafts aids in the differential diagnosis of Griscelli syndrome.[20]

Depending on the type, patients can also be diagnosed by other internal organ abnormalities. Patients with type II GS may exhibit hemiparesis, peripheral facial palsy, spasticity, seizures, psychomotor retardation, and severe retarded psychomotor development, as well as hepatosplenomegaly and jaundice. Furthermore, partial ocular albinism has been observed in some patients, but retinal degeneration has not been reported.

Since Griscelli syndrome is an autosomal recessive disorder, genetic testing should be performed. Prenatal diagnosis of type I and type II can be performed through chorionic villus sampling by the sequencing of the MYO5A or the RAB27A gene.

Management

The treatment and/or management of the disorder depends on the subtype. There is no treatment for patients with type I, and their quality of life depends on the severity of their neurological impairment. For patients with type II, the only real preventive treatment against the development of hemophagocytic lymphohistiocytosis is early bone marrow transplant. Certain studies have used antibiotics and antiviral agents for treatment, reporting mixed results.

REFERENCES

1. Dessinioti C, Stratigos AJ, Rigopoulus D, Katsambas AD. A review of genetic disorders of hypopigmentation: Lessons learned from the biology of melanocytes. *Exp Dermatol.* 2009;18:741–749.

2. Scheinfeld NS. Syndromic albinism: A review of genetics and phenotypes. *Dermatol Online J.* December 2003;9(5):5.

3. Hermansky F, Pudlak P. Albinism associated with hemorrhagic diathesis and unusual pigmented reticular cells in the bone marrow: Report of two cases with histochemical studies. *Blood.* 1959;14:162–169.

4. Data provided by Orphanet (www.orpha.net), the European website providing information about orphan drugs and rare diseases.

5. "HPS most prevalent in persons from northwest Puerto Rico, where the disorder affects one of every 1.800 individuals," according to the data published by NORD, the National Organisation of Rare Disorders, https://rarediseases.org/rare-diseases/hermansky-pudlak-syndrome/

6. Berber I, Erkurt MA, Kuku I et al. Hermansky-Pudlak syndrome: A case report. *Case Rep Hematol.* 2014;2014:249195–6.

7. Ramsay M, Colman MA, Stevens G et al. The tyrosinase-positive oculocutaneous albinism locus maps to chromosome 15q11.2-q12. *Am J Hum Genet.* 1992;51:879–884.

8. Pierson DM, Ionescu D, Qing G et al. Pulmonary fibrosis in Hermansky-Pudlak syndrome: A case report and review. *Respiration.* 2006;73(3):382–395.

9. El-Chemaly S, Young LR. Hermansky-Pudlak syndrome. *Clin Chest Med.* 2016;37(3):505–511.

10. Huizing M, Malicdan MCV, Gochuico BR et al. Hermansky-Pudlak syndrome. In: Adam MP, Ardinger HH, Pagon RA et al. eds. *GeneReviews.* Seattle (WA): University of Washington, Seattle; 2000:1993–2018. https://www.ncbi.nlm.nih.gov/sites/books/NBK1287/

11. Oshima J, Martin GM, Hisama FM. Werner syndrome. In: Adam MP, Ardinger HH, Pagon RA et al., eds. *GeneReviews.* Seattle (WA): University of Washington, Seattle, 2002:1993–2018. https://www.ncbi.nlm.nih.gov/books/NBK1514/

12. Chediak MM. New leukocyte anomaly of constitutional and familial character. *Rev Hematol.* 1952;7:362–367.

13. Higashi O. Congenital gigantism of peroxidase granules: The first case ever reported of qualitative abnormity of peroxidase. *Tohoku J Exp Med.* 1954;59:315–332.

14. Sato A. Chédiak and Higashi's disease: Probable identity of a new leucocytal anomaly (Chédiak) and congenital gigantism of peroxidase granules (Higashi) Tohoku. *J Exp Med.* 1995;61:201–210.

15. Beguez-Cesar AB. Neutropenia crónica maligna familiar con granulaciones atípicas de los leucocitos. *Boletín de la Sociedad Cubana de Pediatría.* 1943;15:900–922.

16. Ajitkumar A, Ramphul K. Chediak Higashi syndrome. [Updated June 10, 2018]. In: *StatPearls [Internet].* Treasure Island (FL): StatPearls Publishing; 2018. https://www.ncbi.nlm.nih.gov/books/NBK507881/

17. Toro C, Nicoli ER, Malicdan MC et al. Chediak-Higashi syndrome. In: Adam MP, Ardinger HH, Pagon RA et al. eds. GeneReviewsSeattle (WA): University of Washington, Seattle; 2009:1993–2018. https://www.ncbi.nlm.nih.gov/books/NBK5188/

18. Solomons HD. Hermansky-Pudlak/Chediak-Higashi syndromes. *Cardiovasc J Afr.* 2012;23(6):312.

19. Dotta L, Parolini S, Prandini A et al. Clinical, laboratory and molecular signs of immunodeficiency in patients with partial oculo-cutaneous albinism. *Orphanet J Rare Dis.* 2013;8:168. Published October 17, 2013.

20. Valente NY, Machado MC et al. Polarized light microscopy of hair shafts aids in the differential diagnosis of Chédiak-Higashi and Griscelli-Prunieras syndromes. *Clinics (Sao Paulo).* August 2006;61(4):327–332.

21. Umeda K, Adachi S. Allogeneic hematopoietic stem cell transplantation for Chediak-Higashi syndrome, *Pediatr Transplant.* March 2016;20(2):271–275.

22. Goding CR. Melanocytes: the new black. *Int J Biochem Cell Biol.* 2007;39:275–279.

23. Griscelli C, Prunieras M. Pigment dilution and immunodeficiency: A new syndrome. *Int J Dermatol.* December 1978;17(10):788–791.

24. Cağdaş D, Ozgür TT, Asal GT, Tezcan I, Metin A, Lambert N, de Saint Basile G, Sanal O. Griscelli syndrome types 1 and 3: Analysis of four new cases and long-term evaluation of previously diagnosed patients. *Eur J Pediatr.* October 2012;171(10):1527–1531.

25. Tardieu M, Rostasy K. Neurological expression of genetic immunodeficiencies and of opportunistic infections. In: *Handbook of Clinical Neurology.* 2013;112:1219–1227. doi:10.1016/B978-0-444-52910-7.00044-1.

26. Ménasché G, Ho CH, Sanal O, Feldmann J, Tezcan I, Ersoy F, Houdusse A, Fischer A, de Saint Basile G. Griscelli syndrome restricted to hypopigmentation results from a melanophilin defect (GS3) or a MYO5A F-exon deletion (GS1). *J Clin Invest.* 2003;112:450–456.

27. Bizario JC, Feldmann J, Castro FA, Ménasché G, Jacob CM, Cristofani L, Casella EB, Voltarelli JC, de Saint-Basile G, Espreafico EM. Griscelli syndrome: Characterization of a new mutation and rescue of T-cytotoxic activity by retroviral transfer of RAB27A gene. *J Clin Immunol.* July 2004;24(4):397–410.

28. Van Gele M, Dynoodt P, Lambert J. Griscelli syndrome: A model system to study vesicular trafficking. *Pigment Cell Melanoma Res.* 2009;22:268–282.

Piebaldism

15

JOVAN LALOŠEVIĆ and MILOŠ NIKOLIĆ

CONTENTS

Introduction	101	Histopathology	103
Epidemiology	101	Differential diagnosis	103
Etiopathogenesis	101	Treatment	103
Clinical presentation	101	References	104

INTRODUCTION

Piebaldism is an uncommon autosomal dominant disorder characterized by congenital white skin (leukoderma) and white hair (poliosis) on the frontal scalp, forehead, ventral trunk, and extremities. This condition has been documented throughout history, from the ancient Egyptians to the slave plantations of South America. The term piebald stems from the Latin word for magpie and is used to describe animals whose bodies are covered in black and white patches.[1]

EPIDEMIOLOGY

Piebaldism is a rare genodermatosis. Its incidence is estimated at less than 1/20,000 newborns.[2]

ETIOPATHOGENESIS

The mast cell growth factor (c-KIT), a tyrosine kinase receptor, is involved in melanoblast expansion, survival, and migration. Mutations leading to reduction in receptors impact the survival and migration of the neural crest-derived melanoblasts, resulting in failure of their colonization at anatomical sites most distant to the neural crest. Another gene required for melanoblast migration and/or survival is the SLUG gene (SNAIL), a zinc finger neural crest transcriptional factor.[3–5]

Piebaldism results from inactivating mutations or deletions of the c-KIT gene, which is mapped on chromosome 4q12, or of the SLUG gene, located on chromosome 8q11. These mutations result in decreased receptor tyrosine kinase signaling, impaired melanoblast development, and a decrease in melanogenesis.[3] The number and functionality of the c-KIT depends on the type and extent of the mutations. Frameshift mutations that result in a null gene product produce melanoblasts with half as many c-KIT receptors and therefore a milder form of the disorder. By contrast, point missense mutations, specifically in the tyrosine kinase domains, produce a nonoperational gene product, which reduces the signal transduction capability to one-fourth and results in a more severe phenotype.[6] Point missense mutations in the KIT ligand-binding domain have been identified in patients and present with extremely mild forms of piebaldism.[7] Patients with piebaldism that have no c-KIT mutations are found to have heterozygous deletions in the SLUG coding region.[8]

CLINICAL PRESENTATION

The most prominent characteristic is the white forelock (poliosis) (Figures 15.1 and 15.2) present in 80%–90% of patients with piebaldism. The white forelock typically appears in a triangular shape and the underlying skin of the scalp also is amelanotic (Figure 15.1). The eyebrows and eyelashes may also be involved[9] (Figure 15.1). Together with poliosis, patients may have leukoderma, classically distributed on the central forehead and anterior trunk (Figure 15.3), with extension on the flanks, anterior aspects of the medial arm, and leg regions (Figure 15.4). Sparing of the dorsal midline (Figure 15.3), hands, feet, and periorificial area is characteristic. Leukoderma is commonly stable throughout life, although additional hyperpigmented macules (Figures 15.3 and 15.4) may develop at or within the margins of the white patches.[10] Also, there are few reports on spontaneous repigmentation in infants, and even more sparse reports on repigmentation in older children and adults.[11,12]

Not unusually, patients with piebaldism may also develop hyperpigmented macules that are not within the boundaries of leukoderma (Figure 15.5). These are café au lait macules (CALMs) and axillary and/or inguinal freckles.[13,14] In contrast to depigmentation, the pathogenesis and genetic mechanism for development of hyperpigmentation in piebaldism remain to be elucidated. One group of authors has postulated that mutation in the KIT proto-oncogene in piebaldism leads to inadequate phosphorylation of Sprouty-related, Ena/vasodilator-stimulated phosphoprotein homology-1 domain-containing protein 1 (SPRED1), a protein that is defective in patients with neurofibromatosis 1 (NF1)-like syndrome, leading to the loss of function. This induces the development of CALMs and intertriginous freckles.[15] In contrast to depigmentation, hyperpigmented lesions like CALMs and freckles are not constant features of piebaldism and their severity does not parallel the severity of the depigmentation. If a patient with piebaldism has

102 Piebaldism

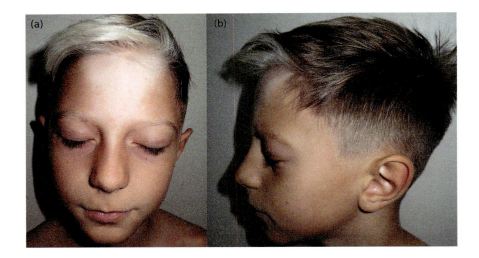

Figure 15.1 (a,b) Characteristic white forelock (poliosis) and underlying triangularly shaped leukoderma on the forehead.

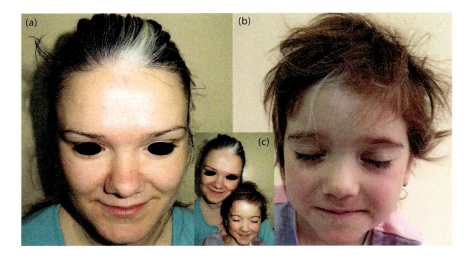

Figure 15.2 (a–c) Mother and daughter with different phenotypes. Mother with a more prominent poliosis and the daughter with a more noticeable frontal leukoderma.

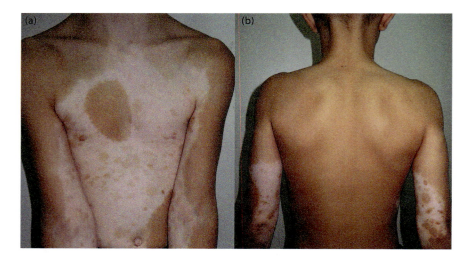

Figure 15.3 (a) Amelanotic macules on the anterior part of the arms and trunk with distinctive hyperpigmented macules within the margins of leukoderma. (b) The characteristic sparring of the dorsal midline.

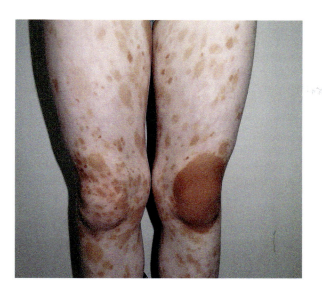

Figure 15.4 Large leukodermatous patches on the anterior aspects of the legs.

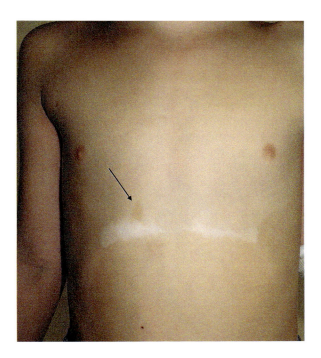

Figure 15.5 Café au lait macule (black arrow) arising outside the leukoderma margins on the trunk.

CALMs and intertriginous freckling, this does not necessarily represent a coexistence of NF1, regardless of the sufficient clinical criteria for the diagnosis of NF1.[16,17]

HISTOPATHOLOGY

Melanocytes are absent or considerably reduced in depigmented patches both by light and electron microscopy. The hyperpigmented macules are characterized by an normal number of melanocytes with plenty of melanosomes in them and in keratinocytes.[9]

DIFFERENTIAL DIAGNOSIS

There are several genetic disorders that feature either poliosis and/or leukoderma. Waardenburg syndrome (WS) is characterized by poliosis and leukoderma in WS types 1–4, heterochromatic irises in types 1 and 2, sensorineural hearing loss in types 1–4, dystopia canthorum in types 1 and 3, musculoskeletal abnormalities of the upper limbs in type 3, and Hirschsprung disease in type 4.[18] Tietze syndrome is also a rare autosomal dominant disorder characterized by congenital deafness and stable congenital leukoderma and poliosis, but no heterochromatic irises.[19] Hypopigmented macules and rarely poliosis have been described in patients with tuberous sclerosis. Even though poliosis occurs in only 20% of patients with tuberous sclerosis, it may be one of the earliest signs of the disease.[20] The previously reported Ziprkowski-Margolis or Woolf syndrome, characterized by hypomelanosis, deafness, and mutism, has now been included in the albinism-deafness syndrome and the gene has been localized to Xq26.3–q27.1, but not identified.[21,22] There are reports of piebaldism phenotype associated with Marfan syndrome, ganglioglioma, glycogen storage disease 1a, and Rubinstein-Taybi syndrome.[23–26]

Poliosis and leukoderma can also be present in certain acquired conditions. They have been commonly associated with vitiligo, more frequently in patients with the segmental form, with eyebrows being most commonly affected.[27] Vogt-Koyanagi-Harada syndrome is a rare multisystem autoimmune disease that affects tissues containing melanin, including the eye, inner ear, meninges, and skin. The disease is characterized by bilateral uveitis associated with vitiligo, poliosis, aseptic meningitis, tinnitus, dysacusis, and alopecia.[28] Alezzandrini syndrome is a condition characterized by unilateral degeneration of the retina, unilateral vitiligo, poliosis, and hearing abnormalities.[29] White hair is often noted with early hair regrowth in alopecia areata (AA). Pigmented hairs are selectively affected in AA and may result in sudden whitening of a salt-and-pepper scalp.[30,31] In sarcoidosis, poliosis can be present on the eyelashes, in the setting of uveitis.[32] Also, it can be a manifestation of chronic blepharitis.[33]

There are single reports on hypopigmented hair arising from an underlying neurofibroma or a melanoma. In the case of melanoma, it was postulated that the depigmentation was probably due to immune destruction of the melanocytes by cytotoxic lymphocytes. In case of neurofibroma, the authors postulated that pathogenesis of poliosis is either due to cytotoxic T cells targeting neurofibroma cross-reacting with the melanocytes of the hair bulbs, or due to neurochemical mediators secreted by neurofibroma, cytotoxic to melanocytes.[34,35]

TREATMENT

Piebaldism is a disease in which depigmented skin areas are unresponsive to topical or light treatment. The nonpigmented patches are at an increased risk of sunburn and skin cancer related to excessive sun exposure; therefore, sunscreen should be used frequently. Topical treatments with makeup or artificial pigmenting agents, for example, dihydroxyacetone (the ingredient used in sunless tanning products) that causes the skin to turn brown/dark by polymerizing the amino acids and amino groups, could be used in patients who are still not old enough for grafting procedures.[36]

Depigmented areas may be treated with autografting of normal skin or melanocytes into amelanotic areas, either by thin split-thickness grafts and minigrafting or with *in vitro* cultured epidermis and suction epidermal grafting.[37,38] A large retrospective study concluded that stable types of leucoderma, that is, segmental vitiligo and piebaldism, responded in most cases with 100% repigmentation, regardless of the surgical method that was used.[39] Phototherapy alone is insufficient, but could be used to prepare the recipient site before cell suspension transplantation or after the transplantation to enhance melanocyte migration.[38,40]

REFERENCES

1. Huang A, Glick SA. Piebaldism in history—"The Zebra People." *JAMA Dermatol.* 2016;152(11):1261.
2. Debbarh FZ, Mernissi FZ. Piebaldisme: A rare genodermatosis. *Pan Afr Med J.* 2017;27:221.
3. Dessinioti C, Stratigos AJ, Rigopoulos D, Katsambas AD. A review of genetic disorders of hypopigmentation: Lessons learned from the biology of melanocytes. *Exp Dermatol.* 2009;18(9):741–1269.
4. Perez-Losada J, Sanchez-Martin M, Rodriguez-Garcia A et al. Zinc-finger transcription factor SLUG contributes to the function of the stem cell factor c-kit signaling pathway. *Blood.* 2002;100(4):1274–1286.
5. Tomita Y, Suzuki T. Genetics of pigmentary disorders. *Am J Med Genet C Semin Med Genet.* 2004;131c(1):75–81.
6. Spritz RA. The molecular basis of human piebaldism. *Pigment Cell Res.* 1992;5(5 Pt 2):340–343.
7. Fleischman RA, Gallardo T, Mi X. Mutations in the ligand-binding domain of the kit receptor: An uncommon site in human piebaldism. *J Invest Dermatol.* 1996;107(5):703–706.
8. Sanchez-Martin M, Perez-Losada J, Rodriguez-Garcia A et al. Deletion of the SLUG (SNAI2) gene results in human piebaldism. *Am J Med Genet A.* 2003;122a(2):125–132.
9. Agarwal S, Ojha A. Piebaldism: A brief report and review of the literature. *Indian Dermatol Online J.* 2012;3(2):144–147.
10. Oiso N, Fukai K, Kawada A, Suzuki T. Piebaldism. *J Dermatol.* 2013;40(5):330–335.
11. Arase N, Wataya-Kaneda M, Oiso N et al. Repigmentation of leukoderma in a piebald patient associated with a novel c-KIT gene mutation, G592E, of the tyrosine kinase domain. *J Dermatol Sci.* 2011;64(2):147–149.

12. Frances L, Betlloch I, Leiva-Salinas M, Silvestre JF. Spontaneous repigmentation in an infant with piebaldism. *Int J Dermatol.* 2015;54(6):e244–e246.
13. Spritz RA, Itin PH, Gutmann DH. Piebaldism and neurofibromatosis type 1: Horses of very different colors. *J Invest Dermatol.* 2004;122(2): xxxiv–xxxv.
14. Sarma N, Chakraborty S, Bhanja DC, Bhattachraya SR. Piebaldism with non-intertriginous freckles: What does it mean? *Indian J Dermatol Venereol Leprol.* 2014;80(2):163–165.
15. Chiu YE, Dugan S, Basel D, Siegel DH. Association of piebaldism, multiple cafe-au-lait macules, and intertriginous freckling: Clinical evidence of a common pathway between KIT and Sprouty-related, Ena/vasodilator-stimulated phosphoprotein homology-1 domain containing protein 1 (SPRED1). *Pediatr Dermatol.* 2013;30(3):379–382.
16. Jia WX, Xiao XM, Wu JB et al. A novel missense KIT mutation causing piebaldism in one Chinese family associated with cafe-au-lait macules and intertriginous freckling. *Ther Clin Risk Manag.* 2015;11:635–638.
17. Nagaputra JC, Koh MJA, Brett M, Lim ECP, Lim HW, Tan EC. Piebaldism with multiple cafe-au-lait-like hyperpigmented macules and inguinal freckling caused by a novel KIT mutation. *JAAD Case Rep.* 2018;4(4):318–321.
18. Pingault V, Ente D, Dastot-Le Moal F, Goossens M, Marlin S, Bondurand N. Review and update of mutations causing Waardenburg syndrome. *Hum Mutat.* 2010;31(4):391–406.
19. Smith SD, Kelley PM, Kenyon JB, Hoover D. Tietz syndrome (hypopigmentation/deafness) caused by mutation of MITF. *J Med Genet.* 2000;37(6):446–448.
20. Sleiman R, Kurban M, Succaria F, Abbas O. Poliosis circumscripta: Overview and underlying causes. *J Am Acad Dermatol.* 2013;69(4):625–633.
21. Jacob AN, Kandpal G, Gill N, Kandpal RP. Toward expression mapping of albinism-deafness syndrome (ADFN) locus on chromosome Xq26. *Somat Cell Mol Genet.* 1998;24(2):135–140.
22. Shiloh Y, Litvak G, Ziv Y et al. Genetic mapping of X-linked albinism-deafness syndrome (ADFN) to Xq26.–q27.I. *Am J Hum Genet.* 1990;47(1):20–27.
23. Bansal L, Zinkus TP, Kats A. Poliosis with a rare association. *Pediatr Neurol.* 2018;83:62–63.
24. Ghoshal B, Sarkar N, Bhattacharjee M, Bhattacharjee R. Glycogen storage disease 1a with piebaldism. *Indian Pediatr.* 2012;49(3):235–236.
25. Herman KL, Salman K, Rose LI. White forelock in Marfan's syndrome: An unusual association, with review of the literature. *Cutis.* 1991;48(1):82–84.
26. Herranz P, Borbujo J, Martinez W, Vidaurrazaga C, Diaz R, Casado M. Rubinstein-Taybi syndrome with piebaldism. *Clin Exp Dermatol.* 1994;19(2):170–172.

27. Hann SK, Lee HJ. Segmental vitiligo: Clinical findings in 208 patients. *J Am Acad Dermatol.* 1996;35(5 Pt 1):671–674.

28. Greco A, Fusconi M, Gallo A et al. Vogt-Koyanagi-Harada syndrome. *Autoimmun Rev* 2013;12(11): 1033–1038.

29. Andrade A, Pithon M. Alezzandrini syndrome: Report of a sixth clinical case. *Dermatology.* 2011;222(1):8–9.

30. Elston DM, Clayton AS, Meffert JJ, McCollough ML. Migratory poliosis: A forme fruste of alopecia areata? *J Am Acad Dermatol.* 2000;42(6):1076–1077.

31. Jalalat SZ, Kelsoe JR, Cohen PR. Alopecia areata with white hair regrowth: Case report and review of poliosis. *Dermatol Online J.* 2014;20(9).

32. Lett KS, Deane JS. Eyelash poliosis in association with sarcoidosis. *Eye (Lond).* 2005;19(9):1015–1017.

33. Bernardes TF, Bonfioli AA. Blepharitis. *Semin Ophthalmol.* 2010;25(3):79–83.

34. Dunn CL, Harrington A, Benson PM, Sau P, James WD. Melanoma of the scalp presenting as poliosis circumscripta. *Arch Dermatol.* 1995;131(5):618–619.

35. Kwon IH, Cho YJ, Lee SH et al. Poliosis circumscripta associated with neurofibroma. *J Dermatol.* 2005;32(6):446–449.

36. Suga Y, Ikejima A, Matsuba S, Ogawa H. Medical pearl: DHA application for camouflaging segmental vitiligo and piebald lesions. *J Am Acad Dermatol.* 2002;47(3):436–438.

37. Thomas I, Kihiczak GG, Fox MD, Janniger CK, Schwartz RA. Piebaldism: An update. *Int J Dermatol.* 2004;43(10):716–719.

38. Njoo MD, Nieuweboer-Krobotova L, Westerhof W. Repigmentation of leucodermic defects in piebaldism by dermabrasion and thin split-thickness skin grafting in combination with minigrafting. *Br J Dermatol.* 1998;139(5):829–833.

39. Olsson MJ, Juhlin L. Long-term follow-up of leucoderma patients treated with transplants of autologous cultured melanocytes, ultrathin epidermal sheets and basal cell layer suspension. *Br J Dermatol.* 2002;147(5):893–904.

40. Lommerts JE, Meesters AA, Komen L et al. Autologous cell suspension grafting in segmental vitiligo and piebaldism: A randomized controlled trial comparing full surface and fractional CO_2 laser recipient-site preparations. *Br J Dermatol.* 2017;177(5):1293–1298.

Waardenburg syndrome

16

CARMEN MARIA SALAVASTRU, STEFANA CRETU, and GEORGE SORIN TIPLICA

CONTENTS

Introduction	107	SOX10	108
Genetic background	107	EDN3 and EDNRB	108
PAX3	107	Clinical findings	108
Microphthalmia-associated transcription factor	107	Cutaneous features	109
SNAI2	108	References	110

INTRODUCTION

Waardenburg syndrome (WS), a genetic condition first described in 1951 by the Dutch ophthalmologist Petrus Johannes Waardenburg,[1] is classified into four subtypes, with several genes involved.[2] Multiple studies have found that the prevalence of the disease ranges between 1 in 20,000 and 1 in 42,000.[1,3–7] The inheritance pattern in WS is usually autosomal dominant, although autosomal recessive cases have been described.[7]

The syndrome associates disabling features, such as hearing loss, found more frequently in WS type II; limb abnormalities in type III; or life-threatening features, as are associated with Hirschsprung disease in type IV. Although they are not the main cause of disability, cutaneous findings are present in all types of WS and their recognition, either in the patients or their family members, can aid in rapidly establishing the correct diagnosis.[1–8]

GENETIC BACKGROUND

The neural crest was first described over 150 years ago.[9] WS is a typical neurocristopathy and its characteristics are due to mutations affecting neural crest cells. These multipotent embryonic cells migrate from the dorsal part of the neural tube and are precursors for several cell lineages: melanocytes, peripheral and enteric neurons and glia, craniofacial chondrocytes, osteoblasts, adrenal chromaffin cells, intermediate cells of the stria vascularis in the cochlea, and certain cells of the heart and thymus.[10–12] All melanocytes, except for those of the retina (derived from the optic cup of the brain), are derived from cells of the neural crest.[9,12] The function of the protein products of the mutated genes can be absent or diminished compared to the wild-type gene, depending on the mutations present and on how much of the original protein was altered.[13] The features present in WS are the result of a reduced level of expression (haploinsufficiency) of different transcription factors.[12] This results in anomalies of the proliferation, survival, migration, and differentiation of the cells derived from the neural crest. These cells, at key moments in their development, express specific genes.

PAX3

Most of the cases of WS type I, if not all, are the result of heterozygous PAX3 mutations. Homozygous or compound heterozygous PAX3 mutations are responsible for severe cases of the WS type III, occasionally resulting in death in early infancy or *in utero*. Mutations can either be inherited in an autosomal dominant manner or occur *de novo*.[10]

In the developing embryo, PAX3 expression coincides with the formation of somites and is switched off as the somites dissociate. It is also expressed in the undifferentiated mesenchyme of the limb buds, explaining the presence of phenotypes such as those seen in WS type III.[7] In addition to their involvement in the development of the melanocyte lineage, PAX3 genes are important for the formation of craniofacial cartilage and bones, hence the reason dystopia canthorum is seen in WS type I, but not in type II, as microphthalmia-associated transcription factor (MITF) is very important for the melanocytic lineage, but not for cell precursors of the cranial cartilage and bones.[9,13,14]

In order for a neural crest cell to follow the pathway to become a melanocyte, PAX3 and MITF need to be expressed,[14] with the MITF expression being regulated by PAX3;[13] the expression of the PAX3 gene is required for melanoblast proliferation, whereas the expression of MITF is important in their survival during and after their migration.[14]

MICROPHTHALMIA-ASSOCIATED TRANSCRIPTION FACTOR

Approximately 15% of WS type II cases are the result of mutations in the MITF gene. Individuals are heterozygotes and the mutations can be inherited in an autosomal dominant manner or occur *de novo*. Microphthalmia-associated transcription factor controls the development and differentiation of melanocytes, osteoclasts, and mastocytes.[10,15] Mutations involving this gene lead to pigmentation loss, microphtalmia, deafness, failure of secondary bone resorption, and a small number of mast cells. The promoter of MITF-M, one of the five known isoforms of MITF, is functional only in cells of the melanocyte lineage. This promoter is upregulated by other transcription factors like PAX3 and SOX10. In

SNAI2

The SNAI2 gene encodes for a zinc-finger transcription factor and is expressed in neural crest cells as they migrate from their original site, important in the migration of these cells, not in their development. *In vivo*, it also interacts with KIT. Mutations in this gene are also responsible for WS type II. In these cases, although MITF is present and transactivates the promoter for SNAI2, the downstream cellular events can no longer follow their usual path, resulting in the phenotype being consistent with WS type II.[16]

SOX10

SOX10 is a transcription factor responsible for the development and preservation of melanocytes, Schwann cells, and enteric ganglion cells, all of which derive from the neural crest cells.[17] The gene is expressed in the developing embryo in neural crest cells that contribute to the formation of the peripheral nervous system and transiently in melanoblasts. In later stages of development, it is also expressed in the central nervous system, reaching a maximum level of expression at this site in the adult life. Among the transcription factors modulated by SOX10 are PAX3 and MITF.[13] Individuals with WS and SOX10 mutations are heterozygotes. In the homozygous state, SOX10 mutations are lethal in early infancy or *in utero*.[10]

EDN3 AND EDNRB

Endothelins (EDNs) are a family of three proteins (EDN1, EDN2, EDN3) functioning as ligands for the endothelin receptor (EDNR). The EDNRB subtype is able to interact with all three members of the EDN family; however, murine studies have suggested that the EDN3 protein is its main ligand.[10,18] The genes encoding EDN3 and EDNRB are important in the proliferation, migration, and differentiation of cell lineages derived from the neural crest.[19] During embryogenesis, EDNRB is expressed for the first time in the cells at the dorsal tip of the neural tube and then in cells of the neural crest.[10] Afterward, it is only expressed by the cells that follow the dorso-ventral migration pathway and then in most of the cellular types derived from them, such as the enteric ganglia. Heterozygous mutations of these genes lead to aganglionic megacolon, a feature of WS type IV. Patients suffering from this condition develop life-threatening functional bowel obstruction.[18,20] Although the genes involved in the pathogenesis of WS have been extensively studied, there are still cases in which the phenotype cannot be explained on the basis of mutations to any of the known genes. This is the case for approximately 70% of WS type II and 35% of WS type IV, as opposed to the majority of WS type I and III cases, where the findings are due to mutations to the PAX3 gene.[10,21] Mutations of the EDNRB gene are estimated to be the cause of 5%–6% of mutations in WS type II. In homozygotes, the mutated genes have complete penetrance, leading to severe phenotypes, whereas in heterozygotes, they have an autosomal dominant mode of transmission, with incomplete penetrance leading to no changes or to partial phenotypes.[22] These are summarized in Table 16.1.

CLINICAL FINDINGS

When the syndrome was first described, Waardenburg characterized it by the following aspects: (1) congenital

Table 16.1 WS subtypes and their mode of inheritance

Type	Genetic mutations involved	Gene product	Mode of inheritance
I	PAX3	**PA**ired bo**X 3** transcription factor	AD
II	MITF	**M**elanocyte **I**nducing **T**ranscription **F**actor	AD
	SNAI2 (SLUG)	**SNAIL** homolog **2** protein	AD
	SOX10	**S**ry **10 bOX** transcription factor	AD
	EDNRB	**END**othelin Receptor type **B**	AD
III	PAX3	**PA**ired bo**X 3** transcription factor	AD
IV	SOX10	**S**ry **10 bOX** transcription factor	AD
	EDN3	**END**othelin 3	AR
	EDNRB	**END**othelin Receptor type **B**	AR

Sources: Farrer LA et al. *Am J Hum Genet.* May 1992;50(5):902; Tamayo ML et al. *Am J Med Genet A.* April 15, 2008;146(8):1026–1031; Milunsky JM. Waardenburg syndrome type I. InGeneReviews® [Internet] 2017 May 4. University of Washington, Seattle. Available from: https://www.ncbi.nlm.nih.gov/books/NBK1531/, accessed on December 2018; Hageman MJ, Delleman JW. *Am J Hum Genet.* September 1977;29(5):468; Read AP, Newton VE. *J Med Genet.* August 1, 1997;34(8):656–665; U.S. National Library of Medicine, National Institutes of Health. Genetics Home Reference: Your guide to understanding genetic conditions. Available from: https://ghr.nlm.nih.gov/condition/waardenburg-syndrome, accessed on December 2018; Pingault V et al. *Hum Mutat.* April 2010;31(4):391–406; Pilon N. *Rare Dis.* January 1, 2016;4(1):4483–4496.

Table 16.2 Variation in clinical features in WS

Site of involvement	Clinical findings	Percentage of affected individuals
Cranio-facial anomalies	High nasal root	52%–100%
	Dystopia canthorum	98%–100%
Hearing loss (>100 dB)	Bilateral or unilateral sensorineural hearing loss	47%–58%
Hair	Synophrys	63%–73%
	White forelock	43%–48%
	Early graying	23%–38%
Skin	Leukoderma	22%–38%
Eyes	Heterochromic irides	15%–31%
	Hypoplastic blue irides	15%–18%

Sources: Farrer LA et al. *Am J Hum Genet*. May 1992;50(5):902; Tamayo ML et al. *Am J Med Genet A*. April 15, 2008;146(8):1026–1031; Milunsky JM. Waardenburg syndrome type I. In GeneReviews® [Internet] 2017 May 4. University of Washington, Seattle. Available from: https://www.ncbi.nlm.nih.gov/books/NBK1531/, accessed on December 2018.

deafness or partial (unilateral) deafness; (2) circumscribed albinism of the frontal head hair (white forelock); (3) lateral displacement of the medial canthi and lacrimal points (dystopia canthorum); (4) partial or total heterochromia iridum; (5) hyperplasia of the medial portions of the eyebrows; and (6) a hyperplastic, broad, and high nasal root.[1] Several investigator groups have studied the penetrance of clinical features found in affected individuals, and a detailed description is available in Table 16.2. Genotype/phenotype correlations are difficult to establish across the different types of WS, as phenotypes vary greatly even between members of the same family.[10]

CUTANEOUS FEATURES

Skin depigmentation

Congenital leukoderma in a child can be the consequence of many processes (Figure 16.1). WS is an uncommon condition in comparison to other diseases such as vitiligo or other genodermatoses, like neurofibromatosis type I or tuberous sclerosis complex.[23,24] Skin findings in WS usually present as hypopigmented macules and patches on the face, trunk, or limbs. The periphery of the lesions may appear hyperpigmented.[5,23] Upon Wood lamp examination, the lesions appear hypopigmented, unlike chalk-white in vitiligo. The hypopigmented lesions of TSC appear early in the course of the disease, and a thorough evaluation should be performed. Lisch nodules of NF1 can be easily differentiated from iris pigmentary anomalies of WS by ophthalmologic examination.[23,24] Severe depigmentation associated with upper limb defects and other clinical features are the result of homozygous mutations or compound heterozygous mutations of the PAX3 gene.[10] Also, this can be found in cases with particular SOX10 variants. Watanabe et al. reported a patient with extensive hypopigmentation carrying a deletion type mutation to this gene.[25]

Hair depigmentation

With age and as a consequence of oxidative stress, newly formed hair follicles are devoid of melanocytes, because their stem cell precursors become dysfunctional, undergoing apoptosis; the process involves the reduction of Bcl-2 gene expression levels in the melanocyte stem cells. This is a proto-oncogene, interacting with other key genes, including MITF.[26] Hair depigmentation in WS includes the presence of a white forelock, usually in the medial part of the forehead and extending toward the posterior, or patches of white hair located in other areas of the scalp.[10,27] The underlying scalp skin and forehead may appear hypopigmented.[5] These features are not present in all cases.

Other clinical findings are early hair graying, usually before the age of 30, and white eyebrows and/or eyelashes.[10] Both early graying and the white forelock are considered, by some authors, forms of partial hair albinism.[28]

Synophrys

Medial confluence of the eyebrows above the nasal bridge is also called synophrys. It is a feature of several genetic syndromes, as well as a normal variation.[29] In WS, it is the

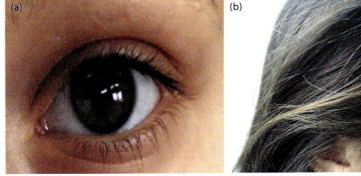
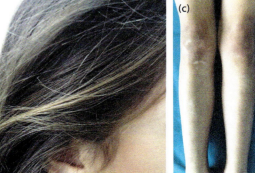

Figure 16.1 (a) Partial/segmental heterochromia; (b) hair hypopigmentation; (c) hypopigmentation of the skin. (Courtesy of Carmen Maria Salavastru.)

result of pathological migration of the cells from the neural crest to the medial region of the face.[28]

Diagnosis

Diagnosis is in most cases clinical, based on major and minor criteria, detailed in Table 16.3, with cutaneous findings being present in all four types.[2–4,7]

The diagnosis for WS type I is established in the presence of two major criteria or one major and two minor. For WS type II, two major criteria are necessary and dystopia canthorum is excluded. In WS type III, also called Klein-Waardenburg, diagnosis is established based on the same criteria as WS I plus musculoskeletal findings. The diagnosis for WS type IV, also known as Shah-Waardenburg, is based on the same criteria as type I plus Hirschsprung disease.[2–5,7]

Family members of the patient can present with features of the syndrome and their examination can prove useful in cases with few clinical findings, especially in very young children and where the diagnosis is difficult to establish. Also, gene testing can prove useful for diagnosis of such cases.

Treatment

No specific treatment is available.

As with many other conditions, a rapid diagnosis is very important in the prognosis of the patient, especially in cases of life-threatening bowel involvement or in those with sensorineural deafness.

REFERENCES

1. Waardenburg PJ. A new syndrome combining developmental anomalies of the eyelids, eyebrows and noseroot with pigmentary anomalies of the iris and head hair and with congenital deafness; Dystopia canthi medialis et punctorum lacrimalium lateroversa, hyperplasia supercilii medialis et radicis nasi, heterochromia iridum totaliis sive partialis, albinismus circumscriptus (leucismus, polioss) et surditas congenita (surdimutitas). *Am J Hum Genet.* September 1951;3(3):195.

2. Zaman A, Capper R, Baddoo W. Waardenburg syndrome: More common than you think! *Clin Otolaryngol.* February 2015;40(1):44–48.

3. Farrer LA, Grundfast KM, Amos J, Arnos KS, Asher JH, Beighton P, Diehl SR, Fex J, Foy C, Friedman TB, Greenberg J. Waardenberg syndrome (WS) type I is caused by defects at multiple loci, one of which is near ALPP on chromosome 2: First report of the WS consortium. *Am J Hum Genet.* May 1992;50(5):902.

4. Tamayo ML, Gelvez N, Rodriguez M, Florez S, Varon C, Medina D, Bernal JE. Screening program for Waardenburg syndrome in Colombia: Clinical definition and phenotypic variability. *Am J Med Genet A.* April 15, 2008;146(8):1026–1031.

5. Milunsky, JM. Waardenburg syndrome type I. InGeneReviews® [Internet] 2017 May 4. University of Washington, Seattle. Available from: https://www.ncbi.nlm.nih.gov/books/NBK1531/, accessed on December 2018.

6. Hageman MJ, Delleman JW. Heterogeneity in Waardenburg syndrome. *Am J Hum Genet.* September 1977;29(5):468.

7. Read AP, Newton VE. Waardenburg syndrome. *J Med Genet.* August 1, 1997;34(8):656–665.

8. U.S. National Library of Medicine, National Institutes of Health. Genetics Home Reference: Your guide to understanding genetic conditions. Available from: https://ghr.nlm.nih.gov/condition/waardenburg-syndrome, accessed on December 2018.

9. Bronner ME, LeDouarin NM. Development and evolution of the neural crest: An overview. *Dev Biol.* June 1, 2012;366(1):2–9.

10. Pingault V, Ente D, Dastot-Le Moal F, Goossens M, Marlin S, Bondurand N. Review and update of mutations causing Waardenburg syndrome. *Hum Mutat.* April 2010;31(4):391–406.

11. Pilon N. Pigmentation-based insertional mutagenesis is a simple and potent screening approach for identifying neurocristopathy-associated genes in mice. *Rare Dis.* January 1, 2016;4(1):4483–4496.

12. Takeda K, Takahashi NH, Shibahara S. Neuroendocrine functions of melanocytes: Beyond the skin-deep melanin maker. *Tohoku J Exp Med.* 2007;211(3):201–221.

Table 16.3 Diagnostic criteria of WS

Major criteria	Minor criteria
Congenital sensorineural hearing loss	Congenital leukoderma
White forelock, hair hypopigmentation	Synophrys and/or medial eyebrow flare
Abnormal pigmentation of the iris: • Complete heterochromia iridum • Partial/segmental heterochromia • Hypoplastic or brilliant blue irides	Broad/high nasal root, low-hanging columella
Dystopia canthorum, W index > 1.95[a]	Underdeveloped alae nasi
First-degree relatives with specific clinical findings	Premature gray hair

Sources: Zaman A et al. *Clin Otolaryngol.* February 2015;40(1):44–48; Farrer LA et al. *Am J Hum Genet.* May 1992;50(5):902; Tamayo ML et al. *Am J Med Genet A.* April 15, 2008;146(8):1026–1031; Milunsky JM. Waardenburg syndrome type I. InGeneReviews® [Internet] 2017 May 4. University of Washington, Seattle. Available from: https://www.ncbi.nlm.nih.gov/books/NBK1531/, accessed on December 2018; Read AP, Newton VE. *J Med Genet.* August 1, 1997;34(8):656–665.

[a] The W index is calculated using the inner canthal distance (a), interpupillary distance (b), outer canthal distance (c) and the following formula:

$W index = X + Y + a/b$, where
$X = (2a-(0.2119c + 3.909))/c$
$Y = (2a-(0.2479b + 3.909))/b$

13. Bondurand N, Pingault V, Goerich DE, Lemort N, Sock E, Caignec CL, Wegner M, Goossens M. Interaction among SOX10, PAX3 and MITF, three genes altered in Waardenburg syndrome. *Hum Mol Genet.* August 12, 2000;9(13):1907–1917.

14. Wang Q, Fang WH, Krupinski J, Kumar S, Slevin M, Kumar P. PAX genes in embryogenesis and oncogenesis. *J Cell Mol Med.* December 1, 2008;12(6a):2281–2294.

15. Shibahara S, Takeda K, Yasumoto KI, Udono T, Watanabe KI, Saito H, Takahashi K. Microphthalmia-associated transcription factor (MITF): multiplicity in structure, function, and regulation. In *Journal of Investigative Dermatology Symposium Proceedings* November 1, 2001 (Vol. 6, No. 1, pp. 99–104). Elsevier.

16. Sánchez-Martín M, Rodríguez-García A, Pérez-Losada J, Sagrera A, Read AP, Sánchez-García I. SLUG (SNAI2) deletions in patients with Waardenburg disease. *Hum Mol Genet.* December 1, 2002;11(25): 3231–3236.

17. Ito Y, Inoue N, Inoue YU, Nakamura S, Matsuda Y, Inagaki M, Ohkubo T, Asami J, Terakawa YW, Kohsaka S, Goto YI. Additive dominant effect of a SOX10 mutation underlies a complex phenotype of PCWH. *Neurobiol Dis.* August 1, 2015;80:1–4.

18. Pla P, Larue L. Involvement of endothelin receptors in normal and pathological development of neural crest cells. *Int J Dev Biol.* June 1, 2003;47(5):315–325.

19. Doubaj Y, Pingault V, Elalaoui SC, Ratbi I, Azouz M, Zerhouni H, Ettayebi F, Sefiani A. A novel mutation in the endothelin B receptor gene in a Moroccan family with Shah-Waardenburg syndrome. *Mol Syndromol.* 2015;6(1):44–49.

20. Charrier B, Pilon N. Toward a better understanding of enteric gliogenesis. *Neurogenesis.* January 1, 2017;4(1):1283–1293.

21. Bergeron KF, Nguyen CM, Cardinal T, Charrier B, Silversides DW, Pilon N. Upregulation of the Nr2f1-A830082K12Rik gene pair in murine neural crest cells results in a complex phenotype reminiscent of Waardenburg syndrome type 4. *Dis Model Mech.* 2016 Nov 1;9(11):1283–93.

22. Issa S, Bondurand N, Faubert E et al. EDNRB mutations cause Waardenburg syndrome type II in the heterozygous state. *Hum Mutat.* 2017, 38(5):581–593.

23. Huggins RH, Janusz CA, Schwartz RA. Vitiligo: A sign of systemic disease. *Indian J Dermatol Venereol Leprol.* January 1, 2006;72(1):68.

24. Que SK, Weston G, Suchecki J, Ricketts J. Pigmentary disorders of the eyes and skin. *Clin Dermatol.* March 1, 2015;33(2):147–158.

25. Watanabe S, Matsudera S, Yamaguchi T, Tani Y, Ogino K, Nakajima M, Yamaguchi S, Sasaki K, Suzumura H, Tsuchioka T. Waardenburg syndrome with isolated deficiency of myenteric ganglion cells at the sigmoid colon and rectum. *Pediatr Rep.* May 24, 2018;10(2).

26. Seiberg M. Age-induced hair greying—The multiple effects of oxidative stress. *Int J Cosmetic Sci.* December 2013;35(6):532–538.

27. Karaman A, Aliagaoglu C. Waardenburg syndrome type 1. *Dermatol Online J.* January 1, 2003;12(3).

28. Pardono E, van Bever Y, van den Ende J, Havrenne PC, Iughetti P, Maestrelli SR, Costa FO, Richieri-Costa A, Frota-Pessoa O, Otto PA. Waardenburg syndrome: Clinical differentiation between types I and II. *Am J Med Genet A.* March 15, 2003;117(3):223–235.

29. Kumar P. Synophrys: Epidemiological study. *Int J Trichology.* July 2017;9(3):105.

Alezzandrini syndrome, Margolis syndrome, Cross syndrome, and other rare genetic disorders

17

ATHANASIOS I. PAVLIDIS and ANDREAS D. KATSAMBAS

CONTENTS

Introduction	113	Differential diagnosis	115
Epidemiology	113	Treatment	115
Pathophysiology	113	References	115
Clinical presentation	114		

INTRODUCTION

Alezzandrini syndrome is a condition of unknown etiology first described by Alezzandrini and Casala in 1959.[1] This syndrome is a rare group of ipsilateral pigmentary changes characterized by poliosis, facial vitiligo, unilateral degenerative retinitis, an atrophic iris, reduced visual acuity, and occasionally deafness.[2]

Ziprkowski-Margolis syndrome is a condition also known as X-linked albinism-deafness syndrome characterized by congenital neural deafness and a severe or extreme piebald-like phenotype with extensive areas of hypopigmentation. This syndrome was first identified by both Ziprkowski and Margolis in 1962, in an Israeli Jewish family of Sephardic origin.[3,4]

Cross syndrome was first identified by Cross et al. in 1967. This syndrome is characterized by hypopigmentation involving skin and hair, intellectual disability, microcephaly, and neurologic and ocular disorders.[5]

Hermansky-Pudlak syndrome (HPS) was first described by Hermansky and Pudlak in 1959 in two unrelated patients.[6] This syndrome is a rare autosomal recessive genetic disorder characterized by oculocutaneous albinism and prolonged bleeding diathesis due to platelet dysfunction. In some individuals, it is related to pulmonary fibrosis, granulomatous colitis, or immunodeficiency.[7,8]

Vici syndrome, first described by Dionisi-Vici and colleagues in 1988,[9] is a severe congenital multisystem disorder characterized by callosal agenesis, cataracts, oculocutaneous hypopigmentation, cardiomyopathy, and a combined immunodeficiency.[10]

Chediak-Higashi syndrome is a rare autosomal recessive disorder characterized by variable degrees of oculocutaneous albinism, recurrent infections, a tendency for mild bleeding, progressive neurologic deterioration, and hemophagocytic lymphohistiocytosis (HLH).[11]

Griscelli syndrome (GS) is a rare autosomal recessive disorder with characteristic pigmentary dilution of the skin and hair. GS was first described by Griscelli and Siccardi in 1978.[12]

EPIDEMIOLOGY

Alezzandrini syndrome is a rare disorder with an unknown prevalence instead of mortality rate. Most patients initially present when they are 12–30 years, and it is not limited to a certain race. Only a few clinical cases in world literature have been described.[13]

The incidence of Ziprkowski-Margolis syndrome is unknown. Few cases are published to date.

The prevalence of Cross syndrome in consanguineous families is in favor of an autosomal recessive inheritance, and it has been suggested that it maps to chromosome 3q27.1q29.[14]

Hermansky-Pudlak syndrome is a rare form of albinism. The prevalence of HPS worldwide is 1 in 500,000–1,000,000 individuals, and it is likely to occur in all ethnic groups, as sporadic cases have been reported in several ethnicities, including Japanese, Finnish, Mexican, and Sri Lankan.[15]

The incidence of Vici syndrome is unknown, and it is likely to be rare but probably underdiagnosed. Since the original description, an increasing number of patients have been reported, with around 50 genetically confirmed cases published to date.[16]

The first case of Chediak-Higashi syndrome was reported in 1943. For the past 20 years, less than 500 cases have been reported worldwide. In China, no more than 50 cases have been reported over the past decades.[11]

The incidence of Griscelli syndrome is unknown. GS usually manifests in persons aged 4 months to 4 years, though the youngest reported is 1 month with no sex predilection.[17]

PATHOPHYSIOLOGY

Alezzandrini syndrome has an unknown etiology. Many theories have been proposed regarding viral or autoimmune processes. As known, melanocytes that originate in the neural crest migrate to the skin, leptomeninges, retinas, uvea, cochleae, and vestibular labyrinths. Any disorder that destroys the melanocytes in the skin also affects other organs and systems such as the eye, ear, and central nervous system.[13]

Margolis syndrome or X-linked albinism-deafness syndrome (ADFN) probably affects the migration of neural crest–derived precursors of melanocytes. A locus at Xq26.3-q27.I has been suggested. The perceptive deafness could be explained by the failure of the nerve cells to migrate from the neural crest to the cochlea.[18]

Cross syndrome, also known as oculocerebral hypopigmentation syndrome (OCHS), is assumed to be autosomal recessive, with its genetic cause still unknown. OCHS maps to chromosome 3q27.1q29.[14]

Hermansky-Pudlak disorder is classified into different subtypes (HPS1–HPS10) based on genetic mutations in different genes. The primary defect in HPS is disruption in the biogenesis of lysosomes and lysosome-related organelles (LROs). LROs include melanosomes, PDG, lamellar bodies of type II pneumocytes, and granule proteins of cytotoxic and suppressor T cells and NK cells. Identification of biallelic pathogenic variants in AP3B1, AP3D1, BLOC1S3, BLOC1S6, DTNBP1, HPS1, HPS3, HPS4, HPS5, or HPS6 confirms the diagnosis using molecular genetic testing if clinical features are inconclusive.[19]

Vici syndrome pathogenesis is caused due to recessive mutations in the ectopic P granules protein 5 (EPG5) gene on chromosome 18q12.3 organized in 44 exons and encoding EPG5. EPG5 is a protein of 2579 amino acids, originally known as KIAA1632, initially identified among a group of genes found to be mutated in breast cancer tissue before its implication in Vici syndrome in 2013. To date, around 40 EPG5 mutations have been identified in families with Vici syndrome, distributed throughout the entire EPG5 coding sequence without clear genotype-phenotype correlations.[20]

In Chediak-Higashi syndrome (CHS), the genetic defect was identified in 1996 and was mapped to human chromosome 1q42–44.[21] The CHS gene was originally called LYST, which contains 53 exons with an open reading frame of 11,406 bp, and encodes for a 3801–amino acid protein, CHS1. Although the exact function of CHS1 remains unknown, it has been thought to play a role in regulating lysosome-related organelle size, fission, and secretion.[22]

In Griscelli syndrome, the three different subtypes are caused by mutations in the Myosin Va (MyoVa) (GS1, Elejalde), small GTPase protein RAB27A (GS2), or melanophil MLPH (GS3) genes, respectively. The protein complex formed by these is essential for the capture and movement of melanosomes in the actin-rich cell periphery of melanocytes.[23]

CLINICAL PRESENTATION

Alezzandrini syndrome is characterized by unilateral tapetoretinal (retinal pigment epithelia) degeneration,

unilateral appearance of facial vitiligo, poliosis, and hearing abnormalities.[13]

In Ziprkowski-Margolis syndrome, males in the same Jewish family showed congenital subtotal nerve deafness and piebaldness. Their skin was characterized by alternating achromatic and hyperpigmented patches, with sharply delineated areas ("leopard skin"), and their hair was white.[18]

The clinical features of patients with Cross syndrome could include skin hypopigmentation silver-gray/white hair, ocular anomalies, microcephaly, hypotonia, ataxia, spasticity, developmental delay/intellectual disability, brain malformation, growth retardation, recurrent urinary tract infections/malformations, heart malformations, vertebral anomalies, osteoporosis, and acetabular hypoplasia.[5,24,25]

Hermansky-Pudlak syndrome (HPS) is characterized by oculocutaneous albinism including reduced iris and retinal pigment, foveal hypoplasia with significant reduction in visual acuity, nystagmus, and a bleeding diathesis that can result in variable bruising; epistaxis; gingival bleeding; postpartum hemorrhage; colonic bleeding; and prolonged bleeding with menses or after tooth extraction, circumcision, and other surgeries. Hair color in HPS ranges from white to brown; skin color ranges from white to olive and is usually a shade lighter than that of other family members. Type 1 HPS is the most common and most severe variant and leads to high-risk cases of pulmonary fibrosis, more common among female patients, a restrictive lung disease due to accumulation of ceroid-lipofuscin in the pulmonary alveolar macrophages and presented by dispnea. Granulomatous colitis is severe in about 15% of affected individuals.[7,26]

Vici syndrome is one of the most extensive inherited human multisystem disorders reported to date, presenting invariably in the first months of life. The five principal diagnostic findings include callosal agenesis, cataracts, cardiomyopathy, hypopigmentation, and combined immunodeficiency; additionally, any organ system can be involved.[23] Profound developmental delay, acquired microcephaly, and marked failure to thrive have recently emerged and are, although nonspecific, as consistently associated as the five main diagnostic features and highly supportive of the diagnosis.[20]

Chediak-Higashi syndrome is classified into three phenotypes. Based on clinical symptoms are childhood, adolescent, and adult forms, with 80%–85% being the childhood form.[27] It is characterized by frequent severe infections and massive hemophagocytic lymphohistiocytosis due to inappropriate cytotoxic activity, which leads to the impaired downregulation of immune responses and sustained activation and proliferation of cytotoxic T lymphocytes and NK cells. HLH often occurs following initial exposure to EBV and has a high mortality rate.[28]

Griscelli syndrome includes three types (GS1, GS2, and GS3). GS1 has characteristic albinism with central nervous system dysfunction without immunological involvement. GS2, the most common, is associated with albinism and a severe immunological impairment and commonly develops hemophagocytic lymphohistiocytosis and recurrent infections. In GS3, patients are associated with partial albinism only.[29,30]

DIFFERENTIAL DIAGNOSIS

The relationship between Alezzandrini syndrome and other syndromes involving vitiligo and eye pathology is uncertain. A close differential is Vogt-Koyanagi-Harada syndrome, characterized by bilateral decoloration of the skin, eyebrows, eyelashes, alopecia, chronic uveitis, and meningoencephalitis.

In Margolis syndrome, similar conditions not associated with deafness should lead to consideration of Chediak-Higashi syndrome.

Hermansky-Pudlak syndrome should be included in the differential diagnosis of patients with inflammatory bowel disease and interstitial lung disease, particularly in the presence of bleeding diathesis and albinism like oculocutaneous albinism (OCA), X-linked ocular albinism (XLOA), Chediak-Higashi syndrome, and Griscelli syndrome.

The differential diagnosis of Vici syndrome includes a number of syndromes with overlapping clinical features, neurological and metabolic disorders with similar CNS abnormalities, and primary neuromuscular disorders with a similar muscle biopsy appearance, like Marinesco-Sjögren syndrome (MSS), congenital cataracts, facial dysmorphism and neuropathy syndrome, Chediak-Higashi syndrome, Hermanksy-Pudlak syndrome type 2, Griscelli syndrome, Elejalde syndrome, Cohen syndrome, and Danon disease.

Chediak-Higashi syndrome must be distinguished from the other two autosomal recessive transmission syndromes, Griscelli syndrome and Elejalde syndrome, both characterized by skin hypopigmentation, silvery-gray hair, central nervous system dysfunction in infancy and childhood, and very large and unevenly distributed granules of melanin in the hair shaft and skin.

In Griscelli syndrome, the absence of giant granules in the nucleated cells makes it possible to differentiate from Chediak-Higashi syndrome.

TREATMENT

For all syndromes and genetic disorders, patients with vitiligo should use a sunscreen to prevent sunburn and subsequent skin cancer. Topical steroids and tacrolimus may be tried on localized areas of vitiligo.[31]

In cases with widespread depigmentation, treatment with psoralen plus ultraviolet A (PUVA) can be provided but with great caution in patients with anterior uveitis because PUVA therapy might aggravate the ocular inflammatory disorder.[32]

For many genetic disorders like Vici syndrome there is currently no cure. Management is essentially supportive, aimed at alleviating the effects of extensive multisystem involvement.[16]

The main treatment for CHS focuses on three fields: supportive management of disease-derived complications, treatment of the accelerated phase or HLH, and hematopoietic stem cell transplantation (HSCT), which has been recognized as the most effective treatment for hematologic and immune defects caused by CHS. The only treatment is allogenic HSCT, but the prognosis is poor.[28]

REFERENCES

1. Casala AM, Alezzandrini AA. Vitiligo, poliosis unilateral con retinitis pigmentaria y hypoacusia. *Arch Argent Dermatol.* 1959;9:449.
2. Alezzandrini AA. Unilateral manifestations of tapeto-retinal degeneration, vitiligo, poliosis, grey hair and hypoacousia. *Ophthalmologica.* 1964;147:409–419.
3. Ziprkowski L, Krakowski A, Adam A et al. Partial albinism and deaf-mutism due to a recessive sex-linked gene. *Arch Derm.* October 1962;86:530–539.
4. Margolis E. A new hereditary syndrome: Sex-linked deaf-mutism associated with total albinism. *Acta Genet.* 1962;12:12–19.
5. Cross HE, McKusick VA, Breen W. A new oculocerebral syndrome with hypopigmentation. *J Pediatr.* March 1967;70:398–406.
6. Hermansky F, Pudlak P. Albinism associated with hemorrhagic diathesis and unusual pigmented reticular cells in the bone marrow: Report of two cases with histochemical studies. *Blood.* February 1959;14:162–169.
7. Pierson DM, Ionescu D, Qing G et al. Pulmonary fibrosis in Hermansky-Pudlak syndrome. A case report and review. *Respir Int Rev Thorac Dis.* 2006;73:382–395.
8. Christensen S, Wagner L, Colema MM. et al. The lived experience of having a rare medical disorder: Hermansky-Pudlak syndrome. *Chronic Illn.* March 2017;13(1):62–72.
9. Vici CD, Sabetta G, Gambarara M et al. Agenesis of the corpus callosum, combined immunodeficiency, bilateral cataract, and hypopigmentation in two brothers. *Am J Med Genet.* January 1988;29(1):1–8.
10. Cullup T, Kho AL, Dionisi-Vici C et al. Recessive mutations in EPG5 cause Vici syndrome, a multisystem disorder with defective autophagy. *Nat Genet.* January 2013;45(1):83–87.
11. Kaplan J, De Domenico I, Ward DM. Chediak-Higashi syndrome. *Curr Opin Hematol.* January 2008;15(1):22–29.
12. Griscelli C, Durandy A, Guy-Grand D et al. A syndrome associating partial albinism and immunodeficiency. *Am J Med.* October 1978;65:691–702.
13. Andrade A, Pithon M. Alezzandrini syndrome: Report of a sixth clinical case. *Dermatology.* February 2011;222(1):8–9.
14. Chabchoub E, Cogulu O, Durmaz B et al. Oculocerebral hypopigmentation syndrome maps to chromosome 3q27.1q29. *Dermatology.* 2011;223(4):306–310.

15. Asztalos ML, Schafemak KT, Gray J et al. Hermansky-Pudlak syndrome: Report of two patients with updated genetic classification and management recommendations. *Pedriatr Dermatol.* November 2017;34(6):638–646.

16. Byrne S, Dionisi-Vici C, Smith L et al. Vici syndrome: A review. *Orphanet J Rare Dis.* February 29, 2016;11:21.

17. Kumar M, Sackey K, Schmalstieg F et al. Griscelli syndrome: Rare neonatal syndrome of recurrent hemophagocytosis. *J Pediatr Hematol Oncol.* October 2001;23(7):464–468.

18. Shiloh Y, Litvak G, Ziv Y et al. Genetic mapping of X-linked albinism-deafness syndrome (ADFN) to Xq26.3-q27.I. *Am J Hum Genet.* July 2006;47(1):20–27.

19. Gahl WA, Brantly M, Kaiser-Kupfer MI et al. Genetic defects and clinical characteristics of patients with a form of oculocutaneous albinism (Hermansky-Pudlak syndrome). *N Engl J Med.* April 30, 1998;338(18):1258–1264.

20. Byrne S, Jansen L, U-King Im JM et al. EPG-related Vici syndrome: A paradigm of neurodevelopmental disorders with defective autophagy. *Brain.* March 2016;139(Pt 3):765–781.

21. Barrat FJ, Auloge L, Pastural E et al. Genetic and physical mapping of the Chediak-Higashi syndrome on chromosome 1q42-43. *Am J Hum Genet.* 1996 Spt;59(3):625–632.

22. Durchfort N, Verhoef S, Vaughn MB et al. The enlarged lysosomes in beige J cells result from decreased lysosome fission and not increased lysosome fusion. *Traffic.* January 2012;13(1):108–119.

23. Menasche G, Ho Chen, Sanal O et al. Griscelli syndrome restricted to hypopigmentation results from a melanophilin defect (GS3) or a MYO5A F exon deletion (GS1). *J Clin Invest.* August 2003;112(3):450–456.

24. Pollazzon M, Grosso S, Papa FT et al. A 9.3 Mb microdeletion of 3q27.3q29 associated with psychomotor and growth delay, tricuspid valve dysplasia and bifid thumb. *Eur J Med Genet.* March 2009–June;52(2–3):131–133.

25. De Jong G, Fryns JP. Oculocerebral syndrome with hypopigmentation (Cross syndrome): The mixed pattern of hair pigmentation as an important diagnostic sign. *Genet Couns.* 1991;2(3):151–155.

26. Garay SM, Gardella JE, Fazzini EP et al. Hermansky-Pudlak syndrome. Pulmonary manifestations of a ceroid storage disorder. *Am J Med.* May 1979;66(5):737–747.

27. Karim MA, Suzuki K, Fukai K et al. Apparent genotype-phenotype correlation in childhood, adolescent, and adult Chediak-Higashi syndrome. *Am J Med Genet.* February 2002;108(1):16–22.

28. Mehta RS, Smith RE. Hemophagocytic lymphohistiocytosis (HLH): A review of literature. *Med Oncol.* December 2013;30(4):740.

29. Minocha P, Choudhary R, Agrawal A et al. Griscelli syndrome subtype 2 with hemophagocytic lympho-histiocytosis: A case report and review of literature. *Intractable Rare Dis Res.* February 2017;6(1):76–79.

30. Dotta L, Parolini S, Prandini A et al. Clinical, laboratory and molecular signs of immunodeficiency in patients with partial oculo-cutaneous albinism. *Orphanet J Rare Dis.* October 2013; 17;8:168.

31. Huggins RH, Janusz CA, Schwartz RA. Vitiligo: A sign of systemic disease. *Indian J Dermatol Venereol Leprol.* January 2006–February;72(1):68–71.

32. Bhatnagar A, Kanwar AJ, Parsad D et al. Comparison of systemic PUVA and NB-UVB in the treatment of vitiligo: An open prospective study. *J Eur Acad Dermatol Venereol.* May 2007;21(5):638–642.

Mosaic hypopigmentation

18

IRENE LATOUR-ÁLVAREZ and ANTONIO TORRELO

CONTENTS

Definition and mechanisms of mosaicism	117	Diagnosis	124
Classic patterns of cutaneous mosaicism	118	Follow-up and treatment	124
Clinical manifestations of mosaic hypopigmentation diseases	118	References	124

DEFINITION AND MECHANISMS OF MOSAICISM

A "mosaic" is an organism composed of two or more cell lines that are genetically different, derived from a genetically homogenous zygote.[1,2] Some mosaic skin disorders exclusively occur sporadically because the underlying mutation, when present in the fertilized egg, is incompatible with life, and then the mutation can only survive in the form of mosaicism (e.g., McCune-Albright syndrome[3] and CLOVES syndrome[4]) in close vicinity to the population of normal cells. The hypothesis of lethal genes surviving by mosaicism has been proved on molecular grounds in several diseases.[1,5] The distinction between mosaicism of lethal (e.g., Proteus syndrome[6]) from nonlethal postzygotic mutations (e.g., neurofibromatosis type 1,[7] tuberous sclerosis[8]) is important because the clinical expression of the mosaic state can be modified. Other factors, such as the timing of mutation during embryo development and the cells affected by the mutation, are also key factors in determining the depth of mosaicism and its clinical expression.

Mosaicism can affect autosomes and X chromosomes and can be classified into two major categories,[1] genomic and epigenetic mosaicism:

1. *Genetic mosaicism (genomic)*: This type of mosaicism is related to changes in the DNA sequence due to mutations (somatic mutation) or chromosomal alterations (half-chromatid mutation, chromosomal nondisjunction, or chimerism). In these postzygotic mutations (somatic mosaicism), the mutation occurs *de novo* during embryonic development. Some authors claim that the term *somatic* is not totally correct. In fact, these mosaic manifestations carry an implicit risk of transmission to the next generation because of simultaneous mosaic involvement of the gonads (gonadal mosaicism).[5,9] Therefore, the term *postzygotic mutation* is preferable.

   Two mechanisms exist for the segmental expression of nonlethal, autosomal traits[10] (Figure 18.1):
   - In type 1 mosaicism, a postzygotic mutation occurs in a normal embryo (wild type); therefore, the cutaneous changes are seen only in a localized segment, corresponding to cells carrying the mutation (only in this segment, the individual is heterozygous,

phenotypically abnormal). Nonlethal dominant mutations appear under this form of mosaicism (e.g., segmental neurofibromatosis or segmental tuberous sclerosis).[1] Recessive mutations may also rarely mimic type 1 mosaicism, in case the embryo is heterozygous for the recessive mutation and a second mutation during embryo development will show a segmental manifestation of the disease.
   - In type 2 mosaicism, an individual heterozygous for a dominant disease (and hence manifesting a dominant disease), may exhibit a more intense expression of the disease in one segment because of an early event of loss of heterozygosity in the affected gene. The individual will show homozygosity in this segment, whereas they will remain heterozygous in the germline.[11] There are several mechanisms of loss of heterozygosity, including second hit mutations, gene conversion, mitotic nondisjunction, mitotic recombination, and point mutation deletion.[12]

2. *Epigenetic or functional mosaicism*: This is due to changes in gene expression (gene activation or silencing).
   - *Lyonization*: In women, functional mosaicism occurs due to random X chromosome inactivation; this mechanism may produce cutaneous manifestations of diseases whose responsible genes are located in the X chromosome. In X-linked recessive diseases, inactivation of the normal allele will produce a linear skin disease in females that is often compatible with life, whereas the areas of the skin where the mutated X chromosome is inactivated will remain normal. In some cases, carrier females may appear completely normal or have minimal manifestations of the disease (e.g., in hypohidrotic ectodermal dysplasia). Furthermore, some genes in the X chromosome skip inactivation and in this case, carrier females will not show any manifestations (e.g., X-linked ichthyosis). However, if the mutation is transmitted to a male embryo, he will suffer a nonsegmental disease affecting the germline.

     In X-linked dominant conditions, most males with only one X chromosome die before birth (e.g.,

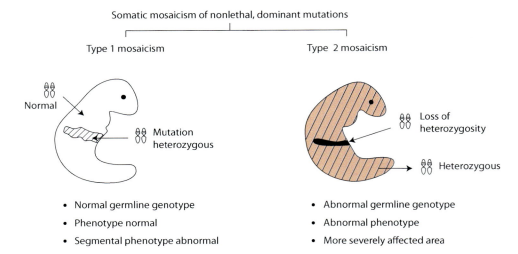

Figure 18.1 Mechanisms for the segmental expression of nonlethal, autosomal disorders.

incontinentia pigmenti) and females will show a segmental skin disease on the areas where the wild-type allele was inactivated. Males can survive in the form of mosaics as a result of extra X chromosome donation (XXY karyotype—Klinefelter syndrome) or due to mosaic postzygotic mutation in the X chromosome or hypomorphic or half-chromatid mutations.[2,12]

- *Epigenetic modification*: This is due to a switch in gene expression, including cytosine methylation and histone modification.[13] This mechanism has, so far, not been demonstrated in humans.

CLASSIC PATTERNS OF CUTANEOUS MOSAICISM

In 1901, Alfred Blaschko described segmental cutaneous lesions following linear patterns as S-figures on the anterior and lateral trunk, linear streaks on extremities, and a V-shape on the central back.[14] These lines are called Blaschko lines after him. Happle, in 2001, described these lines on the cephalic and cervical regions[15] (Figure 18.2).

Mosaic skin lesions can be clinically recognized because they follow fixed patterns described by Happle.[16] These are as follows (Figure 18.3):

- *Type 1*: Blaschko lines. This is the most common type that mirrors the embryonic development of many of the components of the epidermis. Two types of Blaschko lines are recognized:
  - *Type 1a*: Narrow Blaschko lines. Some pigmentary disorders and incontinentia pigmenti are examples of this type.
  - *Type 1b*: Broad Blaschko lines. These frequently appear in segmental pigmentation disorder and in McCune-Albright syndrome.
- *Type 2*: Blocks, flags, segments, or "checkerboard patterns." Alternate areas of skin changes with midline demarcation appear. Examples of this are Becker's nevus or capillary malformations, among many others. This pattern often represents the expansion pattern of mesodermal components of the skin, but, not rarely, pigmentary mosaicism follows this pattern.
- *Type 3*: Phylloid pattern. Streaks and round or oval asymmetric lesions mimicking leaves appear. This pattern is exclusive to hyper- or hypopigmentation disorders, and some cases of phylloid hypopigmentation are due to mosaicism of trisomy 13.
- *Type 4*: Garment-like patterns, with large patches without midline separation. This is typically a migrational patterning that is mostly restricted to melanocytic nevi.
- *Type 5*: Lateralization affecting only one side of the body, with midline demarcation. This pattern is typical, but not restricted to, X-linked mutations.

CLINICAL MANIFESTATIONS OF MOSAIC HYPOPIGMENTATION DISEASES

There are several conditions that can produce a mosaic hypopigmentation. In this chapter, we summarize briefly the most prevalent and important cutaneous manifestations due to a mosaic that can manifest as a hypopigmentation (Table 18.1).

a. *Hypomelanosis following the lines of Blaschko*
   This is the most frequent presentation of hypopigmented mosaicism in children. Various terms have been used to describe this type of dyspigmentation, including hypomelanosis of Ito,[17] nevus achromicus (Figure 18.4), nevus depigmentosus,[18] and blaschkoid dyspigmentation; however, the term linear hypomelanosis is preferred here. Small round or oval patches of hypopigmentation (also called achromic nevus or nevus depigmentosus) most likely represent late-stage mosaicism.

   Linear hypomelanosis is a congenital nonprogressive disorder characterized by hypopigmented skin lesions following Blaschko

Clinical manifestations of mosaic hypopigmentation diseases 119

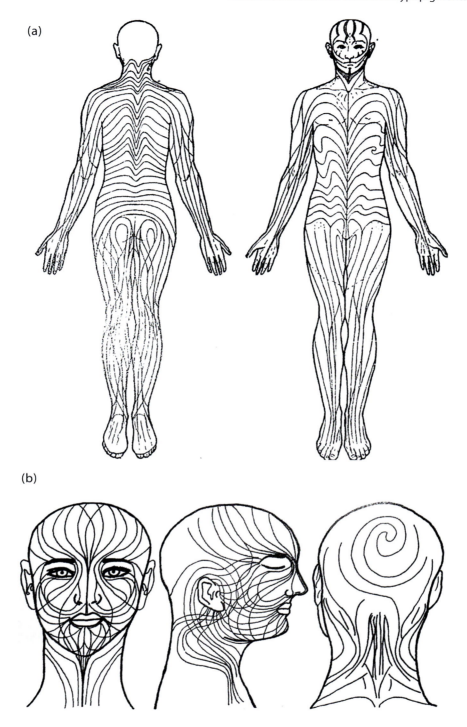

Figure 18.2 Blaschko lines on (a) the body and (b) the head and neck. (From Blaschko A. *Die Nervenverteilung in der Haut in ihre Beziehung zu den Erkrankungen der Haut*. Vienna, Austria, and Leipzig, Germany: Wilhelm Braunmuller; 1901. Happle R. Mosaicism in human skin. *Understanding Nevi, Nevoid Skin Disorders, and Cutaneous Neoplasia*. Springer; 2014. With permission. Happle R, Assim A. *J Am Acad Dermatol*. 2001;44:6125. With permission.)

lines, without a preceding inflammatory phase (Figure 18.5). The hypopigmentation may be evident at the time of birth and remain stable throughout life. However, if the skin is very light, it can be noted later during infancy when the child is exposed to sun.[1,19,20] Lesions appear off-white under Wood lamp rather than the chalk-white color typical of vitiligo. Histopathology studies revealed melanin was decreased in epidermal layers of the hypopigmented lesion compared with perilesional normal skin; however, the number of melanocytes varied depending on the reports (normal or decreased).[19,21]

120 Mosaic hypopigmentation

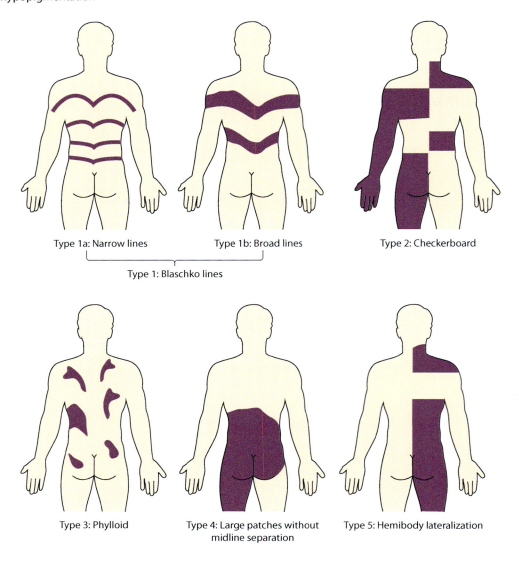

Figure 18.3 Patterns of mosaicism.

This disorder is sometimes associated with extracutaneous defects, including variable neurologic and eye findings.[22] Nevertheless, most patients attended in dermatology consultations showed no association with systemic disease or neurological abnormalities; thus, children with linear hypomelanosis are unlikely to develop serious extracutaneous involvement, especially when lesions are limited to one single segment. Children with linear hypomelanosis who are developing normally and appear normal by the age of 3 usually will not show any related neurologic manifestation of disease.[20] Karyotyping from peripheral blood lymphocytes and skin fibroblasts may detect abnormalities in patients with and without extracutaneous manifestations. The chromosomes involved in the investigated cases of pigmentary mosaicism were 2, 3, 4, 5, 7, 9, 10, 12–16, 18, 20–22, and the sex chromosomes.[23] Mosaic mutations of mTOR have been reported in children with diffuse megalencephaly and hypopigmentary linear mosaicism in skin.[24]

b. *Segmental hypomelanosis arranged in a checkerboard pattern*
   This entity, sometimes named "flag-like hypomelanosis," consists of a unilateral patch of variable shape, with serrated borders, arranged in a checkerboard pattern (Figure 18.6). Leucotrichia may be present when the hypopigmentation appears in rich region of terminal hair, in contrast to linear hypomelanosis. Molecular findings are so far not available.[25]

c. *Epidermal nevus*
   The term *epidermal nevus* includes a heterogeneous group of mosaic lesions and can result as a mutation in many genes including KRT1, KRT10, NRAS, HRAS, BRAF, and FGFR2, among others.[26,27] Clinically, most patients with epidermal nevus will show a linear arrangement of brown, velvety papules. One or multiple lines of Blaschko may be involved. Rarely,

Table 18.1 Comparison of the principal diseases of mosaic hypopigmentation

	Linear hypomelanosis in narrowbands	Segmental hypomelanosis arranged in a checkerboard pattern	Epidermal nevi	Incontinentia pigmenti	Pallister-Killian syndrome	Phylloid hypomelanosis	Conradi-Hünermann-Happle syndrome	Goltz syndrome (focal dermal hypoplasia)
Mutation	Miscellanea Abnormal cytogenetic studies Mutation mTOR	Not available	KRT1, KRT10, NRAS, HRAS, PIK3CA, FGFR2, FGFR3	X-linked dominant disorder, mutation in NEMO gene	Extra isochromosome 12p, limited to fibroblasts	Trisomy or tetrasomy 13 or 13q	Mutation in EBP gene	X-linked dominant disorder, mutation in PORCN gene
Distribution of the hypopigmentation	Blaschko lines	Checkboard pattern	Blaschko lines	Hypopigmented lines	"Atypical" Blaschko lines or any pattern	Phylloid pattern	Blaschko lines	Blaschko lines
Skin surface	Smooth	Smooth	Smooth or warty	Smooth	Smooth	Smooth	Mild scaling Atrophoderma	Smooth Dermal atrophy
Skin features	Nonprogressive, without inflammatory phase	Leucotrichia	Hyper- or hypopigmentation, even pink or yellow	Four consecutive stages of the linear skin lesions: 1) Vesicles 2) Verrucous 3) Hyperpigmented 4) Hypopigmented atrophic lines without eccrine gland and hair follicles	Streaks and spots of hypopigmentation	Asymmetrical round or oval lesions	First weeks of life: linear areas of inflammation and hyperkeratosis Later: atrophy and hypopigmentation, follicular atrophoderma on the scalp, scarring alopecia	Dermal atrophy, fat herniations into the dermis "Raspberry-like" papules in lips and anogenital region
Systemic manifestations	±Neurologic	±Neurologic	±Neurologic	Ectodermal abnormalities (tooth, ocular, and neurologic)	Dysmorphic features, mental retardation	Neurologic defects (absence of the corpus callosum)	Sectorial cataracts, epiphyseal stippling	Eyes, teeth, bones

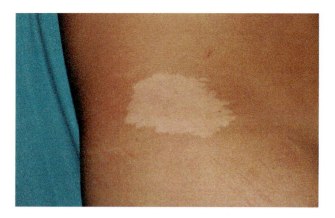

Figure 18.4 Nevus achromicus.

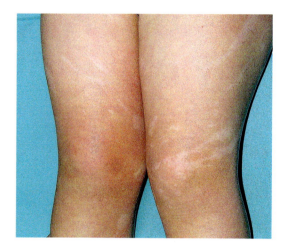

Figure 18.5 Linear hypomelanosis.

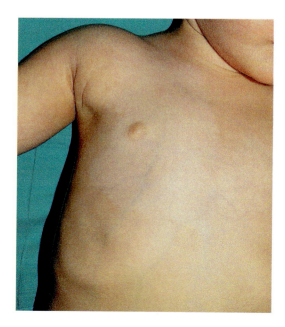

Figure 18.6 Hypomelanosis in a checkerboard pattern.

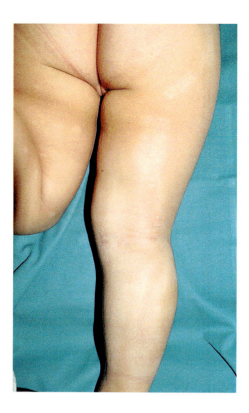

Figure 18.7 Hypopigmented epidermal nevus. Note the hypopigmented lines along the right buttock and velvety papules distributed along the Blaschko lines.

epidermal nevi appear as hypopigmentation along the lines of Blaschko, the so-called hypopigmented epidermal nevus (Figure 18.7). Histopathology will show a moderate degree of acanthosis. Epidermal nevi can appear isolated or associated with extracutaneous, mostly neurologic, abnormalities. Developmental delay, epilepsy, intellectual disability, and focal motor deficits are the principal manifestations observed. When neurological manifestations are present, the epidermal nevus usually affects the scalp or the face; however, it can appear on other skin regions. A careful history should provide information in case of systemic involvement.[28]

d. *Incontinentia pigmenti*

Incontinentia pigmenti (IP) is an X-linked dominant disorder caused by mutations in IKBKG (inhibitor of Kappa light polypeptide gene enhancer in B cells, Kinasa gamma), also known as NEMO (NF-κB essential modulator) located at Xq28. This mutation results in failure to activate NF-κB, which normally protects against TNF-α-induced apoptosis;[29] then, cells with mutations in NEMO are not protected from apoptosis. IP is considered a type of ectodermal dysplasia, with a likelihood of associated tooth, eye, and neurologic involvement.

The Blaschko-linear pattern of the cutaneous manifestations reflects functional mosaicism because of lyonization. IP typically has four consecutive stages: (1) linear erythema and vesicles during the first weeks of life, (2) verrucous linear plaques, (3) hyperpigmented swirls and streaks along lines of Blaschko, and (4) from puberty onward, hypopigmented atrophic lines without eccrine gland and hair follicles[30] (Figures 18.8 and 18.9).

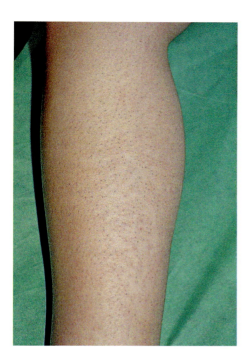

Figure 18.8 Incontinentia pigmenti stage 4. Note hypopigmented atrophic lines without hair follicles.

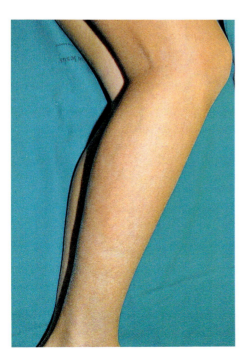

Figure 18.9 Incontinentia pigmenti stage 4. Linear hypopigmented bands.

e. *Pallister-Killian syndrome*
   Pallister-Killian syndrome (PKS) is caused by somatic mosaicism of an extra chromosome, limited to fibroblasts and not present in lymphocytes.[31] PKS is a rare genetic disorder caused by tissue-limited mosaicism tetrasomy of the short arm of chromosome 12, which usually cytogenetically presents as an extra isochromosome 12p.[32]
   The clinical phenotype of PKS includes dysmorphic features (brachycephaly, temporal balding the first years of life, short nose with flat bridge, microstomia, progressive macroglossia, small mandible, and short neck), mental retardation, and other severe systemic manifestations.[32,33] Skin lesions consist of streaks and spots of hypopigmentation along "atypical" Blaschko lines, whereas other lesions do not follow any pattern.[1]

f. *Phylloid hypomelanosis (mosaic trisomy 13)*
   Most cases of phylloid hypomelanosis are caused by mosaic forms of trisomy (or tetrasomy) 13 or 13q.[1,34] A neurocutaneous syndrome consisting of a phylloid pattern of skin pigmentation associated with neurological defects (especially absence of the corpus callosum), colobomas, conductive hearing loss, craniofacial anomalies, and digital malformations has been reported. The hypomelanosis consists of round or oval lesions and large asymmetrical areas reminiscent of the leaves of a begonia, as well as pear-shaped areas or oblong macules.[35]

g. *Conradi-Hünermann-Happle syndrome (X-linked dominant chondrodysplasia punctata)*
   Conradi-Hünermann-Happle syndrome is caused by mutations in a gene that encodes emopamil binding protein, EBP (beta-hydroxysteroid-delta 8, delta 7-isomerase), an enzyme involved in cholesterol biosynthesis.[36] This syndrome includes skin lesions along the Blaschko lines, sectorial cataracts, asymmetric shortening of the proximal limbs, and asymmetric bone defects (epiphyseal stippling). In the first weeks of life, the patient shows linear areas of inflammation and hyperkeratosis; later, these lesions are followed by atrophy and hypopigmentation with rather mild scaling. Scarring alopecia on the scalp following the Blaschko lines and follicular atrophoderma on the scalp, wrists, and hands are also common.[1]

h. *Goltz syndrome*
   Goltz syndrome, also called focal dermal hypoplasia, is a rare genetic X-linked dominant disorder affecting ectodermal and mesodermal structures. It is caused by mutations in PORCN gene, which encodes an O-acyltransferase, which is a regulator of Wnt, an important morphogen in ecto-mesodermal tissue devolopment.[37] The phenotype is variable depending on the proportion and distribution of cells expressing the mutant X chromosome. Clinically, mutation on PORCN is expressed in the eyes (e.g., colobomas,

microphtalmia, cataracts), teeth (e.g., hypodontia, vertical grooving), bones (e.g., limb malformations, osteopathia striata), and skin. The skin lesions are characterized by linear streaks along the lines of Blaschko, with dermal atrophy, fat herniations into the dermis, and hypo- or hyperpigmentation. Erythematous ("raspberry-like") papules may appear in any location, but the anogenital region and lips are the most common.[2]

DIAGNOSIS

Genetic mosaicism is detected by comparing affected with unaffected tissue from the same individual. In mosaic cutaneous disease, genetic analysis of the affected skin can reveal the presence of the mutation, which is not present in normal skin. Sometimes, the mosaic can be expressed in a low percentage of blood cells, especially if the mutation occurs early in embryogenesis. Selection of the appropriate unaffected control tissue is thus important, and in cutaneous mosaic disorders, blood, buccal swabs, or saliva are usually employed.[38]

FOLLOW-UP AND TREATMENT

Although mosaic skin hypopigmentation is usually an isolated manifestation, patients must be followed up in order to rule out association with internal organ involvement. It is important to recognize mosaic hypopigmentation because it may be the first manifestation of a systemic disease. Especially in linear hypopigmentation, if the cutaneous lesions are very extensive, the patient must be examined by an ophthalmologist and neurologist.

Mosaic conditions are usually not heritable. However, the mutation can affect not only the skin but also the gonads (germinal or gonadal mosaicism), and in this case, the mutations can be inherited and expressed constitutionally by subsequent generations.[38,39] Genetic counseling may thus be difficult.[40]

Nowadays, unfortunately, there is no effective treatment for mosaic hypopigmented conditions.

REFERENCES

1. Happle R. Mosaicism in human skin. *Understanding Nevi, Nevoid Skin Disorders, and Cutaneous Neoplasia.* Springer; 2014.
2. Celia Moss. Mosaicism and linear lesion. In: Bolognia JL, Jorizzo JL, Schaffer JV. *Dermatology.* Vol 1. 4th ed. Elsevier; 2018:1004–1025.
3. Happle R. The McCune Albright syndrome: A lethal gene surviving by mosaicism. *Clin Genet.* 1986;29:321–324.
4. Kurek KC, Luks VL, Ayturk UM et al. Somatic mosaic activating mutations in PIK3CA cause CLOVES syndrome. *Am J Hum Genet.* 2012;90:1108–1115.
5. Happle R. The molecular revolution in cutaneous biology: Era of mosaicism. *J Invest Dermatol.* 2017;137:e73–e77.
6. Lindhurst MJ, Sapp JC, Teer JK et al. A mosaic activating mutation in AKT1 associated with the Proteus syndrome. *N Engl J Med.* 2011;365:611–619.
7. Lara-Corrales I, Moazzami M, García-Romero MT et al. Mosaic neurofibromatosis type 1 in children: A single-institution experience. *J Cutan Med Surg.* 2017;21:379–382.
8. Bessis D, Malinge MC, Girard C. Isolated and unilateral facial angiofibromas revealing a type 1 segmental postzygotic mosaicism of tuberous sclerosis complex with c.4949_4982del TSC2 mutation. *Br J Dermatol.* 2018;178:e53–e54.
9. Nagao-Watanabe M, Fukao T, Matsui E et al. Identification of somatic and germline mosaicism for a keratin 5 mutation in epidermolysis bullosa simplex in a family of which the proband was previously regarded as a sporadic case. *Clin Genet.* 2004;66:236e8.
10. Happle R. Segmental forms of autosomal dominant skin disorders: Different types of severity reflect different states of zygosity. *Am J Med Genet.* 1996;66:241–242.
11. Happle R. The concept of type 2 segmental mosaicism, expanding from dermatology to general medicine. *J Eur Acad Dermatol Venereol.* 2018;32:1075–1088.
12. Siegel DH. Cutaneous mosaicism: A molecular and clinical review. *Adv Dermatol.* 2008;24:223–244.
13. Geiman TM, Robertson KD. Chromatin remodeling histone modifications, and DNA methylation-how does it all fit together? *J Cell Biochem.* 2002;87:117–125.
14. Blaschko A. *Die Nervenverteilung in der Haut in ihre Beziehung zu den Erkrankungen der Haut.* Vienna, Austria and Leipzig, Germany: Wilhelm Braunmuller; 1901.
15. Happle R, Assim A. The lines of Blaschko on the head and neck. *J Am Acad Dermatol.* 2001;44:6125.
16. Happle R. Mosaicism in human skin. Understanding the patterns and mechanisms. *Arch Dermatol.* 1993;129:1460–1470.
17. Ito M. Studies of melanin XI. Incontinentia pigmenti achromians: A singular case of nevus depigmentosus systematicus bilateralis. *Tohoky J Exp Med* 1952; 55(Suppl):57–59.
18. Lee HS, Chun YS, Hann SK. Nevus depigmentosus: Clinical features and histopathologic characteristics in 67 patients. *J Am Acad Dermatol.* 1999;40:21–26.
19. Kim SK, Kang HY, Lee ES, Kim YC. Clinical and histopathologic characteristics of nevus depigmentosus. *J Am Acad Dermatol.* 2006;55:423–428.
20. Cohen J 3rd, Shahrokh K, Cohen B. Analysis of 36 cases of Blaschkoid dyspigmentation: Reading between the lines of Blaschko. *Pediatr Dermatol.* 2014;31:471–476.
21. Hogeling M, Fieden IJ. Segmental pigmentation disorder. *Br J Dermatol.* 2010;162:1337–1341.

22. Nehal KS, PeBenito R, Orlow SJ. Analysis of 54 cases of hypopigmentation and hyperpigmentation along the lines of Blaschko. *Arch Dermatol.* 1996;132:1167–1170.

23. Kromann AB, Ousager LB, Ali IKM, Aydemir N, Bygum A. Pigmentary mosaicism: A review of original literature and recommendations for future handling. *Orphanet J Rare Dis.* 2018;13:39.

24. Mirzaa GM, Campbell CD, Solovieff N et al. Association of MTOR mutations with developmental brain disorders, including megalencephaly, focal cortical dysplasia, and pigmentary mosaicism. *JAMA Neurol.* 2016;73:836–845.

25. Torchia D, Happle R. Segmental hypomelanosis and hypermelanosis arranged in a checkerboard pattern are distinct naevi: Flag-like hypomelanotic naevus and flag-like hypermelanotic naevus. *J Eur Acad Dermatol Venereol.* 2015;29:2088–2099.

26. Asch S, Sugarman JL. Epidermal nevus syndromes: New insights into whorls and swirls. *Pediatr Dermatol.* 2018;35:21–29.

27. Garcias-Ladaria J, Cuadrado Rosón M, Pascual-López M. Epidermal nevi and related syndromes— Part 1: Keratinocytic nevi. *Actas Dermosifiliogr.* 2018;109:677–686.

28. Laura FS. Epidermal nevus syndrome. *Handb Clin Neurol.* 2013;111:349–368.

29. Fusco F, Bardaro T, Fimiani G et al. Molecular analysis of the genetic defect in a large cohort of IP patients and identification of novel NEMO mutations interfering with NF-kappaB activation. *Hum Mol Genet.* 2004;13:1763–1773.

30. Greene-Roethke C. Incontinentia pigmenti: A summary review of this rare ectodermal dysplasia with neurologic manifestations, including treatment protocols. *J Pediatr Health Care.* 2017;31:e45–e52.

31. Peltomäki P, Knuutila S, Ritvanen A et al. Pallister-Killian syndrome: Cytogenetic and molecular studies. *Clin Genet.* 1987;31:399–405.

32. Karaman B, Kayserili H, Ghanbari A, Uyguner ZO, Toksoy G, Altunoglu U, Basaran S. Pallister-Killian syndrome: clinical, cytogenetic and molecular findings in 15 cases. *Mol Cytogenet.* 2018;11:45. Published online August 17, 2018. doi:10.1186/s13039-018-0395-z.

33. Wilkens A, Liu H, Park K, Campbell LB, Jackson M, Kostanecka A, Pipan M, Izumi K, Pallister P, Krantz ID. Novel clinical manifestations in Pallister-Killian syndrome: Comprehensive evaluation of 59 affected individuals and review of previously reported cases. *Am J Med Genet A.* 2012;158A:3002–3017.

34. Dhar SU, Robbins-Furman P, Levy ML, Patel A, Scaglia F. Tetrasomy 13q mosaicism associated with phylloid hypomelanosis and precocious puberty. *Am J Med Genet A.* 2009;149A:993–996.

35. Happle R. Phylloid hypomelanosis and mosaic trisomy 13: A new etiologically defined neurocutaneous syndrome. *Hautarzt.* 2001;52:3–5.

36. Braverman N, Lin P, Moebius FF et al. 1999. Mutations in the gene encoding 3 beta-hydroxysteroid-delta 8, delta 7-isomerase cause X-linked dominant Conradi-Hünermann syndrome. *Nat. Genet.* 22:291–294.

37. Clements SE, Mellerio JE, Holden St et al. PORCN gene mutation and the protean nature of focal dermal hypoplasia. *Br J Dermatol.* 2009;160:1103–1109.

38. Lim YH, Moscato Z, Choate KA. Mosaicism in cutaneous disorders. *Annu Rev Genet.* 2017;51:123–141.

39. Bachoo S, Gibbons RJ. Germline and gonosomal mosaicism in the ATR-X syndrome. *Eur J Hum Genet.* 1999;7:933–936.

40. Sachdev NM, Maxwell SM, Besser AG, Grifo JA. Diagnosis and clinical management of embryonic mosaicism. *Fertil Steril.* 2017;107:6–11.

19 Skin disorders causing post-inflammatory hypopigmentation

POLYTIMI SIDIROPOULOU, DIMITRIOS SGOUROS, and DIMITRIS RIGOPOULOS

CONTENTS

Introduction	127	Management	128
Etiology	127	Course and prognosis	129
Pathogenesis	127	Disorders involving hypopigmentation	129
Clinical features	128	Conclusion	132
Histological features	128	References	132
Diagnosis	128		

INTRODUCTION

Post-inflammatory hypopigmentation (PIH) is a common cause of acquired partial or diffuse loss of skin pigmentation. It can occur in all skin types as a result of cutaneous inflammation, injury, or dermatological interventions. However, it is more prominent in dark-skinned or tanned individuals, possibly because of the color contrast with the surrounding normal skin.[1–3]

Hypopigmentation secondary to cutaneous inflammation covers a wide array of etiologies. Several dermatoses, including psoriasis, seborrheic or atopic dermatitis, and pityriasis alba, tend to induce PIH. Atypical presentation of classic diseases such as mycosis fungoides and sarcoidosis may also involve hypopigmentation. Moreover, cutaneous injuries (e.g., burns, chemical peels, cryotherapy) represent other examples of post-inflammatory leukoderma.[1–7]

Causal diagnosis of PIH is often clinically straightforward by determining the distribution and configuration of the primary lesions, if present. Nevertheless, some situations require further investigation, and sometimes a biopsy should be performed.[1–3,6] The most important key to management is to identify and treat the primary cause. Most cases of PIH resolve spontaneously with treatment of the underlying condition; however, it can be permanent as a result of complete destruction of melanocytes.[1,2,4,8]

In this review, the origin, pathogenesis, clinical features, differential diagnosis, and treatment options for PIH are discussed. "Disorders Involving Hypopigmentation" toward the end of this chapter briefly covers some of the common entities involving a hypopigmented phenotype. A detailed description of trauma-induced and iatrogenic hypopigmentation is beyond the scope of this chapter and is not discussed.

ETIOLOGY

PIH can occur following cutaneous inflammation, injury, or dermatological interventions. It covers a broad spectrum of etiologies, thus including a wide differential diagnosis. A large number of inflammatory dermatoses, such as psoriasis (Figure 19.1), seborrheic or atopic dermatitis, pityriasis alba, and lupus erythematosus, may induce PIH. Sarcoidosis, lichen sclerosus, mycosis fungoides, and scleroderma may all present with hypopigmented lesions, as may Hansen disease. In addition, external skin injuries from severe scratching, burns, and irritants, as well as dermatological and cosmetic procedures (e.g., chemical peels, dermabrasion, cryotherapy, laser ablation, intralesional steroid injections) can also lead to PIH.[1–7]

PATHOGENESIS

The underlying mechanisms governing the pathogenesis of PIH remain elusive. The variation in individual

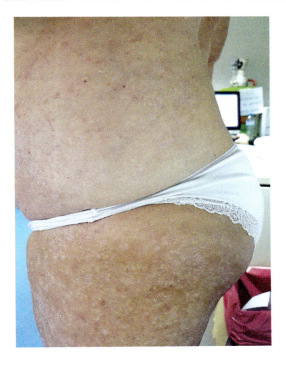

Figure 19.1 PIH with fine scaling due to psoriasis.

melanocyte response to trauma or inflammation is not well understood.[2,8] The term "inherited individual chromatic tendency" has been proposed to describe this variation.[9] Melanocytes can react to cutaneous inflammation or trauma with normal, increased, or decreased melanin production. People with melanocytes susceptible to damage are more prone to develop hypopigmentation.[2,8,9]

Melanogenesis is a complex process involving various steps that determine the skin color (melanosome biogenesis, melanin production, melanosome transport, and transfer to keratinocytes). It is controlled by multiple mediators (e.g., growth factors, cytokines) acting directly or indirectly on melanocytes, keratinocytes, and fibroblasts. Through dysregulation of these processes, cutaneous inflammation can induce abnormal melanocyte-keratinocyte interactions, leading to hypopigmentation.[2,4]

It has been suggested that hypopigmentation is usually associated with a decrease, but not absence, of pigment.[2,4] As tumor necrosis factor (TNF)-α and IL-17 are known to synergistically suppress pigmentation-related signaling and melanin production, it is possible to represent a potential mechanism by which inflammatory dermatoses such as psoriasis are complicated by hypopigmentation.[7] However, when there is severe local inflammation, loss or even death of functional melanocytes occurs, resulting in permanent pigmentary changes.[2,4]

CLINICAL FEATURES

PIH may appear in a localized or diffuse pattern.[1,3,10] The disorders described in this chapter can initially be localized; however, the distribution of hypopigmentation often progresses to involve multiple body surfaces.

The distribution and morphology of hypopigmented lesions usually reflects the area affected by the primary inflammatory condition, and the color ranges from hypopigmentation to depigmentation (reduced or absent melanin skin content).[1,2,8] Complete depigmentation is most commonly seen in the setting of severe atopic dermatitis (AD) and discoid lupus erythematosus (DLE), especially in dark-skinned individuals. Whether this represents koebnerization of vitiligo into areas of inflammation versus the consequence of severe inflammation is controversial.[2,4]

Hypomelanosis usually follows or coexists with the original inflammatory lesions, making the diagnosis straightforward on clinical grounds. However, in some cases, the inflammatory phase is not present, and hypopigmentation may be the only feature. Examples include mycosis fungoides (MF), lichen sclerosus (LS), morphea (localized sleroderma), systemic sclerosis (generalized scleroderma), and sarcoidosis.[2–4]

HISTOLOGICAL FEATURES

In general, histopathology of PIH is rarely diagnostic. A skin biopsy of the hypopigmented lesions shows nonspecific findings, including decreased epidermal melanin, superficial lymphohistiocytic infiltration, and presence of melanophages in the upper dermis.[2,12]

DIAGNOSIS

Since the causes of PIH are different and heterogeneous, establishing the correct diagnosis requires a thorough history and physical examination, the use of special lighting techniques, such as Wood's lamp, and sometimes a biopsy of the abnormally pigmented skin.[1,10–12]

Apart from the aforementioned clinical features, the presence of other morphological signs, such as scaling, epidermal atrophy, alopecia, induration, and infiltration, may address the underlying condition. The presence of epidermal changes is a clue toward skin diseases that disrupt the normal turnover of the epidermis. The presence of fine scaling may be suggestive of pityriasis alba. If hypopigmentation is related to epidermal atrophy, LS, morphea, and the hypopigmented variant of MF are to be considered. If induration occurs, it indicates the presence of dense collagen, which characterizes LS and morphea.[2,3,12]

Further investigation is determined by the suspected diagnosis. Wood's lamp testing can be used to further refine the diagnostic approach and differentiate between hypopigmented and depigmented skin. Wood's lamp accentuates depigmented lesions (complete pigment loss) but does not enhance hypopigmented lesions (partial pigment loss).[2,7,12] Confocal laser scanning microscopy may further facilitate distinction between different hypomelanotic conditions based on the melanin content and distribution patterns. Melanophages are present in PIH, but undetectable in vitiligo and nevus depigmentosus. However, the contents of melanin and dermal papillary rings vary with the degree of the inflammation.[2]

A skin biopsy is not always mandatory to establish the diagnosis. In some cases, histology is less specific and the diagnosis is made primarily on a clinical basis. In certain dermatoses, however, there may be some histopathological evidence that can reveal the primary cause of PIH, such as in MF, LE, and sarcoidosis. Hypopigmentation associated with epidermal changes (e.g., atrophy), induration, sensory changes, alopecia, or refractory to conventional treatment should be considered for biopsy. Pathology can also be of value in eliminating entities that can be confused with common hypopigmentary disorders such as vitiligo.[2,4,6,12]

MANAGEMENT

Identifying and controlling or preventing the underlying etiology is the key step in managing PIH. Once the primary inflammatory condition is effectively treated, PIH usually resolves over time. Current treatment modalities include topical medications, phototherapy, laser, surgical grafting techniques, and cosmetic camouflage.[1,2,4,12]

Topical corticosteroids and/or calcineurin inhibitors have been found to be beneficial in treating PIH when lesions are limited. Although the exact mechanisms of action remain elusive, those agents may affect inflammatory cells. Sun or ultraviolet (UV) exposure (UVA or UVB phototherapy, PUVA) may lead to repigmentation if melanocytes in the affected areas are still functional and may be of value when lesions are widespread. Overexposure, however, may accentuate the color contrast due to tanning of the surrounding skin. Both the 308-nm excimer laser and the ablative fractional CO_2 laser have been used to stimulate melanogenesis with favorable outcomes. However, regular subsequent treatment is usually needed to maintain the results. In cases of amelanotic leukoderma with total melanocyte loss, transplantation techniques such as epidermal or melanocyte grafting may be considered and seem to be the most promising procedures to repigment extensive hypopigmented areas. In addition, cosmetic cover-ups for camouflage, including high-coverage makeup, tanning products, and tattooing, may be an alternative option in order to decrease the color disparity with the normal skin. However, all therapeutic approaches are hampered by the fact that the pathophysiology of PIH remains poorly understood.[2,4,8,12]

Sun protection, including the use of a broad-spectrum sunscreen, can be of great value depending on the underlying disease. In some cases, hypopigmented lesions are susceptible to sun damage and will become more obvious with tanning of the surrounding normal skin. On occasion, however, hypopigmentation may improve with sun exposure, as happens in the context of psoriasis.[12]

COURSE AND PROGNOSIS

The severity of pigment loss is related to the extent and degree of the inflammation. PIH is usually self-limited and improves or resolves spontaneously within a few weeks or months if the primary cause is ceased. However, depigmentation induced by severe inflammation (e.g., LE, scleroderma) may require years to become repigmented, and may become permanent due to irreversible melanocyte destruction.[2,4,8]

DISORDERS INVOLVING HYPOPIGMENTATION
Pityriasis alba

Pityriasis alba (PA), a common benign condition, typically occurs during childhood and adolescence, affecting 1% of the general and 9.9% of the pediatric population. Although its pathogenesis remains unknown, it is included among PIH disorders. Excessive sun exposure, skin dryness, and atopic predisposition are strongly implicated in the development of PA. Clinically, the condition is characterized by ill-defined, round to oval, slightly scaly macules and patches with mild to moderate hypopigmentation. The lesions vary in size from 0.5 to 3 cm, but larger lesions can also occur. The face, especially the malar region, is the most frequent site of involvement, but lesions can occasionally develop on the neck, trunk, and extremities. This dermatosis is usually asymptomatic, but some patients complain of itching and burning. Under Wood's lamp examination, the lesions are enhanced. Histopathology of the affected skin reveals subacute spongiotic dermatitis along with reduced numbers of active melanocytes and a decrease in the number and size of melanosomes. Topical corticosteroids may be beneficial, but emollients seem to be equally effective. Recent data reported perfect results with topical calcineurin inhibitors (pimecrolimus, tacrolimus) as well as calcipotriol. Sun protection is of the utmost importance. The hypopigmented patches often remain stable for several months or years and may become more apparent during the summer period when the surrounding skin is tanned. The condition usually, but not always, resolves spontaneously after puberty.[4–6,10,13]

Dermatitis/eczema

PIH is frequently seen in association with atopic dermatitis, as well as with other forms of eczema, especially in patients with colored skin. Although AD or atopic diathesis is occasionally related to vitiligo vulgaris, patients may also develop PIH manifested as ill-defined white patches with eczema (Figure 19.2a,b). The decrease in pigmentation can be attributed to a disruption in melanogenesis secondary to the inflammatory process or to the application of potent topical corticosteroids. In the latter case, pigmentary changes are more common and intense.[12,14] An extremely inflammatory form of vitiligo, called vitiligo with inflammatory raised border, can also arise as a consequence of severe AD.[15] Interestingly, the severity of AD seems to be higher if leukoderma occurs. The levels of eosinophil counts, SCORAD, CCL17/TARC, and LDH tend to be higher in AD cases with associated leukoderma compared to nonleukoderma patients, indicating that the incidence of leukoderma may be dependent on the severity

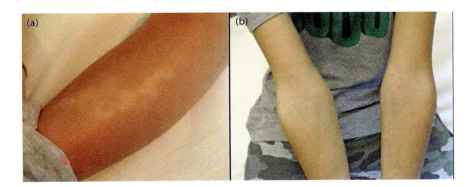

Figure 19.2 (a, b) PIH following resolution of AD eruption. (a) Localized leukoderma on the dorsum of the right shin in a 9-year-old girl. (b) Post-inflammatory hypopigmented vitiligo-like lesions on the bilateral antecubital region in a 12-year-old boy with eczema.

of AD.[14] Seborrheic dermatitis is another common and often difficult-to-treat cause of PIH, particularly in patients with darker skin phototypes.[16]

Lupus erythematosus

Hypopigmentation or depigmentation is commonly seen in LE as a result of the destruction of the basal layer homing melanocytes. In discoid LE, skin lesions begin as dull-red macules or indurated plaques that develop pigment changes. Hypomelanosis favors the center of the lesions and is usually surrounded by an irregular rim of hyperpigmentation. Cutaneous atrophy and scarring almost always coexist (Figure 19.3a–c). In chronic scarring DLE cases, the pigmentary changes are persistent. Histologically, in addition to decreased epidermal melanocytes, features that help to establish the diagnosis include epidermal atrophy, basal vacuolar degeneration, a dense inflammatory infiltration consisting mainly of CD123+ plasmacytoid dendritic cells, pigmentary incontinence, and fibrosis. Hypopigmentation is also frequently encountered in the center of annular lesions of subacute LE, but is usually reversible.[1,4,10,17]

Lichen sclerosus

Lichen sclerosus is a common cause of PIH and typically affects middle-aged women in their 50s and 60s. This chronic mucocutaneous disorder of unclear etiology is delineated by violaceous erythema and ivory- or porcelain-white depigmentation, mainly involving the genitals. However, the inflammatory phase may be clinically undetectable, and hypopigmentation can be the sole feature. The pathogenesis of LS-associated leukoderma remains unknown, but it results in hypomelanotic or amelanotic keratinocytes. Three possible mechanisms have been suggested: reduced melanin production, melanocyte decrease or loss, and blocked transfer of melanosomes to keratinocytes. LS manifests with anogenital and extragenital features. Typical lesions consist of well-demarcated porcelain-white patches or plaques with irregular borders, and varying degrees of sclerosis (Figure 19.4a–c). Additional changes include epidermal atrophy, follicular plugging, and, in the anogenital region, purpura. On occasion, extragenital LS can present as guttate leukoderma. Genital involvement may cause pruritus, dysuria, dyspareunia, and a burning sensation, while extragenital lesions

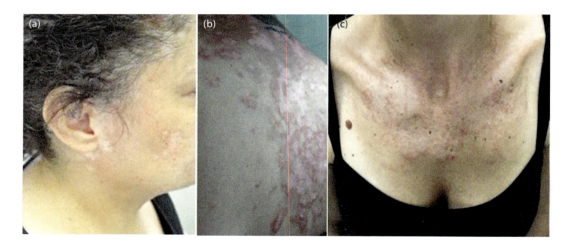

Figure 19.3 (a–c) Clinical appearance of leukoderma in DLE lesions. Well-demarcated hypopigmented slightly atrophic patches with atrophy involving the face and scalp of a 58-year-old woman (a), the back of a 27-year-old woman (b), and the neck and upper chest area of a 46-year-old woman (c).

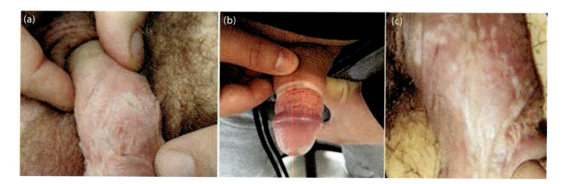

Figure 19.4 (a–c) LS-associated leukoderma presenting irregular ivory- or porcelain-white penile patches and plaques in three male patients.

are often asymptomatic. If LS is left untreated, scarring and progression to squamous cell carcinoma (SCC) can occur. LS should be considered in any patient with genital vitiligo-like depigmentation. Although the clinical evaluation usually provides a straightforward diagnosis, a histologic confirmation may be sought to rule out SCC and its precursors. Ultra-high-potency topical corticosteroids represent the mainstay of treatment and can achieve complete resolution of skin texture and color. Male circumcision can be curative in some patients. Surgical referral is necessary if complications occur (e.g., phimosis, meatal stenosis, urethral stricture), or with symptoms refractory to treatment. Long-term follow-up every 6–12 months is highly recommended to monitor for disease recurrence, progression, or development of malignancy.[1,3,4,6,12]

Scleroderma

Hypopigmentation is not uncommon in lesions of morphea and systemic sclerosis (SS). Hypomelanotic changes described in the setting of SS include a mixture of hypo- and hyperpigmentation in areas of chronic sclerosis, for example, the hands, and a characteristic vitiligo-like phenotype in both sclerotic and nonsclerotic skin. The latter early feature of SS is characterized by circumscribed areas of depigmentation with perifollicular pigment retention, forming a "salt-and-pepper" appearance. The epidermal melanocytes disappear in the interfollicular regions but are retained in the near vicinity of hair follicles. This peculiar leukoderma resembles repigmenting vitiligo and usually involves the retro-auricular region, scalp, forehead, chest, and/or trunk. When such leukoderma presents, SS must be excluded, as it is only known to occur in two other settings: overlap syndromes (that may include SS) and scleromyxedema. Hypopigmented lesions may also be seen in morphea or localized scleroderma. In a subset of children, early juvenile localized scleroderma (JLS) or hypopigmented morphea manifests with depigmented lesions that mimic, both clinically and histologically, vitiligo, resulting in a protracted diagnosis and treatment. A reciprocal distribution of CD34+ and FXIIIa+ cells (i.e., significant decrease or absence of FXIIIa+ and CD34+ cells in the papillary and reticular dermis, respectively, and increased FXIIIa+ cells in areas of fibrosis) can help distinguish early JLS from vitiligo. The origin and pathogenesis of scleroderma-associated pigmentary disturbances are elusive. Early diagnosis and adequate treatment are pivotal in preventing disfiguring progression and require a multidisciplinary approach.[1,3,4,10,12]

Sarcoidosis

The skin is one of several organs potentially affected by sarcoidosis, a multisystem idiopathic disease characterized by noncaseating granulomas. Cutaneous involvement is protean and occurs in up to one-third of patients (25%–30%). Although the true incidence of leukoderma in sarcoidosis is unknown, hypopigmented patches are one of the less typical presentations. Hypopigmented sarcoidosis is mainly reported in darkly pigmented individuals, especially of South African origin, with a female-to-male ratio of approximately 2:1. Skin lesions consist of circumscribed or poorly marginated, irregular, hypochromic papules or plaques distributed extensively on limbs and trunk, and they may not be indurated. In addition, hypomelanosis surrounding dermal nodules may be seen. The lesions are asymptomatic, favor the extremities, and display no other secondary changes. Histopathology is similar to classic sarcoidosis, with noncaseating granulomas expanding in the dermis. By electron microscopy, a vacuolated appearance in some melanocytes as well as a decreased number of melanosomes within keratinocytes is observed.[3,4,6]

Mycosis fungoides

Although typical MF (erythematous patches, plaques, and nodules) can induce PIH, there is a variant in which hypomelanotic lesions are the only or main characteristic. This type of MF prevails in the juvenile setting, especially in patients with dark skin, and in the pediatric population. Hypopigmented MF (HMF) presents with scaly hypomelanotic patches that may be pruritic with loss of hair of the affected skin and develop on the trunk and extremities (Figure 19.5). Typical MF lesions such as erythema and slight infiltration are usually, but not always, present concurrently. Histologically, epidermotropism of atypical T lymphocytes is seen, a picture similar to that of classic MF. Electron microscopy demonstrates decreased numbers of melanosomes within epidermal keratinocytes,

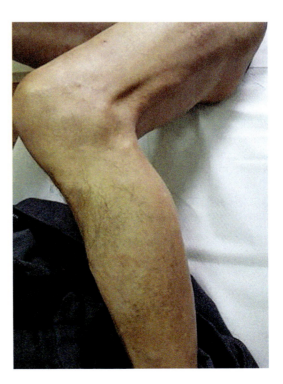

Figure 19.5 Hypopigmented MF showing macular hypomelanosis with ill-defined borders expanding on the legs with characteristic concomitant focal hair loss.

whereas numerous morphologically normal melanosomes are present in melanocytes. This finding is suggestive of a defect in melanosomal transfer. Clinically, HMF may mimic vitiligo, PA, leprosy, and pityriasis versicolor. In a high level of suspicion, such a diagnosis should be carefully considered in any young patient presenting with persistent hypopigmented patches, especially over the trunk and sun-protected areas. Assessment of lymph nodes and routine histology and immunophenotyping may guide diagnosis. Successful treatment, including photo(chemo) therapy or topical nitrogen mustard, usually results in repigmentation.[3,4,6,12,18–20]

CONCLUSION

This chapter addresses PIH, a significant disease group among pigmentary skin disorders that can be particularly distressing for cosmetic reasons and may also be associated with underlying malignancies or systemic disease. Enhancing dermatologists and other clinicians' experience in recognizing the key clinical features can greatly improve diagnostic accuracy, reduce unnecessary interventions, and prevent disabling complications.

REFERENCES

1. Saleem MD, Oussedik E, Picardo M et al. Acquired disorders with hypopigmentation: A clinical approach to diagnosis and treatment. *J Am Acad Dermatol.* 2019;80:1233–1250.e10. doi: 10.1016/j.jaad.2018.07.070
2. Vachiramon V, Thadanipon K. Postinflammatory hypopigmentation. *Clin Exp Dermatol.* 2011;36:708–714. doi: 10.1111/j.1365-2230.2011.04088.x.
3. Tey HL. Approach to hypopigmentation disorders in adults. *Clin Exp Dermatol.* 2010;35:829–834. doi: 10.1111/j.1365-2230.2010.03853.x.
4. Passeron T, Ortonne J. Vitiligo and other disorders of hypopigmentation. In: Callen J, ed. *Dermatology* by Jean L. Bolognia, Julie V. Schaffer, and Lorenzo Cerroni, 4th ed. China: Elsevier; 2018:1103–1106.
5. Nicolaidou E, Katsambas AD. Pigmentation disorders: Hyperpigmentation and hypopigmentation. *Clin Dermatol.* 2014;32:66–72.
6. Patel AB, Kubba R, Kubba A. Clinicopathological correlation of acquired hypopigmentary disorders. *Indian J Dermatol Venereol Leprol.* 2013;79:376–382.
7. Disturbances of Pigmentation. In: James W, ed. *Andrews' Diseases of the Skin: Clinical Dermatology,* 12th ed. China: Elsevier; 2016:856, 870.
8. Hartmann A, Bröcker EB, Becker JC. Hypopigmentary skin disorders: Current treatment options and future directions. *Drugs.* 2004;64:89–107.
9. Ruiz-Maldonado R, Orozco-Covarrubias ML. Post-inflammatory hypopigmentation and hyperpigmentation. *Semin Cutan Med Surg.* 1997;16:36–43.
10. Mollet I, Ongenae K, Naeyaert JM. Origin, clinical presentation, and diagnosis of hypomelanotic skin disorders. *Dermatol Clin.* 2007;25:363–371, ix. doi: 10.1016/j.det.2007.04.013.
11. Plensdorf S, Livieratos M, Dada N. Pigmentation disorders: Diagnosis and management. *Am Fam Physician.* 2017;96:797–804.
12. Tey HL. A practical classification of childhood hypopigmentation disorders. *Acta Derm Venereol.* 2010;90:6–11.
13. Engin RI, Cayir Y. Pigmentation disorders: A short review. *Pigment Disord.* 2015;2:6. doi: 10.4172/2376-0427.1000189.
14. Kuriyama S, Kasuya A, Fujiyama T et al. Leukoderma in patients with atopic dermatitis. *J Dermatol.* 2015;42:215–218.
15. Sugita K, Izu K, Tokura Y. Vitiligo with inflammatory raised borders, associated with atopic dermatitis. *Clin Exp Dermatol.* 2006;31:80–82.
16. Lopez I, Ahmed A, Pandya AG. Topical PUVA for post-inflammatory hypopigmentation. *J Eur Acad Dermatol Venereol.* 2011;25:742–743.
17. Connective tissue diseases. In: James W, ed. *Andrews' Diseases of the Skin: Clinical Dermatology,* 12th ed. China: Elsevier; 2016:153–162.
18. Amorim GM, Niemeyer-Corbellini JP, Quintella DC et al. Hypopigmented mycosis fungoides: A 20-case retrospective series. *Int J Dermatol.* 2018;57:306–312.
19. Castano E, Glick S, Wolgast L et al. Hypopigmented mycosis fungoides in childhood and adolescence: A long-term retrospective study. *J Cutan Pathol.* 2013;40:924–934.
20. Furlan FC, Sanches JA. Hypopigmented mycosis fungoides: A review of its clinical features and pathophysiology. *An Bras Dermatol.* 2013;88:954–960.

Infectious and parasitic causes of hypopigmentation

20

SERENA GIANFALDONI, ALEKSANDRA VOJVODIC, NOOSHIN BAGHERANI,
BRUCE R. SMOLLER, BALACHANDRA ANKAD, LEON GILAD, ARIEH INGBER,
FABRIZIO GUARNERI, UWE WOLLINA, and TORELLO LOTTI

CONTENTS

Pityriasis versicolor	133		Treponematoses	139
Leprosy	135		References	141
Onchocerciasis	139			

PITYRIASIS VERSICOLOR

Introduction

Pityriasis versicolor (PV) is a common benign superficial fungal skin disease,[1-3] characterized by scaly hyper- and hypopigmented skin lesions[4]. It is caused by lipophilic yeasts from the genera *Malassezia* (previously named *Pityrosporum orbiculare*), which are members of the skin microflora.[1-7]

Epidemiology

PV affects up to 40% of the population, especially in tropical regions. Teenagers and young adults are frequently afflicted.[7-12] *Malassezia* colonies on the skin begin immediately after birth and increase with age[4] and *Malassezia* is seen as normal skin flora in 75%–98% of healthy adults.[5] Distribution of various species of *Malassezia* shows differences based on geographical situation,[4,13] seasonal variation,[9] ethnicity,[13-14] body site, age, gender,[4,12,15] different sampling techniques, and culture media.[12]

Etiopathogenesis

Malassezia yeasts are the causative factor for developing PV. These are divided into about 14 species, among which *M. furfur, M. globosa, M. sympodialis, M. slooffiae, M. restricta,* and *M. obtuse* have been isolated from the skin of patients with PV.[4] *M. globosa* is the most common species cultured from PV lesions.[3,4,12,14,15]

PV is associated with increased activity of sebaceous glands.[8] *Malassezia* species are dimorphic fungi which upon conversion from yeast to mold or mycelial phase can result in their penetration and invasion of the stratum corneum, with consequent PV.[4,5] Individual factors include genetic predisposition, hyperhidrosis, long-term corticosteroid administration,[8,11,14,16] broad-spectrum antibiotic therapy,[11] occlusive dressing,[8] administration of topical oily agents, malnutrition, chronic infections, and pregnancy.[14]

Cell-mediated immunity plays an important role in the skin equilibrium of *Malassezia* species.[7,16] Monocyte-derived dendritic cells play a great role in binding and phagocytizing virulent fungal organisms in immunocompetent cases.[14] It seems that in cases with recurrent and disseminated pityriasis versicolor (RDPV), an underlying reduced cellular immunity can be a predisposing factor in development of disease.[7]

The role of humoral-mediated immunity against *Malassezia* infections is debatable. In a study on patients with atopic dermatitis, the role of *Malassezia* in promoting production of T helper 2 (Th2)-type cytokine profile, including interleukin 4 (IL-4) and IL-10 and expression of *Malassezia*-specific IgE antibodies, was demonstrated.[17]

The pathogenesis of hypopigmented lesions is different from that of hyperpigmented ones. The former is caused by damage of melanocytes, inhibition of tyrosinase by *Malassezia*-produced dicarboxylic acid and inflammation.[14] Activation of complement factors via direct and alternative pathways plays a role in production of the inflammation.[16]

Clinical features

PV is a superficial pigmentary noninflammatory dermatosis.[4] It is characterized by hypopigmented, hyperpigmented, or erythematous scaly, oval, and round macules and patches (Figures 20.1 through 20.3).[1,4,8,14] The follicular type of PV has been described[18] (Figure 20.4). Its color ranges from white to brown and black.[3,16] The term "versicolor" refers to these various colors, which can be seen simultaneously in the same patient. These lesions can coalesce, forming irregular and large patches.[8,14] Gentle scraping produces a mild scaling, which helps in establishing the diagnosis.[14]

The lesions of PV are mostly asymptomatic, but pruritus has been reported in some cases.[11,16] The trunk, including the chest and upper back, neck, proximal upper extremities,[2,11] abdomen, and inguinal areas are the sites that are most commonly involved by this disease.

134   Infectious and parasitic causes of hypopigmentation

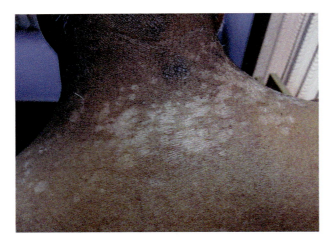

Figure 20.1 Pityriasis versicolor with hypopigmented patches with fine scaling, more evident by stretching the skin. (Courtesy of Prof. Balachandra Ankad; Department of Dermatology, SN Medical College, Rajiv Gandhi University of Health Sciences, Bengaluru, India.)

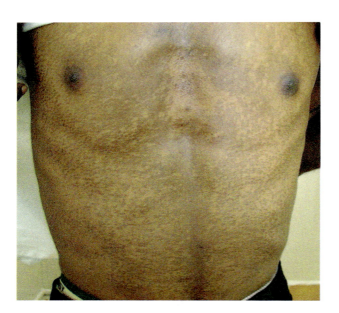

Figure 20.2 Hyperpigmented variant of pityriasis versicolor showing brown macules coalescing into patches. (Courtesy of Prof. Balachandra Ankad; Department of Dermatology, SN Medical College, Rajiv Gandhi University of Health Sciences, Bengaluru, India.)

Histopathology

A biopsy is not needed unless, in atypical cases, other skin diseases should be excluded. Histologically, PV shows hyperkeratosis, acanthosis,[9,19] spongiosis, exocytosis, reticular degeneration, hydropic degeneration of basal layer,[18] hyperpigmentation of basal layer,[19] melanin incontinence,[9] epidermal thinning, and mononuclear cell infiltration, mainly of lymphocytes and histiocytes. Short hyphae and budding yeast cells are seen in the stratum corneum[9] (Figure 20.5).

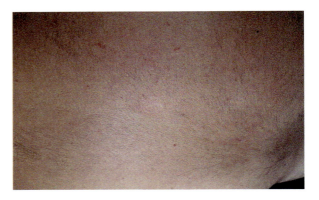

Figure 20.3 Pityriasis versicolor with pink scaly patches. (Courtesy of Prof. Balachandra Ankad; Department of Dermatology, SN Medical College, Rajiv Gandhi University of Health Sciences, Bengaluru, India.)

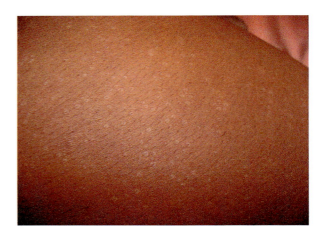

Figure 20.4 Follicular variant of PV showing hypopigmented macules with follicular distribution. (Courtesy of Prof. Balachandra Ankad; Department of Dermatology, SN Medical College, Rajiv Gandhi University of Health Sciences, Bengaluru, India.)

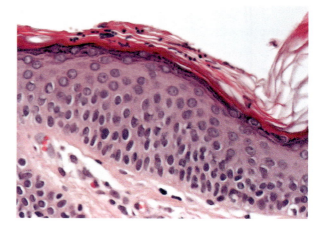

Figure 20.5 Multiple yeast forms within the stratum corneum characterize pityriasis versicolor. (Courtesy of Prof. Bruce R. Smoller; University of Rochester, School of Medicine and Dentistry, USA.)

Diagnosis

Diagnostic methods of PV include:

- *Clinical examination*: It forms the basis of diagnosis.[7,8,15] Zileris sign[3] or "evoked scale" sign is a marker for the clinical diagnosis and is defined as producing fine desquamation through stretching or scraping the skin. This sign confirms fragility of the stratum corneum in PV lesions.[9]
- *Wood's lamp examination*: Under Wood's lamp, yellowish or golden fluorescence may be seen.[8]
- *Direct microscopy*: In direct microscopic assessment of scaling lesions, treatment with 10%–20% KOH is performed.[5] In this method, finding round spores and short curved hyphae with a spaghetti-and-meatballs appearance is typical for diagnosing PV.[5,7,14] Porto's method is finding collections of round or oval cells in association with short hyphae of bizarre forms.[3]
- *Culture*: *Malassezia* can be cultured in slants of Sabouraud's dextrose agar and Sabouraud's dextrose in mixture with sterile olive oil for isolating lipophilic species.[5] Leeming–Notman agar or modified Dixonagar is another media for *Malassezia* culture.[12]
- *Molecular studies*: Molecular methods such as the PCR-based restriction fragment length polymorphism (RFLP) technique are used for identification and differentiation of different species of *Malassezia*.[5,20]

Differential diagnosis

The differential diagnoses of PV include: seborrheic dermatitis, erythrasma, secondary syphilis, mycosis fungoides,[14] pityriasis alba, leprosy, vitiligo,[9,14] pityriasis rubra pilaris,[18] post-kala-azar dermal leishmaniasis, idiopathic guttate hypomelanosis, lichen sclerosus et atrophicus, lichen planus depigmentosus, nevus depigmentosus, sarcoidosis, confluent and reticulated papillomatosis, and pityriasis rosea.[14]

Prognosis

PV is a benign condition with a high rate of relapse.[5] It tends to relapse in approximately 60% and 80% of patients during the first and second years of treatment, respectively.[1,5,16,21]

In immunocompromised patients, the recurrence frequency is higher and systemic therapy for PV may be required.[14]

Treatment

Although PV is a benign condition, cosmetic reasons and pruritus, particularly in more widespread extension, may require therapy including systemic azoles or topical agents such as azoles, terbinafine, zinc pyrithione, selenium sulfide, and ciclopiroxolamine.[16,21,22]

LEPROSY

Introduction

Leprosy, or Hansen disease, is a chronic granulomatous infection involving primarily peripheral nerves, skin, and mucosa of the upper respiratory tract and eyes, potentially resulting in irreversible disabilities and deformities if left untreated. It also may involve joints, lymph nodes, bone marrow, and internal organs.

Leprosy is caused by an intracellular bacterium called *Mycobacterium leprae* (*M. leprae*), a weakly acid-fast bacillus (AFB). It is contagious; however, the exact mechanism of transmission is not known. It is believed to spread via droplets from the nose or mouth or rarely by direct skin contact with lesions of infected individuals.[23-25] Among people exposed to *M. leprae*, 95% are not susceptible to infection, while among the 5% who become infected, only 1% shows the disease. Hence, it appears that hosts' genetic predisposition and impaired immune system play a critical role in disease development.[26,27]

Epidemiology

Currently, it is distributed all over the world, particularly in Southeast Asia, Africa, and Latin America. Although its prevalence has significantly decreased secondary to introduction of the multiple drug therapy (MDT), more than 200,000 new patients have been reported annually over the globe.[28]

Classification

According to the Ridley-Jopling classification criteria, histopathological changes, skin-slit smear assessment (SSS), and bacteria index (BI), leprosy is divided into five types: tuberculoid leprosy (TT), borderline tuberculoid (BT), mid-borderline (BB), borderline lepromatous (BL), and lepromatous leprosy (LL). Indeterminate leprosy (IL) is considered the initial presentation of the disease.[23,28,29]

The World Health Organization (WHO) divides leprosy into paucibacillary (PB) and multibacillary (MB), based on the number of skin lesions, presence of nerve involvement, and identification of bacilli on slit-skin smear.[23,30]

Pure neuritic leprosy (PNL) is seen in 4%–8% of leprosy cases; it is a type of leprosy with exclusively neural involvement without skin manifestations.[31]

In the course of leprosy, and before, during, and after initiation of MDT, patients may show inflammatory episodes, so-called lepra reactions. Lepra reactions are classified into three types: type 1 reaction (reversal reaction/RR/downgrading), type 2 reaction (such as erythema nodosum leprosum/ENL/upgrading), and Lucio phenomenon (LP).[29,32]

Clinical features

Based on *M. leprae*–specific cell-mediated immunity, leprosy has a wide spectrum of clinical manifestations, ranging from more nerve involvement and its consequent anesthesia and deformities to more skin lesions. Among the nerves, the ulnar, median, lateral popliteal, posterior tibial, and greater auricular ones are commonly involved.[33] The clinical features of the most frequent types of leprosy include:

- *IL*: It is usually characterized by one or two hypopigmented lesions with ill-defined borders and impaired temperature sensation. No peripheral nerve thickening is seen. Erythema, infiltration, and impairment of pain and/or touch perception show its progression to other clinical types.[23]

- *TT*: It is characterized by a small number of round hypopigmented and erythematous macules and patches with well-defined populated borders,[28,29] atrophic centers, and hair loss. Impairment of temperature, pain, and touch sensation has been reported[23] (Figure 20.6).
- *BT*: It is manifested as hypopigmented plaques of different size and number. The number varies from 5 to 20. Asymmetrical distribution is characteristic. Bigger lesions are more common as compared to smaller lesions. Involvement of peripheral nerves is very common and crucial in this type. Sensation over the patches is lost[23] (Figure 20.7).
- *BL*: It is characterized by numerous patches arranged in an almost symmetrical pattern. The number of smaller lesions is higher than that of larger lesions. Its clinical features are common with BB and LL. Normal skin areas along with infiltrations are seen in BB (Figures 20.8 and 20.9). Without treatment, it can progress to subpolar lepromatous leprosy (LLp). Peripheral nerves are commonly involved.[23]

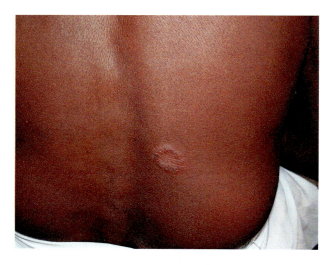

Figure 20.6 TT showing well-defined plaque with peripheral activity and central clearing. (Courtesy of Prof. Balachandra Ankad; Department of Dermatology, SN Medical College, Rajiv Gandhi University of Health Sciences, Bengaluru, India.)

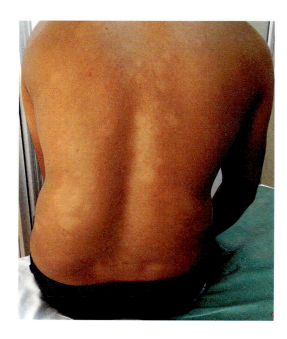

Figure 20.8 BL with well-to ill-defined patches and plaques (note the greater number of larger patches and the infiltrated border extending peripherally). (Courtesy of Prof. Balachandra Ankad; Department of Dermatology, SN Medical College, Rajiv Gandhi University of Health Sciences, Bengaluru, India.)

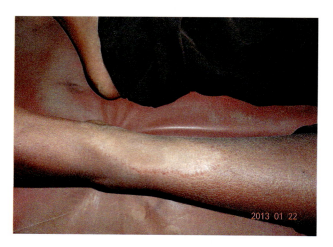

Figure 20.7 BT showing well- to ill-defined plaque on the left leg. Note the infiltrated border extending peripherally. (Courtesy of Prof. Balachandra Ankad; Department of Dermatology, SN Medical College, Rajiv Gandhi University of Health Sciences, Bengaluru, India.)

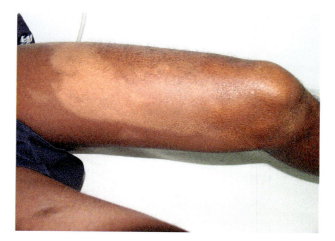

Figure 20.9 A 45-year-old Ethiopian male with BL downgrading from BB, presented with a hypopigmented sharply demarcated lesion. (Courtesy of Prof. Leon Gilad; the Lepers Hospital, Department of Dermatology, Hadassah University Hospital, Hebrew University, Jerusalem, Israel.)

- *LL*: It is characterized by symmetrically widespread erythematous, hypopigmented and edematous macules and infiltrated nodules, madarosis, xerosis, edema of the extremities, cyanosis of the palmar and plantar regions, and plantar trophic ulcers (Figure 20.10). Lepromatous macules have poorly defined borders and no loss of sensation. Local nerve enlargement is not characteristic. In addition to macules, nodules, plaques, or diffuse infiltration of skin are observed. Such infiltration on the face results in "leonine facies." Nose septum perforation and total collapse of the nose are the result of advanced LL. Papules are common on the hard palate. Nerve involvement is characteristically symmetrical and exhibits a stocking-glove distribution, unrelated to the location of skin lesions.[23] In addition to skin manifestations, systemic involvement including eyes, bones, testicles, and solid organ involvement have been reported in LL.
- *Type 1 reaction*: It is seen in borderline leprosy.[29] It is the leading cause for hospitalization of leprosy patients and is accompanied by lifelong neurological complications.[30] RR is characterized by skin and nerve inflammation, which include exacerbation of preexisting skin lesions, appearance of new skin lesions, induration, and erythema. Lesions are tender. Neurological dysfunction is reported in 50% of patients.[34]
- *Type 2 reaction*: It is seen more commonly in BL and LL types. ENL is characteristically manifested by tender erythematous nodules along with constitutional and systemic features including fever, malaise, and arthralgia (Figure 20.11). Rare and atypical manifestations of ENL

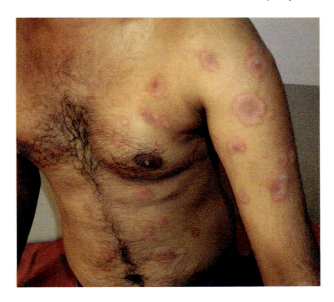

Figure 20.11 ENL in a case with LL showing erythematous, tender nodules on the extremities, abdomen, and chest. (Courtesy of Prof. Balachandra Ankad; Department of Dermatology, SN Medical College, Rajiv Gandhi University of Health Sciences, Bengaluru, India.)

include ulceration, pustule formation, bullous lesion, livedo reticularis, and erythema multiforme- and Sweet syndrome-like features.[29]
- *LP*: It is a rare reactional state seen exclusively in Lucio leprosy. LP is characterized by vascular thrombosis and skin ulceration and necrosis.[35]

Leprosy in children is an indicator of being in prolonged contact with a person with untreated disease, particularly in the family and with active infection in the community.[25]

Diagnosis

To achieve control and eradication of leprosy, its accurate diagnosis and prompt therapy initiation would be optimal.[36] Hansen disease is diagnosed based on clinical presentation, and the diagnosis is confirmed by skin or nerve biopsy and acid fast staining. Serological tests lack sensitivity and specificity and are not used to diagnose leprosy.[37] The diagnosis of leprosy remains based on the presence of at least one of three cardinal signs:[38]

i. Definite loss of sensation in a pale (hypopigmented) or reddish skin patch
ii. Thickened or enlarged peripheral nerve with loss of sensation and/or weakness of the muscles supplied by that nerve
iii. Presence of acid-fast bacilli in a slit-skin smear

- *Physical examination*: Hypopigmented macules characteristic of leprosy can guide in the diagnosis of leprosy. Other important signs and symptoms in physical examination are related to neurological involvement, which includes thickened peripheral nerve, dysesthesia, and motor disorders.[39]

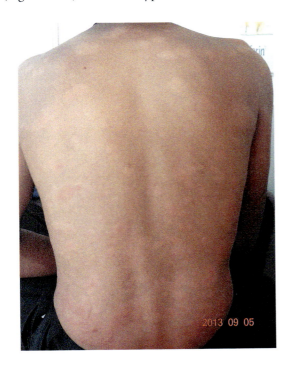

Figure 20.10 LL showing numerous small patches (note the symmetrical distribution). (Courtesy of Prof. Balachandra Ankad; Department of Dermatology, SN Medical College, Rajiv Gandhi University of Health Sciences, Bengaluru, India.)

- *Microbiological evaluation*: Staining techniques like Ziehl-Neelsen and Fite-Faraco are performed on specimens derived through SSS, nasal swabs, and formalin-fixed paraffin embedded tissue.[23]
- *Histopathology of cutaneous lesion*[23]
    - IL: Nonspecific periadnexal and peri- and/or intraneural inflammatory infiltration.
    - TT: Thickened nerve, enlarged funicles. Well-formed epithelioid cell granulomas, predominant component of epithelioid cells with vesicular slipper shaped nuclei, collar of lymphocytes, occasional giant cell, foci of necrosis, no foamy histiocytes, and seldom AFB in Wade Fite stain (Figures 20.12 and 20.13).
    - BT: Loose endoneurial granulomas, intermingled lymphocytes, many Langhans-type giant cells, and occasional AFB in Wade Fite stain.
    - BB: Admixture of scattered epithelioid cells, lymphocytes, and foamy histiocytes; no well-formed granulomas or necrosis; and easily identified AFB in Wade Fite stain.
    - BL: Minimally thickened nerve, intense endoneurial infiltrate of foamy histiocytes, a few lymphocytes, no epithelioid histiocytes, no necrosis, no giant cells, and abundant AFB.
    - LL: Diffuse and intense foam cell infiltrate, no lymphocytes, no epithelioid histiocytes, no necrosis, no giant cells, and numerous AFB (Figure 20.14).
- *Molecular method*: Polymerase chain reaction is used for the detection of AFB and is sensitive and specific, particularly for diagnosing neural involvement.[31]
- *Nerve biopsy*: Although it is the gold standard for diagnosis of PNL,[39] because of probability of nerve destruction and consequent disabilities, it has limited use. Furthermore, its histopathologic interpretation needs highly specific skills.[33] Fine-needle aspiration cytology (FNAC) of the nerves is a relatively less aggressive alternative to nerve biopsy whose results are comparable with nerve biopsy.[39]

Other methods

- *Imaging techniques*: Ultrasonography, color Doppler, and magnetic resonance imaging are used for detecting nerve involvement in the course of leprosy or its reactions.[33]
- *Nerve and muscle testing*: Nerve conduction studies have limited use in diagnosis of leprosy because they fail to recognize leprosy as an exact cause of neuropathy.[33]
- *Mitsuda skin test orlepromin skin test*: It is intradermal injection of heat-killed *M. leprae* and assessment of the skin induration at the injection site after 21 days (A51). It is positive in 57%–100% of PNL cases. Because of its poor diagnostic value, it is used along with other studies.[39]

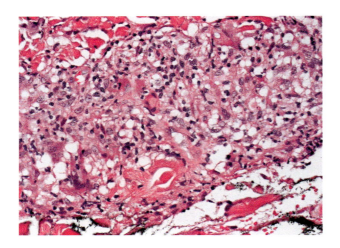

Figure 20.12 Granuloma with surrounding lymphocytes and plasma cells present surrounding dermal nerves in TT. (Courtesy of Prof. Bruce R. Smoller; University of Rochester, School of Medicine and Dentistry, USA.)

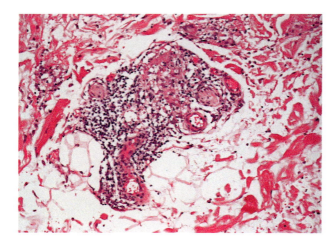

Figure 20.13 A well-formed granuloma is present in TT. (Courtesy of Prof. Bruce R. Smoller; University of Rochester, School of Medicine and Dentistry, USA.)

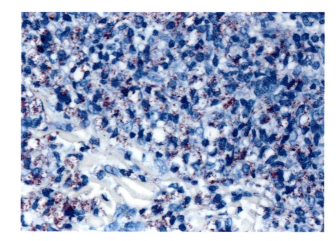

Figure 20.14 A Fite stain demonstrates multiple organisms in LL. (Courtesy of Prof. Bruce R. Smoller; University of Rochester, School of Medicine and Dentistry, USA.)

Differential diagnosis

Differential diagnosis of leprosy includes sarcoidosis, pityriasis versicolor, systemic lupus erythematosus, dermatomyositis granuloma annulare, and cutaneous tuberculosis.[23]

Treatment and prognosis

Leprosy is a curable disease. Disability is prevented if diagnosed and treated early. According to WHO guidelines, treatment includes multiple (two or three) drugs, and the duration of treatment, dose, and number of antibiotics depend on the type of leprosy (PB or MB) and age of the patient: adult or child. A three-drug regimen of rifampicin, dapsone, and clofazimine is recommended for a duration of 6 months for PB leprosy and 12 months for MB leprosy.[38]

Prompt diagnosis and initiating the MDT can prevent long-term disabilities.[38] PNL can result in severe disabilities.[39]

ONCHOCERCIASIS
Introduction

Onchocerciasis, also known as "river blindness," is a parasitic disease caused by the filarial nematode *Onchocerca volvulus*.[40,41] Its burden and socioeconomic consequences are significant: estimated loss of 1 million disability-adjusted life-years (healthy life-years lost due to disability and mortality), because of cutaneous manifestations, severe visual impairment (500,000 cases), blindness (270,000 cases), parasite-induced immunosuppression, epilepsy, and social stigmatization, all leading to a decrease of a host's life expectancy, although onchocerciasis is not lethal per se.[42]

Onchocerca volvulus is an almost exclusively human parasite (isolated cases reported in chimpanzees, gorillas, cynomolgus monkeys). Blackflies of the genus *Simulium*, living and breeding near fast-flowing, aerated water streams (e.g., rivers), are its vectors and obligate intermediate hosts.[43,44]

Epidemiology

Onchocerciasis is endemic in tropical areas, mainly Sub-Saharan countries, where more than 99% of patients live. Estimated cases were 37 million in 2006.[42] Thanks to extensive long-term public health intervention, that figure is now halved, and four previously endemic countries are disease free.[40]

Pathogenesis

Microfilariae invade mainly skin and eyes. Tissue damage is most often due to inflammation triggered by molecules from parasite death.[45,46]

Clinical features

Early signs of infection include fever, neuralgic pain in joints, and temporary hives on trunk and face. Onchocerciasis is initially characterized by itch, often intense and widespread. This is followed, in 3–36 months, by erythematous exanthema, with numerous small (1–3 mm), round papular elements, sometimes with superficial and/or apical desquamation (acute papular onchodermatitis). Evolution is to chronic papular onchodermatitis and lichenified onchodermatitis, with possible hypertrophic, verrucous, and/or eczema-like aspects, xerosis, and hyperpigmentation. Late skin lesions include hypo-/atrophy, hypo-/depigmentation ("leopard skin"), and onchocercomas (fibrous, mobile, asymptomatic nodules, located at bony prominences in areas of *Simulidae* bites and containing adult nematodes).[40,41,43]

Asymptomatic axillary, inguinal, or femoral lymphadenopathy may occur. The clinical picture-defined "hanging groins" include femoral lymphadenopathy, inguinal hernia, hydrocele, elephantiasis of external genitals, and inguinal folds of inelastic, atrophic skin.[43]

Peculiar cutaneous manifestations of onchocerciasis are *mal morado*, characterized by thickened, smooth, pale pink skin and leprosy-like "leonine facies"; *erisipela de la costa*, erysipeloid form involving face and neck; and *sowda*, with lichenoid, hyperpigmented, unilateral leg lesions associated with intense itch and inguinal lymphadenopathy.

Eye involvement may cause punctuate/sclerosing keratitis, iridocyclitis, uveitis, or active optic inflammation, and result in visual impairment, glaucoma, or blindness.[45]

Laboratory workup

Blood exams show hypereosinophilia and elevated erythrosedimentation rate, total IgE and IgG.[40,41] During acute papular onchodermatitis, histopathology shows microfilariae in the upper dermis, with infiltration of macrophages, eosinophils and neutrophils around dead or degenerating ones, but little reaction against live ones. Ortho-parakeratotic hyperkeratosis, acanthosis and dermal fibrosis are characteristic of chronic papular onchodermatitis. Microfilariae can also be detected by examining skin-snip biopsies incubated in saline solution for 30 minutes.[44,47]

Treatment

Ivermectin (microfilaricidal), administered once or, preferably, twice yearly for the lifespan of adult worms (10–15 years), or as long as evidence of skin or eye infection exists, is the treatment of choice.[40,48] Adjustment of treatment strategy is required for patients with high blood levels of *Loa loa*, to avoid possibly severe adverse events.[48] Because of bactericidal effects on *Wolbachia*, doxycyclin is indirectly lethal for adult *Onchocerca volvulus*, offering a new, promising therapeutic approach.[49]

TREPONEMATOSES
Introduction

Treponematoses are chronic bacterial infections caused by the spirochetal organisms of the *Treponema* species. The agents of human treponematoses include four closely related members of the genus Treponema: three subspecies of *Treponema pallidum* plus *Treponema carateum*. *T. pallidum* subsp. *pallidum* causes venereal syphilis, while *T. pallidum* subsp. *pertenue*, *T. pallidum* subsp. *endemicum*, and *T. carateum* are the agents of the endemic treponematoses yaws, bejel, and pinta, respectively. All human treponematoses share remarkable similarities in pathogenesis and clinical manifestations, consistent with the high genetic and antigenic relatedness of their etiological pathogens.[50,51]

Endemic treponematoses: Yaws, pinta, bejel

Epidemiology

Yaws is caused by *Treponema pallidum* subspecies *pertenue*. It affects mainly children aged under 15 years who live in poor communities in warm, humid, and tropical forested areas of Africa, Asia, Latin America, and the Pacific Islands.[50–52]

Transmission of endemic treponematoses is due to skin-to-skin contact for all three diseases and mucous membrane contact in the case of bejel.

Clinical manifestations

The clinical manifestations of endemic treponematoses occur in three distinct stages: primary lesions, dissemination, and late manifestations. In yaws, the primary lesions are either a localized papilloma or a solitary ulcer 2–5 cm in diameter that may be mistaken for cutaneous leishmaniasis, tropical ulcer, or pyoderma. Yaws skin ulcers are typically circular in shape and have central granulating tissue and elevated edges. The ulcers are often painless and rarely produce a discharge with malodor.[50–52]

The pinta primary lesion is an itchy, scaly papule or plaque that expands to greater than 10 cm but does not ulcerate. In bejel, the primary lesion is seldom seen because of its small size and location within the oral and oropharyngeal mucosa. Primary lesions in yaws and pinta are most commonly found on the exposed lower extremities, but also on the buttocks, arms, hands, and face.[50–52]

Secondary skin lesions of yaws are polymorphous, affecting the skin with papulosquamous lesions resembling other dermatoses such as psoriasis, mycosis, or crusted scabies. Secondary yaws lesions usually heal spontaneously after 3 to 6 months, though infectious relapses may occur for up to 5 years. The differential diagnosis therefore includes vitiligo, erythema dyschromicumperstans, and leprosy.[50,53]

Late changes of endemic treponematoses are osteo-periostitis (yaws, bejel) with diffuse cortical thickening followed by bone deformation.

Diagnostic tests

Treponemes may be identified in a wet preparation of material obtained from primary lesions by dark-field microscopy. Direct fluorescent antibody tests using anti–*T. pallidum* antibodies can distinguish pathogenic treponemal infections from saprophyte treponemes. The skin pathology of the silver impregnation technique is largely similar to that of venereal syphilis. The early lesions of yaws and bejel show epidermal hyperplasia with collections of neutrophils and a typical plasmocytic

dermal infiltrate. In early bejel, granulomas consisting of epithelioid cells and multinuclear giant cells may be present. In early pinta lesions, there is loss of melanin in basal cells and liquefaction degeneration. Epidermal atrophy and the presence of many melanophages in the dermis are typical findings of late-stage pinta.[54,55]

Serologic tests are rarely available in those countries where endemic treponematoses are abundant. The serological tests used to diagnose endemic treponematoses are the same as those used to diagnose syphilis: Nontreponemal agglutination tests, rapid plasma regain (RPR), or Venereal Disease Research Laboratory (VDRL) are positive in untreated cases; treponemal tests TPHA, *Treponema pallidum* particle agglutination (TPPA), and FTA-Abs are more specific, but remain positive for life.[56,57]

Rapid point-of-care (PoC) treponemal tests have become available in the form of immunochromatographic strips; these can be used with whole blood and do not require refrigeration.[58,59]

Treatment

For the treatment of yaws, the WHO recommends a single oral dose of azithromycin (30 mg/kg, with a maximum of 2 g). Benzathine penicillin as a single intramuscular dose of 1.2 million units (MU) of BPG for people aged over 10 years, and 0.6 MU for children less than 10 years of age, for those patients who "clinically fail on azythromycin" or are allergic to azithromycin.[60]

Syphilis

Introduction

Syphilis is a sexually transmitted disease caused by the bacterium *Treponema pallidum* subsp. *pallidum*. Infection can be transmitted by sexual contact and to the unborn child through the placenta at any gestational stage. In exceptional cases, syphilis can be transmitted at birth through the child's contact with the birth canal when there are maternal genital lesions (direct transmission).

Clinical manifestations

Acquired (by sexual contact) syphilis is divided into early and late syphilis. Early syphilis is further divided into primary, secondary, and early latent syphilis. Late syphilis includes late latent and tertiary syphilis.[61]

Primary syphilis is usually manifested by an ulcer in the anogenital region (or the mouth) with regional lymphadenopathy. Secondary syphilis usually develops 9–12 weeks after primary disease and is characterized by bacteriaemia and a broad spectrum of variable muco-cutaneous manifestations. Untreated, secondary syphilis can show a relapsing course for about 1 year before the latency phase emerges. Secondary syphilis is usually characterized by a non-itching skin rash that can be macular or papular. The rash may be generalized but has a predilection for the palms and soles. Fever, generalized lymphadenopathy, arthritis, hepatitis, splenomegaly, and glomerulonephritis are possible manifestations of secondary syphilis.[62]

Leucoderma syphiliticum encompasses a spectrum of hypochromic lesions that may emerge during the course of secondary syphilis. The lesions are round to oval, nonscaling, slightly raised, and well demarcated and can be scattered over the trunk.[63] Hypopigmented macules surrounded by pigmented areas and localized around the neck are referred to as the "necklace of Venus."

Diagnostic tests

Syphilis is diagnosed by demonstration of *Treponema pallidum* in the mucosal lesions (by dark-field examination or polymerase chain reaction) and by serological tests.[64]

Treatment

For early syphilis in adults and adolescents, the WHO and European guidelines recommend benzathine penicillin G (BPG), 2.4 million units once intramuscularly.[64–66]

When BPG cannot be used (due to penicillin allergy) or is not available, doxycycline 100 mg twice daily orally for 14 days or ceftriaxone 1 g intramuscularly once daily for 10–14 days, or, in special circumstances, azithromycin 2 g once orally are the alternatives. Doxycycline is preferred over ceftriaxone due to its lower cost and oral administration, but should not be used in pregnant women. There are reports of treatment failure due to azithromycin resistance of *T. pallidum*.[66]

In pregnant women with early syphilis, BPG G 2.4 million units once intramuscularly is the treatment of choice. Alternatively, procaine penicillin can be used, 1.2 million units intramuscularly once daily for 10 days. When penicillin cannot be used or is unavailable, erythromycin 500 mg orally four times daily for 14 days, ceftriaxone 1 g intramuscularly once daily for 10–14 days, or azithromycin 2 g once orally may be used.

REFERENCES

1. Balevi A, Üstüner P, Kakşi SA et al. Narrow-band UV-B phototherapy: An effective and reliable treatment alternative for extensive and recurrent pityriasis versicolor. *J Dermatolog Treat* 2018;29(3):252–255.
2. Gobbato AA, Babadópulos T, Gobbato CA et al. A randomized double-blind, non-inferiority Phase II trial, comparing dapaconazoletosylate 2% cream with ketoconazole 2% cream in the treatment of pityriasis versicolor. *Expert Opin Investig Drugs* 2015;24(11):1399–1407.
3. Santana JO, Azevedo FL, Campos Filho PC. Pityriasis versicolor: Clinical-epidemiological characterization of patients in the urban area of Buerarema-BA, Brazil. *An Bras Dermatol* 2013;88(2):216–221.
4. Prohic A, JovovicSadikovic T, Krupalija-Fazlic M et al. *Malassezia* species in healthy skin and in dermatological conditions. *Int J Dermatol* 2016; 55(5):494–504.
5. Elshabrawy WO, Saudy N, Sallam M. Molecular and phenotypic identification and speciation of *Malassezia* yeasts isolated from Egyptian patients with pityriasis versicolor. *J ClinDiagn Res* 2017;11(8):DC12–DC17.

6. Lee KH, Kim YG, Bang D et al. Scanning electron microscopy of *Malassezia furfur* in tinea versicolor. *Yonsei Med J* 1989;30(4):334–338.
7. Romero-Sandoval K, Costa AA, Teixeira Sousa MG et al. Recurrent and disseminated pityriasis versicolor: A novel clinical form consequent to *Malassezia*-host interaction?. *Med Hypotheses* 2017;109:139–144.
8. Ibekwe PU, Ogunbiyi AO, Besch R et al. The spectrum of *Malassezia* species isolated from students with pityriasis versicolor in Nigeria. *Mycoses* 2015;58(4):203–208.
9. Gaitanis G, Magiatis P, Hantschke M et al. The *Malassezia* genus in skin and systemic diseases. *ClinMicrobiol Rev* 2012;25(1):106–141.
10. Pakran J, Riyaz N. Interesting effect of *Malassezia* spp. infection on dermatoses of other origins. *Int J Dermatol* 2011;50(12):1518–1521.
11. Rad F, Nik-Khoo B, Yaghmaee R et al. Terbinafin 1% cream and ketoconazole 2% cream in the treatment of pityriasis versicolor: A randomized comparative clinical trial. *Pak J Med Sci* 2014;30(6):1273–1276.
12. Rasi A, Naderi R, Behzadi AH et al. *Malassezia* yeast species isolated from Iranian patients with pityriasis versicolor in a prospective study. *Mycoses* 2010;53(4):350–355.
13. Boralevi F, Marco-Bonnet J, Lepreux S et al. Hyperkeratotic head and neck *Malassezia* dermatosis. *Dermatology* 2006;212(1):36–40.
14. Kallini JR, Riaz F, Khachemoune A. Tinea versicolor in dark-skinned individuals. *Int J Dermatol* 2014;53(2):137–141.
15. Prohic A, Ozegovic L. *Malassezia* species isolated from lesional and non-lesional skin in patients with pityriasis versicolor. *Mycoses* 2007;50(1):58–63.
16. Gupta AK, Kogan N, Batra R. Pityriasis versicolor: A review of pharmacological treatment options. *Expert OpinPharmacother* 2005;6(2):165–178.
17. Kröger S, Neuber K, Gruseck E et al. Pityrosporumovale extracts increase interleukin-4, interleukin-10 and IgE synthesis in patients with atopic eczema. *ActaDermVenereol* 1995;75(5):357–360.
18. Darling MJ, Lambiase MC, Young RJ. Tinea versicolor mimicking pityriasisrubra pilaris. *Cutis* 2005;75(5):265–267.
19. Mostafa WZ, Assaf MI, Ameen IA et al. Hair loss in pityriasis versicolor lesions: A descriptive clinicopathological study. *J Am AcadDermatol* 2013;69(1):e19–e23.
20. Gaitanis G, Velegraki A, Frangoulis E et al. Identification of *Malassezia* species from patient skin scales by PCR-RFLP. *ClinMicrobiol Infect* 2002;8(3):162–173.
21. Zawar V, Chuh A. Case report on *Malassezia* infection of palms and fingernails—Speculations on cause for therapeutic failure in pityriasis versicolor. *J Eur Acad Dermatol Venereol* 2009;(2):171–172.
22. Nasarre J, Umbert P, Herrero E et al. Therapeutic efficacy and safety of the new antimycotic

sertaconazole in the treatment of pityriasis versicolor. *Arzneimittelforschung* 1992;42(5A):764–767.

23. Cruz RCDS, Bührer-Sékula S, Penna MLF et al. Leprosy: Current situation, clinical and laboratory aspects, treatment history and perspective of the uniform multidrug therapy for all patients. *An Bras Dermatol* 2017;92(6):761–773.

24. Reibel F, Cambau E, Aubry A. Update on the epidemiology, diagnosis, and treatment of leprosy. *Med Mal Infect* 2015;45(9):383–393.

25. Daniel OJ, Adejumo OA, Oritogun KS et al. Spatial distribution of leprosy in Nigeria. *Lepr Rev* 2016;87(4):476–485.

26. Wang N, Wang Z, Wang C et al. Prediction of leprosy in the Chinese population based on a weighted genetic risk score. *PLoS Negl Trop Dis* 2018;12(9):e0006789.

27. Campos de Carvalho J, Araújo MG, Alves Coelho-Dos-Reis JG et al. Phenotypic and functional features of innate and adaptive immunity as putative biomarkers for clinical status and leprosy reactions. *Microb Pathogpii* 2018;S0882-4010(18)30305-X.

28. Centers for Disease Control and Prevention (CDC). Hansen's disease (Leprosy). Available at: https://www.cdc.gov/leprosy/about/about.html. Accessed on March 20, 2019.

29. Suryawati N, Saputra H. Erythema nodosum leprosum presenting as Sweet's syndrome-like reaction in a borderline lepromatous leprosy patient. *Int J Mycobacteriol.* April 2018–June;7(2):191–194.

30. World Health Organization (WHO). Leprosy. Available at: https://www.who.int/lep/disease/en/. Accessed on March 20, 2019.

31. Narang T, Vinay K, Kumar S et al. A critical appraisal on pure neuritic leprosy from India after achieving WHO global target of leprosy elimination. *Lepr Rev* 2016;87(4):456–463.

32. Secchin-De-Andrade PJ, De Andrea Vilas-Boas, Hacker M et al. Corticosteroid therapy in borderline tuberculoid leprosy patients co-infected with HIV undergoing reversal reaction: A clinical study. *Lepr Rev* 2016;87(4):516–525.

33. Gupta S, Bhatt S, Bhargava SK et al. High resolution sonographic examination: A newer technique to study ulnar nerve neuropathy in leprosy. *Lepr Rev* 2016;87(4):464–475.

34. Hattori M, Motegi S, Amano H et al. Borderline lepromatous leprosy: Cutaneous manifestation and type 1 reversal reaction. *Acta DermVenereol* 2016;96(3):422–423.

35. Rocha RH, Emerich PS, Diniz LM et al. Lucio's phenomenon: Exuberant case report and review of Brazilian cases. *An Bras Dermatol* 2016;91(5 suppl 1): 60–63.

36. Rao PN. Global leprosy strategy 2016–2020: Issues and concerns. *Indian J Dermatol Venereol Leprol.* January 2017–February ;83(1):4–6.

37. Centers for Disease Control and Prevention (CDC). Leprosy. Laboratory Diagnostics. Available at: https://www.cdc.gov/leprosy/health-care-workers/laboratory-diagnostics.html. Accessed on March 20, 2019.

38. World Health Organization (WHO). Guidelines for the diagnosis, treatment and prevention of leprosy. Executive summary. Available at: http://www.searo.who.int/entity/global_leprosy_programme/approved-guidelines-leprosy-executives-summary.pdf?ua=1. Assessed on March 20, 2019.

39. Thapa M, Sendhil Kumaran M, Narang T et al. A prospective study to validate various clinical criteria used in classification of leprosy: A study from a tertiary care center in India. *Int J Dermatol* 2018;57(9):1107–1113.

40. World Health Organization (WHO). *Onchocerciasis— Fact Sheet.* WHO, 2018. Available at: http://www.who.int/news-room/fact-sheets/detail/onchocerciasis. Accessed on September 9, 2018.

41. Veraldi S. Oncocercosi. In: *Dermatologia di importazione*, 2nd edition (Veraldi S and Caputo R, eds). Milano: Poletto Editore, 2000: 203–209.

42. Basáñez MG, Pion SD, Churcher TS et al. River blindness: A success story under threat? *PLoS Med* 2006;3:e371.

43. The Australian Society for Parasitology. *Onchocerca.* The Australian Society for Parasitology, 2018. Available at: http://parasite.org.au/para-site/text/onchocerca-text.html. Accessed on September 9, 2018.

44. Saint André AV, Blackwell NM, Hall LR et al. The role of endosymbiotic *Wolbachia* bacteria in the pathogenesis of river blindness. *Science* 2002;295:1892–1895.

45. Hall LR, Pearlman E. Pathogenesis of onchocercal keratitis (River blindness). *Clin Microbiol Rev* 1999;12:445–453.

46. McKechnie NM, Gürr W, Yamada H et al. Antigenic mimicry: *Onchocerca volvulus* antigen-specific T cells and ocular inflammation. *Invest Ophthalmol Vis Sci* 2002;43:411–418.

47. Stingl P. Onchocerciasis: Developments in diagnosis, treatment and control. *Int J Dermatol* 2009;48:393–396.

48. Van Laethem Y, Lopes C. Treatment of onchocerciasis. *Drugs.* 1996;52:861–869.

49. Hoerauf A, Specht S, Marfo-Debrekyei Y et al. Efficacy of 5-week doxycycline treatment on adult *Onchocerca volvulus. Parasitol Res* 2009;104: 437–447.

50. Giacani L, Lukehart SA. The endemic treponematoses. *ClinMicrobiol Rev.* 2014;27:89–115.

51. Turner TB, Hollander DH. *Biology of the Treponematoses.* Geneva: World Health Organization, 1957.

52. Mitjà O, Hays R, Ipai A et al. Osteoperiostitis in early yaws: Case series and literature review. *Clin Infect Dis* 2011;52:771–774.

53. Mitjà O, Šmajs D, Bassat Q. Advances in the diagnosis of endemic treponematoses: Yaws, bejel, and pinta. *PLoS Negl Trop Dis.* 2013;7:e2283.

54. Hasselmann CM. Comparative studies on the histopathology of syphilis, yaws, and pinta. *Br J Venereal Dis* 1957;33:5–e2212.

55. Fuchs J, Milbradt R, Pecher SA. Tertiary pinta: Case reports and overview. *Cutis* 1993;51:425–430.

56. Garner MF, Backhouse JF, Daskolopolous G, Walsh JL. Treponema pallidum haemagglutination test for yaw; comparison with the TPI and FTA-ABS tests. *Br J Vener Dis* 1972;48:479–482.

57. Menke HE, Veldkamp J, Brunings EA et al. Comparison of cardiolipin and treponemal tests in the serodiagnosis of yaws. *Br J Vener Dis* 1979;55:102–104.

58. Jafari Y, Peeling RW, Shivkumar S et al. Are *Treponema pallidum* specific rapid and point-of-care tests for syphilis accurate enough for screening in resource limited settings? Evidence from a meta-analysis. *PLOS ONE* 2013;8:e54695.

59. Yin YP, Chen XS, Wei W et al. A dual point-of-care test shows good performance in simultaneously detecting non-treponemal and treponemal antibodies in patients with syphilis—A multi-site evaluation study in China. *Clin Infect Dis* 2013;56:659–665.

60. World Health Organization (WHO). Yaws. Available at: https://www.who.int/news-room/fact-sheets/detail/yaws. Accessed on March 20, 2019.

61. Hook EW 3rd. Syphilis. *Lancet* 2017;389:1550–1557.

62. Freitas DMM, Azevedo A, Pinheiro G, Ribeiro R. Psoriasiform papules, condylomalata, lung nodules and hepatitis: The enormous variability of secondary syphilis manifestations. *BMJ Case Rep.* 2017;2017:pii: bcr-2017–219408. doi: 10.1136/bcr-2017–219408.

63. Eyer-Silva WA, Martins CJ, Silva GARD et al. Secondary syphilis presenting as leukoderma syphiliticum: Case report and review. *Rev Inst Med Trop Sao Paulo* 2017;59: e74.

64. Janier M, HegyiV, Dupin N et al. 2014 European guideline on the management of syphilis. *J Eur Acad Dermatol Venereol* 2014;28:1581–1e93.

65. WHO. *Guidelines for the Treatment of* Treponema pallidum *(Syphilis).* Geneva: World Health Organization, 2016.

66. Stamm LV. Syphilis: Antibiotic treatment and resistance. *Epidemiol Infect* 2015;143:1567–1574.

Melanoma leukoderma

21

ALEXANDER J. STRATIGOS, POLYTIMI SIDIROPOULOU, and DOROTHEA POLYDOROU

CONTENTS

Introduction	145	Prognosis	147
Pathogenesis	145	References	147
Clinical picture	145		

INTRODUCTION

Skin depigmentation occurs in 2%–16% of melanoma patients either spontaneously or during/after immunotherapy as a result of strong antimelanoma immunity directed against shared melanocyte differentiation antigens.[1,2,3] It is commonly known as melanoma-associated leukoderma (MAL), but also referred to as melanoma-associated hypopigmentation (MAH), melanoma-associated depigmentation (MAD), or melanoma-associated vitiligo (MAV).[2,4]

MAL can develop in association with primary, recurrent, or metastatic melanoma.[1] Although it may precede melanoma detection, in most cases (79.5%), depigmentation occurs after the diagnosis of melanoma.[3,5] Moreover, in recent years, MAL is increasingly documented in advanced metastatic melanoma patients undergoing treatment with adoptive immune-based therapies with biological response modifiers and/or vaccine strategies.

Immune-based regimes reported to induce MAL include programmed cell death 1 (PD-1; e.g., pembrolizumab, nivolumab) or cytotoxic T-lymphocyte-associated antigen 4 (CTLA-4; e.g., ipilimumab) antibodies (Figure 21.1a,b), BRAF/MEK inhibitors (e.g., vemurafenib, dabrafenib), IL-2, IFN-α, tumor-infiltrating lymphocytes specific for tyrosinase-, gp100-, or TYRP1-derived antigens or peptide vaccines based upon these antigens.[1,3,6–8]

PATHOGENESIS

Although the pathogenesis of MAL still remains elusive, it is considered an immune-driven manifestation illustrating the immunogenic nature of melanoma.[1] Melanoma has traditionally been described as an "immunogenic tumor" that commonly overexpresses several melanocyte differentiation antigens, including Melan-A/MART-1, tyrosinase, TRP-1, TRP-2, and/or gp100, regardless of tumor stage. The immune response elicited against such antigens shared by normal and malignant melanocytes links melanoma and its associated leukodermas.[8]

According to the most prevalent hypothesis, humoral and cell-mediated immune responses targeting melanocyte cross-reactive antigens are involved in modulating an enhanced cytotoxic activity against both tumor cells and normal melanocytes.[3,11] Although autoantibodies are commonly found in melanoma patients, growing evidence points toward an important role for cellular immune reactions. Considering the presence of clonally expanded melanocyte-specific T lymphocytes with identical Vp regions in a primary melanoma and a depigmented halo surrounding the tumor, it has been speculated that MAL results from a cytotoxic T-cell cross-reaction targeting antigenic determinants like MART-1 and gp100 expressed by both healthy and malignant melanocytes.[6]

Such spontaneous or therapy-induced antitumor immunity is responsible for normal melanocyte recognition and attack as well. This is clinically evident as depigmentation either within the melanoma (regression), around melanocytic nevi/melanoma (halo phenomenon), or in a distant site (vitiligo-like depigmentation).[8] It has been suggested that melanoma regression, halo phenomenon, and vitiligo-like lesions are distinct in pathogenesis. Some authors believe that a locally effective immune response against melanoma cells is responsible for the partial or complete regression of the tumor, while the halos and the vitiliginoid phenotype are rather the consequence of the incidental immune destruction of normal epidermal melanocytes.[3,8]

CLINICAL PICTURE

Melanoma can be associated with local or diffuse depigmenting changes. Several types of leukodermas have been described in the setting of melanoma:[3,5,6]

- Spontaneous melanoma regression—Depigmentation associated with spontaneous regression of the tumor (primary, recurrent, or metastatic).
- Halo phenomenon—A localized depigmentation surrounding benign melanocytic nevi or the melanoma.
- Vitiligo-like depigmentation in sites remote from the primary tumor.

Spontaneous melanoma regression

Depigmentation due to melanoma regression is uncommon in older adults.[1] In this process, fibrous stroma progressively replaces the dermal portion of the tumor. From a clinical perspective, areas of tumor depigmentation with white, red, blue, or gray color may be the visible effect of spontaneous regression. However, complete resolution is considered very rare, with approximately 40 cases reported in the literature.[7–9]

Melanoma of unknown origin may represent partially or fully regressed primary tumors.[8] It has been well documented that metastatic melanoma has no detectable primary site in 4%–10% of cases.[1] Melanoma should be considered in adults presenting with a depigmented macule or patch and a history consistent with regression of a pigmented neoplasm. Skin depigmentation associated with a palpable lymph node in the appropriate lymphatic distribution may also be suggestive of a regressed primary melanoma.[1] Depigmentation at the site of a pigmented lesion in adults thus warrants a thorough history and physical investigation aimed at suspicious melanocytic lesions.

Halo phenomenon

The appearance of a rim (halo) of hypopigmentation or depigmentation around a pigmented lesion most commonly occurs in children and young adults surrounding benign acquired melanocytic nevi (halo nevus or Sutton nevus). However, the halo phenomenon can rarely be seen around melanoma. Careful examination of the central lesion is therefore required. The halo of melanoma is more irregular than that of the halo nevus, and the patients are usually older. The sudden appearance of multiple halos around benign melanocytic nevi in older adults may also be a sign of unknown melanoma. Moreover, halos can occur around sites of cutaneous metastatic deposits. Although melanoma-associated halos are rare, individuals beyond 40 years with new-onset halo nevi should be thoroughly examined for melanoma (cutaneous and ocular).[3,6,8]

Vitiligo-like depigmentation

Melanoma-associated vitiligo may represent an important differential diagnosis of vitiligo vulgaris.[5] The occurrence of vitiligo-like lesions in melanoma patients is a well-known even if puzzling and yet poorly understood phenomenon. The risk of developing vitiligo has been estimated to be 7- to 10-fold higher in subjects with melanoma compared with the general population.[8] Although the clinical appearance may be similar, MAL cannot be classified as a subtype of vitiligo according to the Vitiligo Global Issues Consensus Conference.[2,5,11]

The clinical differences and similarities between melanoma-associated and vitiligo vulgaris are not well defined and the literature is contradictory. Some authors consider them identical, while others claim that melanoma-associated vitiligo exhibits a more varied clinical spectrum of manifestations.[10] It is common that patients with MAL have a significantly higher age at onset of depigmentation than vitiligo patients. The median age at onset of MAL is 53–55 years, whereas vitiligo rarely develops in individuals over 50 years of age.[1,2,5,8]

Conflicting data are also reported regarding the distribution pattern of depigmented lesions in MAL versus vitiligo. In the majority of patients, MAL displays a symmetric bilateral distribution corresponding to classic vitiligo, developing in patients with typically no previous history of vitiligo (Figure 21.1). However, atypical clinical presentations of MAL have already been described with mostly hypopigmented macules with irregularly-shaped and not well-demarcated borders as well as confetti-like figuration contrary to vitiligo vulgaris.[5,8,10]

Additional findings that may be suggestive of MAL include the absence of a Koebner phenomenon, a negative vitiligo family history, no gender predilection, and depigmentation localized on photoexposed areas.[1,5] Furthermore, MAL lesions are generally refractory to topical corticosteroids and UV phototherapy.[4] While auto-antibodies against gp-100 and tyrosinase are commonly found in both diseases, serum antibodies against melanoma antigen recognized by T-cells 1 (MART1) are only present in MAL and undetectable in vitiligo. Thus, the presence of MART-1 antibodies may serve as a useful biomarker in order to distinguish MAL from vitiligo and indicate that differences in immunity are involved.[1,2,5]

Interestingly, the clinical features of melanoma-associated vitiligo have been supported to differ depending on the time onset of depigmentation, before or after the detection of melanoma. Vitiligo occurring before melanoma tends to involve younger patients and is mainly generalized with well-defined, round-shaped, milk-white lesions predominantly located on the face, upper limbs, and feet, a picture similar to that of the vulgaris form. In contrast, the clinical pattern of vitiligo appearing after melanoma is distinct from that

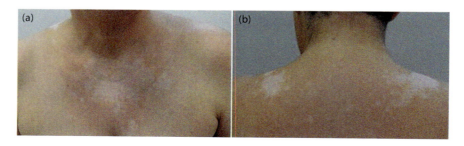

Figure 21.1 (a, b) Vitiligo-like lesions in a 49-year-old woman undergoing anti-PD1 immunotherapy with nivolumab for melanoma.

of vitiligo vulgaris, including pale-colored lesions with not well-demarcated, irregularly shaped borders mainly located on the face and upper trunk.[10]

PROGNOSIS

Although the prognostic impact on the clinical course of melanoma remains a subject of debate, several studies demonstrated that MAL portends a favorable clinical outcome in melanoma patients with significantly enhanced 5-year survival.[3] Given the fact that the antigens recognized by cytotoxic T cells in MAL are common to normal and malignant melanocytes, MAL may represent a marker of antimelanoma immunity. The development of skin depigmentation over the course of immunotherapy is also considered a sign predictive of prolonged efficacy and thus better prognosis.[1,12] Clinical trials of immune-based therapies in advanced metastatic melanoma (stage III-IV) correlated MAL with a durable response and survival benefits, implicating an immune-modulating effect against metastatic disease. It is interesting to note that this prognostic value seems to be independent of the time onset of MAL (before or after melanoma diagnosis). Moreover, no survival differences were found in association with the therapeutic regime.[10]

REFERENCES

1. Saleem MD, Oussedik E, Schoch JJ et al. Acquired disorders with depigmentation: A systematic approach to vitiliginoid conditions. *J Am Acad Dermatol*. 2018. pii: S0190-9622(18)32506-4. doi:10.1016/j.jaad.2018.03.063. [Epub ahead of print].
2. Teulings HE, Willemsen KJ, Glykofridis et al. The antibody response against MART-1 differs in patients with melanoma-associated leucoderma and vitiligo. *Pigment Cell Melanoma Res*. 2014;27:1086–1096.
3. Vyas R, Selph J, Gerstenblith MR. Cutaneous manifestations associated with melanoma. *Semin Oncol*. 2016; 43: 384–389.
4. Teulings HE, Lommerts JE, Wolkerstorfer A et al. Vitiligo-like depigmentations as the first sign of melanoma: A retrospective case series from a tertiary vitiligo centre. *Br J Dermatol*. 2017;176:503–506.
5. Lommerts JE, Teulings HE, Ezzedine K et al. Melanoma-associated leukoderma and vitiligo cannot be differentiated based on blinded assessment by experts in the field. *J Am Acad Dermatol*. 2016;75:1198–1204.
6. Passeron T, Ortonne J. Vitiligo and Other Disorders of Hypopigmentation. In: Callen J, editor. *Dermatology by Jean L. Bolognia, Julie V. Schaffer, and Lorenzo Cerroni*, 4th ed. China: Elsevier, 2018:1108–1109.
7. Ben-Betzalel G, Baruch EN, Boursi B et al. Possible immune adverse events as predictors of durable response to BRAF inhibitors in patients with BRAF V600-mutant metastatic melanoma. *Eur J Cancer*. 2018;101:229–235.
8. Naveh HP, Rao UN, Butterfield LH. Melanoma-associated leukoderma—Immunology in black and white? *Pigment Cell Melanoma Res*. 2013;26:796–804.
9. Spring IR, de Wet J, Jordaan HF et al. Complete spontaneous regression of a metastatic acral melanoma with associated leukoderma. *JAAD Case Rep*. 2017;3:524–528.
10. Quaglino P, Marenco F, Osella-Abate S et al. Vitiligo is an independent favourable prognostic factor in stage III and IV metastatic melanoma patients: results from a single-institution hospital-based observational cohort study. *Ann Oncol*. 2010;21:409–414.
11. Ezzedine K, Lim HW, Suzuki T et al. Revised classification/nomenclature of vitiligo and related issues: The Vitiligo Global Issues Consensus Conference. *Pigment Cell Melanoma Res*. 2012;25:E1–13.
12. González R, Torres-López E. Immunological basis of melanoma-associated vitiligo-like depigmentation. *Actas Dermosifiliogr*. 2014;105:122–127.

Halo nevi

22

CHRISTINA STEFANAKI

CONTENTS

Halo nevi   149

References   151

HALO NEVI

Definition

Halo nevus (HN), also termed Sutton's nevus or leukoderma acquisitum centrifugum, is a benign melanocytic nevus surrounded by an achromic rim that simulates a halo, resulting in regression of the nevus.[1]

Epidemiology

The estimated incidence of HN in the population is around 1%, and there is no predilection for sex or race.[1,2] Children and young adults are predominately affected, with an average age of onset of 15 years.[1,3,4] Stress and puberty have been mentioned as major triggering factors for halo nevi, and a familial tendency has been reported.[5–7] The occurrence of halo nevi has been associated with sun exposure and sunburn, probably because of an increased accentuation of tanned skin contrasting with the depigmented halo.[5] Drugs, such as tocilizumab, an antibody directed against the interleukin (IL)-6 receptor, and anti-TNF-α therapies may also trigger the appearance of multiple halo nevi.[8,9] Those patients who develop halo nevi have in general an increased number of melanocytic nevi, and the halo phenomenon usually presents in multiple lesions in 25%–50% of patients (Figure 22.1), usually on nevi localized on the back.[2,5–7,10]

Clinical features

The appearance of the central melanocytic nevus in halo nevi varies and lesions range from flat to raised and dark brown to pink colored. The surface of the nevus may be crusted or scaly. In typical halo nevi, the central nevus has all the features of a benign melanocytic lesion, measures <5 mm, and has well-defined and smooth borders and homogenous color. The depigmented halo is occasionally preceded by erythema, lasting from weeks to months. The white halo usually is symmetric, with a uniform width ranging from a few millimeters up to several centimeters. Uncommonly, the halo may be asymmetric, although surrounding a benign nevus.[10]

Histologic features

Most commonly compound nevi are involved, although junctional or dermal nevi may be affected as well.[11] Both congenital (Figure 22.2) and acquired nevi may present the halo phenomenon, less commonly compound Spitz nevi and blue nevi.[5–7,12–14] Studies have described variability in the melanocytic atypia of halo nevi; however, although halo nevi arise from a variety of histologic types of nevi, most are not dysplastic.[2,15]

Histopathologically, in the fully evolved stages, a heavy, lichenoid lymphocytic infiltrate within the dermis is noticed, with nevus cells arranged in nests or singly among the inflammatory cells. The lichenoid infiltrate can be so dense that nevus cells are difficult to distinguish from surrounding lymphocytes without special stains. The whitish halo shows an absence of melanin and melanocytes in the basal layer.[11]

Dermoscopy—Reflectance confocal microscopy

Wood's lamp examination may help to enhance the halo, particularly in fair-skinned individuals and to detect multiple lesions. On dermoscopy, the central nevus in halo nevi typically demonstrates the globular and/or homogeneous pattern and the surrounding halo is white and structureless.[16] Less often, the central nevus component may display a reticular pattern.[11] In the case where the central nevus has disappeared, then a reddish central pigmentation, eventually revealing visible vessels from the dermal vascular plexus, may be present. Reflectance confocal microscopy (RCM) of HN has been previously described in two studies, and some atypical features, also seen in atypical melanocytic lesions and malignant melanoma, were observed in most patients evaluated.[11,17] These atypical features included pagetoid cells, non-edged papilla, junctional thickening, nucleated cells in the dermal papillae, and plump bright cells, possibly due to local inflammation.[11,17]

Clinical course

After the development of a halo nevus, its subsequent course is variable and may regress partially or totally, leading to the presence of only the halo. It is described that at least 50% of patients eventually have total disappearance of the central nevus.[5,16] Before disappearance, the central nevus may become irregular and pink. Halo nevi typically persist for a decade or longer and rarely may persist indefinitely. A subgroup may eventually return to normal-appearing skin, but even these lesions persist for an average of 7.8 years.[11] In one study, 51.5% of halo nevi followed up sequentially with digital dermoscopy demonstrated a decrease in halo size, whereas 27.3% showed an enlargement.[16] However, the

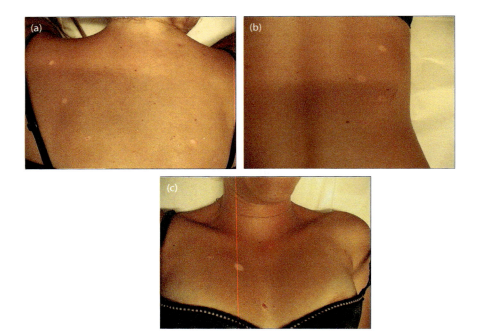

Figure 22.1 (a) Multiple halo nevi on the upper back of a young woman. (b) Multiple halo nevi on the lower back of the same woman. (c) Multiple halo nevi on the chest of the same woman.

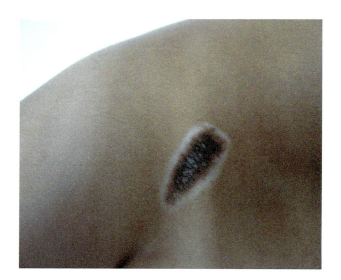

Figure 22.2 Halo medium-sized congenital nevus on the trunk of a girl.

dermoscopic pattern of the nevus remained unchanged as it became smaller. Given that a lesion that displays extensive regression at baseline could eventually completely regress during follow-up and subsequently would no longer be detectable at the next visit, digital dermoscopic follow-up of HN is not recommended, as it does not provide additional diagnostic information compared with a good clinical dermoscopic correlation at baseline.[16]

Differential diagnosis

Halo nevi should be differentiated from nonmelanocytic tumors demonstrating a halo such as dermatofibromas or seborrheic keratosis, among others, and mainly from melanoma presenting with a halo.[10] Although the halo phenomenon is most common in benign melanocytic nevi, there are reports of HN in individuals with a family and/or personal history of melanoma and melanomas with halo.

However, halo melanomas are rare; they occur in adults, demonstrate a more irregular halo, and on dermoscopy exhibit the typical melanoma-specific patterns, including a multicomponent pattern, an atypical pigmented network, irregular dots and globules, irregular streaks, blotches, blue-white veil, and atypical vascular structures.[16,18,19]

Halo nevi and vitiligo—Pathogenesis

HN may be associated with atopic dermatitis or with autoimmune disorders such as vitiligo and Hashimoto thyroiditis.[5] Whether halo nevi should be considered a sign of vitiligo or a risk factor for developing vitiligo is still under debate. Differences in the genetic background have been demonstrated. HLA-DR3 has a negative association and HLA-DR4 and DR53 a positive association with vitiligo, whereas this could not be demonstrated in vitiligo patients with halo nevi.[20] Vitiligo and halo nevi share similar pathophysiological pathways, as both exhibit a strong cytotoxic T-cell reaction, which suggests an immunological reaction against the same melanocyte-specific targets.[14] Whether vitiligo with or without halo nevi constitute different subgroups with differences in degree, mode, or type of surface auto(self)-antigen expression in the initial stage of the disease remains to be elucidated. It has been speculated that if only halo nevi are present, an abnormal auto-antigen expression, originating primarily from melanocytic nevi, is triggering the immune response, while in vitiligo, the auto-antigen originates from normal epidermal melanocytes.[21] According to Van Geel et al.,[21] in cases where both vitiligo and halo nevi are present, the primary immune reaction can be directed to nevoid autoantigens, followed by an immune reaction against shared autoantigens, antigen cross-reactivity, or an epitope spreading phenomenon between nevoid melanocytes and epidermal melanocytes, which might be faster or easier in patients with genetic susceptibility to vitiligo or autoimmune diseases. On the other hand, a second etiopathological pathway might exist in which halo nevi can induce a cytotoxic T-cell-mediated immune reaction against shared antigens between normal melanocytes and nevoid melanocytes in patients without the genetic susceptibility to vitiligo, as seen in melanoma-associated leucoderma.[21]

Some studies point to marked differences in the pathophysiology between halo nevi and vitiligo. Schallreuter et al.[22] observed high H_2O_2 levels in vitiligo skin, which causes impairment of pterin-4a-carbinol-amine dehydratase (PCD), whereas they found upregulated PCD activity in halo nevi. They suggest that low PCD activity leads to oxidation of pterins and causes the characteristic bluish-white fluorescence of vitiligo skin, which is not detectable in halo nevi.[22]

Halo nevi and vitiligo—Clinical

Several case reports have been published regarding the development of vitiligo simultaneously or shortly after the occurrence of a halo naevus.[23–25]

The presence of halo nevi in vitiligo patients ranges in different studies between 1% and 47%.[5,21] However, some cases of extensive vitiligo clearly spare melanocytic nevi.[26]

It has been demonstrated that the presence of halo nevi in patients with vitiligo significantly reduces the risk of associated autoimmune diseases, and the age of onset of vitiligo was significantly lower when compared with vitiligo patients without halo nevi.[21,27] On the other hand, patients with only halo nevi showed less frequently the presence of a Koebner phenomenon and family history of vitiligo.[21]

Body surface area involvement by vitiligo has been found to be lower in patients with both vitiligo and HN, and the trunk tended to be more frequently involved.[20,27] On the contrary, involvement of the hands and feet by vitiligo was negatively associated with HN.[20,27] The question arises whether an increased number of HN increases the risk of vitiligo. Certain investigators have found fewer HN in vitiligo patients,[21] while others demonstrated an association between multiple HN and vitiligo.[28]

Although halo nevi are in general more frequently reported in combination with generalized vitiligo, the concomitant presence of halo nevi with segmental vitiligo has also been described in 1%–6.4% of patients.[29] A controversy exists as to whether there is a link between the progression of segmental vitiligo to mixed vitiligo and the initial presence of halo nevi; some authors have found

an association,[26] while others have not.[5] Interestingly, discrete depigmentations at distance from halo nevi have been described in a limited subset of patients with multiple halo nevi.[5]

Regarding the presence of halo nevi and the prognosis of vitiligo, it has been demonstrated that the presence of a halo nevus does not significantly alter the risk of disease progression and rate of treatment.[30]

Management

The management of the patient with halo nevi should be individualized. All patients should be questioned about family or personal history of melanoma, vitiligo, and autoimmune diseases. Each halo nevus should be inspected carefully for signs of atypia, and a full-body examination is mandatory for vitiligo and in older patients for the presence of melanoma. Only halo nevi with clinical signs of atypia, suggesting a melanoma, need to be removed surgically. Young patients may be reassured, whereas patients aged more than 40 with new onset of halo nevi should be examined very carefully for melanoma.

REFERENCES

1. Aouthmany M, Weinstein M, Zirwas MJ, Brodell RT. The natural history of halo nevi: A retrospective case series. *J Am Acad Dermatol.* 2012;67:582–586.
2. Weyant G, Chung C, Helm K. Halo nevus: Review of the literature and clinicopathologic findings. *Int J Dermatol.* 2015;54:30–447.
3. Haliasos EC, Kerner M, Jaimes N et al. Dermoscopy for the pediatric dermatologist; Part III: Dermoscopy of melanocytic lesions. *Pediatr Dermatol.* 2012; doi:10.1111/pde.12041.
4. Zalaudek I, Manzo M, Ferrara G, Argenziano G. A new classification of melanocytic nevi based on dermoscopy. *Expert Rev Dermatol.* 2008;3:477–489.
5. Van Geel N, Speeckaert R, Lambert J et al. Halo naevi with associated vitiligo-like depigmentations: Pathogenetic hypothesis. *J Eur Acad Dermatol Venereol.* 2012;26: 755–761.
6. MacKie RM. Disorders of the cutaneous melanocyte: halo naevus. In: Burns T, Breathnach S, Cox N, Griffith C, eds. *Rook's Textbook of Dermatology.* Vol 2. 7th ed. Oxford, England: Blackwell Scientific Publications, 2004: 1–39.
7. Herd RM, Hunter JA. Familial halo naevi. *Clin Exp Dermatol.* 1998;23:68–69.
8. Kuet K, Goodfield M. Multiple halo naevi associated with tocilizumab. *Clin Exp Dermatol.* 2014;39:717–719.
9. Thivi Maruthappu T, Leandro M, Morris M. Deterioration of vitiligo and new onset of halo naevi observed in two patients receiving adalimumab. *Dermatologic Therapy* 2013;26:370–372.
10. Rabinovitz HS, Barnhill R. Benign melanocytic neoplasms: halo nevus. In: Bolognia JL, Jorizzo JL, Schaffer JV, eds. *Dermatology.* Vol 2. 3rd ed. Elsevier, 2012;1851–1880.

11. Larre Borges A, Zalaudek I, Longo C et al. Melanocytic nevi with special features: Clinical-dermoscopic and reflectance confocal microscopic-findings. *J Eur Acad Dermatol Venereol*. 2014;28:833–845.

12. Kerr OA, Schlofield O. Halo congenital nevi. *Pediatr Dermatol*. 2003;20:541–542.

13. Harvell JD, Meehan SA, LeBoit PE. Spitz's nevi with halo reaction: A histopathologic study of 17 cases. *J Cutan Pathol*. 1997;24:611–619.

14. Zeff RA, Freitag A, Grin CM, Grant-Kels JM. The immune response in halo nevi. *J Am Acad Dermatol*. 1997;37:620–624.

15. Mooney MA, Barr RJ, Buxton MG. Halo nevus or halo phenomenon? A study of 142 cases. *J Cutan Pathol*. 1995;22: 342–348.

16. Kolm I, Di Stefani A, Hofmann-Wellenhof R et al. Dermoscopy patterns of halo nevi. *Arch Dermatol*. 2006;142:1627–1632.

17. Schwartz RJ, Vera K, Navarrete N, Lobos P. *In vivo* reflectance confocal microscopy of halo nevus. *J Cutan Med Surg*. 2013;17:33–38.

18. Argenziano G, Soyer HP, Chimenti S et al. Dermoscopy of pigmented skin lesions: Results of a consensus meeting via the Internet. *J Am Acad Dermatol*. 2003;48:679–693.

19. Zalaudek I, Argenziano G, Ferrara G et al. Clinically equivocal melanocytic skin lesions with features of regression: A dermoscopic-pathological study. *Br J Dermatol*. 2004;150:64–71.

20. De Vijlder HC, Westerhof W, Schreuder GM et al. Difference in pathogenesis between vitiligo vulgaris and halo nevi associated with vitiligo is supported by an HLA study. *Pigment Cell Res*. 2004;17: 270–274.

21. Van Geel N, Vandenhaute S, Speeckaert R et al. Prognostic value and clinical significance of halo naevi regarding vitiligo. *Br J Dermatol*. 2011;164:743–749.

22. Schallreuter KU, Kothari S, Elwary S et al. Molecular evidence that halo in Sutton's naevus is not vitiligo. *Arch Dermatol Res*. 2003;295:223–228.

23. Kim HS, Goh BK. Vitiligo after halo formation around congenital melanocytic nevi. *Pediatr Dermatol*. 2009;26: 755–756.

24. Itin PH, Lautenschlager S. Acquired leukoderma in congenital pigmented nevus associated with vitiligo depigmentation. *Pediatr Dermatol*. 2002;19: 73–75.

25. Stierman SC, Tierney E, Shwayder TA. Halo congenital nevocellular nevi associated with extralesional vitiligo: Case series with review of the literature. *Pediatr Dermatol*. 2009;26: 414–424.

26. Ezzedine K, Diallo A, Leaute-Labreze C et al. Halo naevi and leukotrichia are strong predictors of the passage to mixed vitiligo in a subgroup of segmental vitiligo. *Br J Dermatol*. 2012;166:539–544.

27. Ezzedine K, Diallo A, Léauté-Labrèze C et al. Halo nevi association in nonsegmental vitiligo affects age at onset and depigmentation pattern. *Arch Dermatol*. 2012;148:497–502.

28. Patrizi A, Bentivogli M, Raone B et al. Association of halo nevus/i and vitiligo in childhood: A retrospective observational study. *J Eur Acad Dermatol Venereol*. 2013;27:e148–e152.

29. van Geel NA, Mollet IG, De Schepper S et al. First histopathological and immunophenotypic analysis of early dynamic events in a patient with segmental vitiligo associated with halo nevi. *Pigment Cell Melanoma Res*. 2010;23:375–384.

30. Cohen BE, Mu EW, Orlow SJ. Comparison of childhood vitiligo presenting with or without associated halo nevi. *Pediatr Dermatol*. 2016;33:44–48.

Drug-induced hypopigmentation

23

KATERINA DAMEVSKA, SUZANA NIKOLOVSKA, RAZVIGOR DARLENSKI, LJUBICA SUTURKOVA, and TORELLO LOTTI

CONTENTS

Introduction	153	Topical drugs	155
Systemic drugs	153	References	156

INTRODUCTION

Drug-induced hypopigmentation refers to the development of skin and/or hair hypopigmentation or depigmentation associated with the use of a medication. This adverse drug reaction is assumed to be relatively rare, and is most commonly associated with topical agents.[1] However, the increasing use of target therapies will make the observation of these side effects more frequent.

Drug-induced hypopigmentations can be particularly difficult to diagnose and differentiate from vitiligo. Thus, if a patient presents with unexplained hypomelanosis, drugs should be included in the differential diagnosis as a possible cause.

SYSTEMIC DRUGS

Targeted antineoplastic agents

Various cutaneous adverse events of targeted therapy have been reported, nevertheless pigmentary changes associated with these treatments have received less attention.[2] Dai et al. identified 36 clinical trials involving 8052 patients that reported on pigmentary adverse events associated with targeted therapies.[3] The overall incidence of pigmentary changes was 17.7%, with the lowest incidence noted with pazopanib (0.7%) and the highest with sunitinib (75%). In pediatric patients, pigmentary abnormalities were reported in 13% of patients receiving imatinib, dasatinib, and cabozantinib.[4] However, the pigmentary changes did not represent a negative prognostic factor, nor imply the necessity for treatment discontinuation.[3]

Tyrosine kinase inhibitors

According to their molecular mechanism of action, tyrosine kinase inhibitors (TKIs) directly or indirectly target the crucial modulators of pigmentation, namely c-KIT and its ligand stem cell factor (SCF). Thus, it is not surprising that interference with this pathway results in pigmentary anomalies. In most cases, the depigmentation due to TKIs is reversible, suggesting that these drugs might determine a temporary dysfunction of melanocytes rather than having a cytotoxic effect. It is not completely clear why TKIs may cause both hypo- or hyperpigmentation. In one series, 3.6% of patients treated with imatinib experienced hyperpigmentation.[5] Both hair lightening and hair darkening have been reported during TKI treatment.[6] In part, the different effects of TKIs on melanin production could be explained by the inhibiting activity of these drugs on other receptors, such as vasoactive endothelial growth factor receptor (VEGFR) or platelet-derived growth factor receptor (PDGFR).[6]

Imatinib

Imatinib is an oral TKI that inhibits Bcr-Abl, PDGFR, and c-Kit. Localized or diffuse, in the majority of cases, reversible depigmentation has been observed in 15%–25% of patients.[5,7] The fact that the depigmentation is frequent and dose-dependent suggests that it is due to a direct pharmacological effect of imatinib.[7] Cases of cutaneous, hair, nail, or gingival pigmentation,[5–8] as well as repigmentation of vitiligo lesions,[9] have also been described.

Dasatinib

Dasatinib is another TKI that targets the Bcr-Abl tyrosine kinase, c-Kit, PDGFR, and Src family kinases. In reported cases, hypopigmentation began 1 to 6 months following treatment initiation, appears to be dose dependent, and has a predilection for the head and neck. Repigmentation began within 8 weeks of drug cessation.[10] Cases of reversible hair depigmentation have been described using ≥100 mg daily of dasatinib.[11]

Pazopanib

Pazopanib is a second-generation TKI with multiple targets including VEGFR, PDGFR, c-Kit, and FGFR. Goyal et al. reported a series of patients with breast cancer treated with pazopanib in combination with radiation. Two patients (17%) experienced hair lightening, one of whom also had skin hypopigmentations outside of the treatment field.[12] Sideras et al. observed that at least half of patients treated with pazopanib developed both hair and skin hypopigmentation, with some patients experiencing hypopigmentation to a degree otherwise encountered only in albinism. The authors speculated that the potent dual inhibition of c-Kit and PDGFR by pazopanib may account for this phenomenon.[13]

154 Drug-induced hypopigmentation

Sunitinib

Sunitinib is an orally bioavailable molecule that inhibits multiple receptor tyrosine kinases, including VEGFR-2, PDGFR, and c-Kit receptor. Sunitinib is associated with many cutaneous side effects, including acral erythema, bullous dermatosis, edema, stomatitis, subungual splinter hemorrhages, hand-foot syndrome, leukotrichia,[14] and depigmentation of the face.[15]

Sorafenib

Sorafenib is a multitarget TKI that inhibits VEGFR 1–3, BRAF, and RET tyrosine kinase. To date, only one case of reversible generalized depigmentation has been described during treatment with sorafenib.[16]

Immune checkpoint inhibitors

Immune checkpoint inhibitors (ICIs) may target cytotoxic T-lymphocyte antigen 4, programmed cell death 1 (PD-1), or its ligand (PD-L1). The activation of the immune system may lead to a spectrum of immune-related adverse events (irAEs), including vitiligo-like depigmentation. The cumulative incidence of depigmentation in melanoma patients receiving ICI ranges from 9.6% to 25%.[17,18] According to Larsbal et al.,[19] these depigmentations are clinically and biologically distinct from vitiligo. Some studies suggest that patients with metastatic melanoma (MM) have shown an association between depigmentation following ICI treatment, and beneficial clinical outcomes.[17–20] Hypopigmentation is not a common side effect in patients with other cancers who receive ICI.[21]

Pembrolizumab

Pembrolizumab is a selective humanized monoclonal IgG4 antibody that binds to the PD-1 receptor and blocks its interaction with PD-L1. Vitiligo-like depigmentation is a well-described side effect of pembrolizumab. Of 67 patients with MM who received pembrolizumab, 17 (25%) developed hypopigmentation. The time to onset of hypopigmentation ranged from 52 to 453 days. Complete or partial response to treatment was associated with a higher occurrence of hypopigmentation (71% vs 28%; P = 0.002). The authors concluded that these visible irAEs could be associated with the clinical benefit to pembrolizumab.[18] In contrast to ordinary vitiligo, patients did not report any personal or family history of vitiligo, thyroiditis, or other autoimmune disorders.[19] The most common involved skin sites in post anti-PD1 depigmentation are sun-exposed areas (Figure 23.1).

Recently, Wolner et al.[22] described a patient with MM treated with pembrolizumab who subsequently developed lightening of the skin, poliosis, and fading of solar lentigines, seborrhoeic keratoses, and melanocytic nevi.

Nivolumab

Nakamura et al.[23] reviewed stage III or IV melanoma patients treated with anti-PD-1 antibody nivolumab. Of 35 patients, 9 (25.7%) developed vitiligo-like depigmentation. The time to onset ranged from 2 to 9 months after the initiation of treatment. The objective response rate was higher in patients with depigmentation than in patients without (44.4% vs 7.7%; P = 0.027). Depigmentation was significantly associated with better overall survival. These observations suggest that the occurrence of depigmentation during nivolumab treatment may be associated with favorable outcomes. Nivolumab has recently been reported to induce hypopigmentation in a patient with a nonmelanoma malignancy.[24]

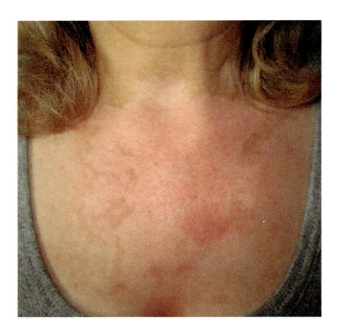

Figure 23.1 Pembrolizumab-induced depigmentation in a patient with metastatic melanoma. There was no personal or family history of vitiligo.

Durvalumab

Durvalumab is an IgG1 monoclonal antibody that binds to PD-1 and CD80, allowing T cells to recognize tumor cells. In the combined safety database (n = 1414), immune-mediated rash occurred in 220 patients (15.6%), and 4 patients (0.3%) developed hypopigmentation.[25]

Antimalarial drugs

Chloroquine is classically associated with bluish-black or gray pigmentation of the skin and mucosa, attributed to the deposition of the drug in the affected tissues. Case reports suggest that chloroquine can also cause depigmentation[26] and bleaching of hair pigment.[27] Depigmented patches are most prominent on sun-exposed areas, starting a few months after initiation of chloroquine therapy and readily reversible after cessation of the drug.

Hematopoietic stem cell transplantation

A population-based study found newly acquired vitiligo-like depigmentation in 1% of hematopoietic stem cell transplantation (HSCT) recipients.[28] In another study, 15 (5.3%) participants with vitiligo were identified among 282 patients with chronic GvHD. Pigmentary changes

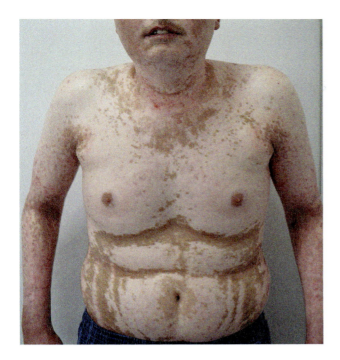

Figure 23.2 Leucoderma in chronic GvHD 24 months after allogeneic hematopoietic stem cell transplantation. There was no personal or family history of vitiligo.

developed in a median of 41 months after transplantation.[29] Allogeneic HSCT-associated leucoderma has been reported as localized disease, generalized involvement (Figure 23.2), and total leukoderma. T-cell recognition of foreign melanocyte antigens may elicit a persistent immune response against host melanocytes.[30]

Miscellaneous

Rare cases of drug-induced hypopigmentation have been reported from anticonvulsants, ganciclovir, arsenic-based antineoplastic drugs, interferon-a, proton pump inhibitors, levodopa, psoralens, and psoralen-UVA (PUVA) photochemotherapy.[1,31–33]

TOPICAL DRUGS

Topical glucocorticosteroids

Hypopigmentation after use of topical corticosteroids (TCS) may occur, but is more noticeable in dark-skinned individuals.[34] According to an FDA report, depigmentation or discoloration is the second most frequent adverse event in the pediatric population, observed in 30 of 202 patients.[35] Depigmentation occurs regularly with prolonged treatment and is dependent on the chemical nature of the drug, the vehicle, and the site of its application (Figure 23.3). These lesions are generally reversible upon discontinuation of steroid therapy. It has been postulated that TCS probably interferes with the synthesis of melanin by smaller melanocytes.

Several case reports have documented local hypopigmentation after intralesional, periocular, or intraarticular injection of steroids.[36–38] Triamcinolone

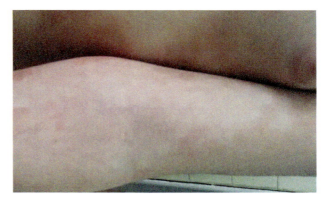

Figure 23.3 Hypopigmentation due to topical steroid abuse in the treatment of flexural eczema.

acetonide causes hypopigmentation more frequently than other steroids.[38] As a macromolecule with suspended crystals, triamcinolone can spread along lymphatic channels and proximal veins, causing ill-defined, linear, stellate, or angulated hypopigmented macules. Differentiation from segmental vitiligo is based on a history of intralesional injection and the pattern and ill-defined border of the lesion. Corticosteroid-induced hypopigmentation can be seen after single or multiple injections and, in the majority of cases, resolves after a few months. Probably the main mechanism of action is reversible inhibition of the function of melanocytes.[37]

Topical imiquimod

A few case reports have documented vitiligo-like depigmentation and poliosis associated with imiquimod treatment. This side effect has been reported in imiquimod treatment of genital warts (Figure 23.4), verruca vulgaris,

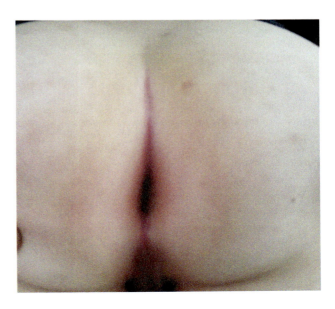

Figure 23.4 Imiquimod-induced hypopigmentation following treatment of perianal warts in a child.

molluscum contagiosum, basal cell carcinoma, lentigo maligna, and extramammary Paget disease.[39–41] Depigmentation is rarely associated with imiquimod use for the treatment of actinic keratoses, which may be due to the twice-weekly dosing regimen.[40]

Duration of therapy to onset of pigment loss ranges from 7 to 28 weeks. Hypopigmentation is confined to the treated area and may be transient or long lasting. The possible mechanisms of hypopigmentation include cytotoxic T lymphocyte-mediated immune reaction, increased sensitivity of melanocytes to oxidative stress, and local apoptosis of melanocytes.[42]

Topical immunotherapy

Repeated applications of diphenylcyclopropenone (DPCP), dinitrochlorobenzene, and squaric acid dibutylester (SADBE) stimulate an immune response and may potentially be useful in the treatment of alopecia areata and recalcitrant warts. Few studies report leucoderma as a side effect of treatment with DPCP[43] and SADBE.[44] Leukoderma may be related to a direct cytotoxic effect on the melanocytes or may represent a Koebner phenomenon to individuals predisposed to vitiligo.[45] Topical immunotherapy should be discontinued at the earliest sign of pigment loss. Repigmentation may occur with application of topical steroids and/or phototherapy, but complete recovery is uncertain.[45]

Transdermal patch

Ghasri et al.[46] identified 51 cases of chemical leukoderma associated with the use of methylphenidate transdermal system. The time to onset ranged from 2 months to 4 years after the initiation of treatment. In most cases, the hypopigmentation was limited to the areas around where the patch was rotated. However, seven patients also reported leucoderma on parts of the body where the patch was never applied; three cases reported continued spread of leukoderma after treatment was discontinued. In 2015, the FDA added a warning to the drug label that permanent loss of skin color may occur with use of the methylphenidate transdermal system.[47]

Recently, Prakash and Chand[48] described a case of leukoderma at the application site of dopamine agonist rotigotine, formulated in a silicone-based transdermal system.

Miscellaneous

Streaky hypopigmentation has been reported as an adverse effect of intralesional injection with lignocaine. The pattern of the hypopigmentation suggests that it is the result of the local spread of the drug along the cutaneous lymphatic vessels.[49]

A number of other topical drugs have been associated with hypopigmentation, including thiotepa, tretinoin, arsenic- and mercury-containing preparations, trichloroacetic acid, benzoyl peroxide, benzyl alcohol, physostigmine, retinoic acid, hydrogen peroxide, carmustine, and liquid amyl nitrite.[1,50–52]

Several cases of depigmentation have been reported at injection sites of paraffin,[53] interferon beta-1a,[54] and botulinum toxin A.[55]

REFERENCES

1. Nicolaidou E, Katsambas AD. Pigmentation disorders: Hyperpigmentation and hypopigmentation. *Clin Dermatol.* January 2014–February;32(1):66–72.
2. Ross JS, Schenkein DP, Pietrusko R et al. Targeted therapies for cancer 2004. *Am J Clin Pathol.* October 2004;122(4):598–609.
3. Dai J, Belum VR, Wu S et al. Pigmentary changes in patients treated with targeted anticancer agents: A systematic review and meta-analysis. *J Am Acad Dermatol.* 2017;77(5):902–910.e2.
4. Belum VR, Washington C, Pratilas CA et al. Dermatologic adverse events in pediatric patients receiving targeted anticancer therapies: A pooled analysis. *Pediatr Blood Cancer.* 2015;62(5):798–806.
5. Arora B, Kumar L, Sharma A et al. Pigmentary changes in chronic myeloid leukemia patients treated with imatinibmesylate. *Ann Oncol.* 2004;15(2):358–359.
6. Mariani S, Abruzzese E, Basciani S et al. Reversible hair depigmentation in a patient treated with imatinib. *Leuk Res.* 2011;35(6):e64–e66.
7. Valeyrie L, Bastuji-Garin S, Revuz J et al. Adverse cutaneous reactions to imatinib (STI571) in Philadelphia chromosome-positive leukemias: A prospective study of 54 patients. *J Am Acad Dermatol.* 2003;48:201–206.
8. Balagula Y, Pulitzer MP, Maki RG, Myskowski PL. Pigmentary changes in a patient treated with imatinib. *J Drugs Dermatol.* 2011;10:1062.
9. Han H, Yu YY, Wang YH. Imatinibmesylate-induced repigmentation of vitiligo lesions in a patient with recurrent gastrointestinal stromal tumors. *J Am Acad Dermatol.* 2008;59:S80–S83.
10. Brazzelli V, Grasso V, Barbaccia V et al. Hair depigmentation and vitiligo-like lesions in a leukaemic paediatric patient during chemotherapy with dasatinib. *Acta Derm Venereol.* 2012;92:218–219.
11. Fujimi A, Ibata S, Kanisawa Y et al. Reversible skin and hair depigmentation during chemotherapy with dasatinib for chronic myeloid leukemia. *J Dermatol.* January 2016;43(1):106–107.
12. Goyal S, Shah S, Khan AJ et al. Evaluation of acute locoregional toxicity in patients with breast cancer treated with adjuvant radiotherapy in combination with pazopanib. *ISRN Oncol.* 2012;2012:896202.
13. Sideras K, Menefee ME, Burton JK et al. Profound hair and skin hypopigmentation in an African American woman treated with the multi-targeted tyrosine kinase inhibitor pazopanib. *J Clin Oncol.* July 1, 2010;28(19):e312–e313.
14. Hartmann JT, Kanz L. Sunitinib and periodic hair depigmentation due to temporary c-KIT inhibition. *Arch Dermatol.* 2008;144:1525–1526.

15. Al Enazi MM, Kadry R, Mitwali H. Skin depigmentation induced by sunitinib treatment of renal cell carcinoma. *J Am Acad Dermatol.* November 2009;61(5):905–906.

16. Hussain SZ, Asghar A, Ikram M, Islam N. Development of skin hypopigmentation in a patient with metastatic papillary carcinoma thyroid treated with Sorafenib. *BMC Endocrine Disorders.* 2013;13:29.

17. Freeman-Keller M, Kim Y, Cronin H et al. Nivolumab in resected and unresectable metastatic melanoma: Characteristics of immune-related adverse events and association with outcomes. *Clin Cancer Res.* February 15, 2016;22(4):886–894.

18. Hua C, Boussemart L, Mateus C et al. Association of vitiligo with tumor response in patients with metastatic melanoma treated with pembrolizumab. *JAMA Dermatol.* 2016;152:45–51.

19. Larsabal M, Marti A, Jacquemin C et al. Vitiligo-like lesions occurring in patients receiving anti-programmed cell death-1 therapies are clinically and biologically distinct from vitiligo. *J Am Acad Dermatol.* May 2017;76(5):863–870.

20. Teulings HE, Limpens J, Jansen SN et al. Vitiligo-like depigmentation in patients with stage III–IV melanoma receiving immunotherapy and its association with survival: A systematic review and meta-analysis. *J Clin Oncol.* 2015;33:773–781.

21. Postow MA, Sidlow R, Hellmann MD. Immune-related adverse events associated with immune checkpoint blockade. *N Engl J Med.* January 11, 2018;378(2):158–168.

22. Wolner ZJ, Marghoob AA, Pulitzer MP et al. A case report of disappearing pigmented skin lesions associated with pembrolizumab treatment for metastatic melanoma. *Br J Dermatol.* January 2018;178(1):265–269.

23. Nakamura Y, Tanaka R, Asami Y et al. Correlation between vitiligo occurrence and clinical benefit in advanced melanoma patients treated with nivolumab: A multi-institutional retrospective study. *J Dermatol.* February 2017;44(2):117–122.

24. Yin ES, Totonchy MB, Leventhal JS. Nivolumab-associated vitiligo-like depigmentation in a patient with acute myeloid leukemia: A novel finding. *JAAD Case Rep.* 2017 2;3(2):90–92.

25. Imfinzi significantly reduces the risk of disease worsening or death in the Phase III PACIFIC trial for Stage III unresectable lung cancer. AstraZeneca; May 12, 2017. https://www.astrazeneca.com/media-centre/press-releases/2017. Accessed July 31, 2017.

26. Martín-García RF, del R Camacho N, Sánchez JL. Chloroquine-induced, vitiligo-like depigmentation. *J Am Acad Dermatol.* June 2003;48(6):981–983.

27. Donovan JC, Price VH. Images in clinical medicine. Chloroquine-induced hair hypopigmentation. *N Engl J Med.* 2010;363:372.

28. Bae JM, Choi KH, Jung HM et al. Subsequent vitiligo after hematopoietic stem cell transplantation: A nationwide population-based cohort study from Korea. *J Am Acad Dermatol.* March 2017;76(3):459–463.

29. Zuo RC, Naik HB et al. Risk factors and characterization of vitiligo and alopecia areata in patients with chronic graft-vs-host disease. *JAMA Dermatol.* 2015;151(1):23–32.

30. Tan AW, Koh LP, Goh BK. Leucoderma in chronic graft-versus-host disease: Excellent repigmentation with noncultured cellular grafting. *Br J Dermatol.* 2011;165(2):435–437.

31. Mimouni D, David M, Feinmesser M et al. Vitiligo-like leucoderma during photochemotherapy for mycosis fungoides. *Br J Dermatol.* 2001;145:1008–1014.

32. Zhu H, Hu J, Chen L et al. J. The 12-year follow-up of survival, chronic adverse effects, and retention of arsenic in patients with acute promyelocytic leukemia. *Blood.* 2016 15;128(11):1525–1528.

33. Holla AP, Kumar R, Parsad D, Kanwar A. Proton pump inhibitor induced depigmentation in vitiligo. *J Cutan Aesthet Surg.* January 2011;4(1):46–47.

34. Hengge UR, Ruzicka T, Schwartz RA, Cork MJ. Adverse effects of topical glucocorticosteroids. *J Am Acad Dermatol.* 2006;54:1–15.

35. Weaver J. Postmarketing safety review—PID D010141. Drugs: Topical corticosteroids. FDA Web site. July 9, 2001. Available at: http://www.fda.gov/ohrms/dockets/ac/03/briefing/3999B1_21_Weaver-Memo%2007-09-01.pdf. Accessed on May 5, 2019.

36. Gupta AK, Rasmussen JE. Perilesional linear atrophic streaks associated with intralesional corticosteroid injections in a psoriatic plaque. *Pediatr Dermatol.* 1987;4:259–260.

37. Shah CP, Rhee D, Garg SJ. Eyelid cutaneous hypopigmentation after sub-tenon triamcinolone injection after retinal detachment repair. *Retin Cases Brief Rep.* 2012 Summer;6(3):271–272.

38. Salvatierra AR, Alweis R. Permanent hypo-pigmentation after triamcinolone injection for tennis elbow. *J Commun Hosp Int Med Perspect.* July 6, 2016;6(3):31814.

39. Kwon HH, Cho KH. Induction of vitiligo-like hypopigmentation after imiquimod treatment of extramammary Paget's disease. *Ann Dermatol.* 2012;24:482–484.

40. Burnett CT, Kouba DJ. Imiquimod-induced depigmentation: Report of two cases and review of the literature. *Dermatol Surg.* 2012;38:1872–1875.

41. Kim NH, Lee JB, Yun SJ. Development of vitiligo-like depigmentation after treatment of lentigo maligna melanoma with 5% imiquimod cream. *Ann Dermatol.* August 2018;30(4):454–457.

42. Mashiah J, Brenner S. Possible mechanisms in the induction of vitiligo-like hypopigmentation by topical imiquimod. *Clin Exp Dermatol.* 2008;33:74–76.

43. Hatzis J, Gourgiotou K, Tosca A, Stratigos J. Vitiligo as a reaction to topical treatment with diphencyprone. *Dermatologica.* 1988;177:146–148.

44. Nasca MR, Micali G, Pulvirenti N et al. Transient leucoderma appearing in an untreated area following contact immunotherapy for alopecia areata. *Eur J Dermatol*. March 1998;8(2):125–126.

45. Ganzetti G, Simonetti O, Campanati A et al. Phototherapy as a useful therapeutic option in the treatment of diphenylcyclopropenone-induced vitiligo. *Acta Derm Venereol*. November 2010;90(6): 642–643.

46. Ghasri P, Gattu S, Saedi N, Ganesan AK. Chemical leukoderma after the application of a transdermal methylphenidate patch. *J Am Acad Dermatol*. June 2012;66(6):e237–e238.

47. Center for Drug Evaluation and Research. FDA Drug Safety Communication: FDA reporting permanent skin color changes associated with use of Daytrana patch (methylphenidate transdermal system) for treating ADHD. U.S. Food and Drug Administration, FDA. www.fda.gov/Drugs/DrugSafety/ucm452244.htm.

48. Prakash N, Chand P. Chemical leukoderma: A rare adverse effect of the rotigotine patch. *Mov Disord Clin Pract*. 2017;4(5):781–783.

49. Yadav S, Gupta S, Kumar R, Dogra S. Streaky hypopigmentation following lignocaine injection: An unusual side effect. *J Cutan Aesthet Surg*. January 2012;5(1):61–62.

50. Harben DJ, Cooper PH, Rodman OG. Thiotepa-induced leukoderma. *Arch Dermatol*. 1979;115(8):973–974.

51. Zackheim HS, Epstein EH Jr, McNutt NS et al. Topical carmustine (BCNU) for mycosis fungoides and related disorders: A 10-year experience. *J Am Acad Dermatol*. 1983;9(3):363–374.

52. Vine K, Meulener M, Shieh S, Silverberg NB. Vitiliginous lesions induced by amyl nitrite exposure. *Cutis*. March 2013;91(3):129–136.

53. Kim SW, Han TY, Lee JH et al. A case of vitiligo associated with paraffin injection. *Annals of Dermatology*. 2014;26(6):775–776.

54. Coghe G, Atzori L, Frau J et al. Localized pigmentation disorder after subcutaneous pegylated interferon beta-1a injection. *Mult Scler*. February 2018;24(2):231–233.

55. Roehm PC, Perry JD, Girkin CA, Miller NR. Prevalence of periocular depigmentation after repeated botulinum toxin a injections in African American patients. *J Neuroophthalmol*. March 1999;19(1):7–9.

Hypopigmentation from chemical and physical agents

24

KATERINA DAMEVSKA, IGOR PEEV, RANTHILAKA R. RANAWAKA, and VIKTOR SIMEONOVSKI

CONTENTS

Introduction	159	Hypopigmentation from physical agents	161
Chemical leukoderma	159	References	162

INTRODUCTION

Hypopigmentation from chemical and physical agents represents a post-inflammatory hypopigmentation, a reactive hypomelanosis that develops following external insults to the skin. It is most prominent among dark-skinned individuals, as the contrast between affected and nonaffected skin is more noticeable.[1] In fair-skinned individuals, these lesions may require Wood's lamp illumination to become obvious.

Physical and chemical agents can alter skin pigmentation in various ways. Whether the end result is a gain or loss of melanocyte activity depends on the nature of the inciting agent, while host susceptibility is equally important. The term "individual chromatic tendency" was initially coined by Ruiz-Maldonado to describe this inherited chromatic tendency.[1]

Occasionally, both hyperpigmentation and hypopigmentation will occur in the same individual.

Among physical causes, heat, cold, and ionizing and nonionizing radiation are known to alter skin pigmentation. Skin damage with post-inflammatory leukoderma can be caused by a great variety of chemicals.[2]

CHEMICAL LEUKODERMA

Chemical leukoderma, also known as occupational or contact leukoderma, is an acquired hypopigmentary disorder after a single or multiple exposures to melano-cytotoxic or depigmenting chemicals.[3]

The first case of chemical leukoderma was reported in 1939 in tannery workers who had experienced total loss of pigmentation from their hands and forearms. Additional studies confirmed that agerite alba, a monobenzyl ether of hydroquinone (HQ), added in rubber gauntlet gloves was indeed the culprit.[2] Since then, numerous chemicals causing chemical leukoderma have been reported (Table 24.1). Phenols and aromatic or aliphatic catechol-derivatives as well as sulfhydryl compounds are common culprits.[4]

Chemical leukoderma is mostly an industrial hazard. However, it can also occur from exposure to common

Table 24.1 Chemicals reported to induce hypopigmentation

Hydroquinone (HQ)
Monobenzyl ether of HQ
Monomethyl ether of HQ
Monoethyl ether of HQ
p-Tertiary amylphenol
p-Phenyl phenol
p-Octylphenol
p-Nonylphenol
Buthylhydroxytoluene (BHT)
Buthylhydroxyanisole (BHA)
p-Cresol (4-methylphenol)
Para-tertiary butylphenol formaldehyde resin (PTBP)
p-Methylcatechol
p-Isopropylcatechol
Pyrocatechol (1,2-benzenediol)
Diisopropyl fluorophosphates
β-mercaptoethylamine hydrochloride (cysteamine)
N-(2-mercaptoethyl)-demethylamine hydrochloride
Sulfanolic acid
Cystamine dihydrochloride
3-Mercaptopropylamine hydrochloride

Source: Adapted from Bonamonte D et al. *Dermatitis.* 2016;27(3):90–9.

consumer products. Many substituted phenols were used as antioxidants or rust inhibitors in the manufacture of plastics, resins, lubricants, petroleum products, photographic chemicals, insecticides, printing inks, disinfectants, synthetic rubber, paints, deodorants, and germicides.[2,3,5] Some of the most common chemicals that cause chemical leukoderma are formaldehyde, azo dyes, and para-phenylenediamine (PPD).

Skin-lightening agents

Hypopigmentation is a recognized effect of skin-lightening products. The most important indications for the use of lightening agents in the White population are melasma, dyschromia of photoageing, and post-inflammatory hyperpigmentation (PIH). The practice of skin bleaching for a cosmetic purpose is becoming more common in non-White populations throughout the world. The prevalence of voluntary depigmentation among different population groups ranges from 25% to 67%. Included are the active principles of HQ, glucocorticoids, mercury iodide, plant extracts, and caustic agents.[6]

Hydroquinone

Hydroquinone is the most commonly used bleaching agent and the gold standard for treatment of hyperpigmentation. Chronic adverse effects include exogenous ochronosis, cataract, colloid milia, nail pigmentation, impaired wound healing, and fish odor. There are infrequent reports of confetti-like, 1–3 mm hypopigmented macules.[7]

Mequinol

Monomethyl ether of HQ, also known as *p*-hydroxyanisole or mequinol, produces side effects like burning, contact dermatitis, and ochronosis. Recently, a case of irregular leukoderma following mequinol was described.[8]

Rhododendrol

Rhododendrol, 4-(4-hydroxyphenyl)-2-butanol, a naturally occurring phenolic compound in plants such as *Acer nikoense* and *Betula platyphylla*, was developed as a tyrosinase (TYR) inhibitor for lightening cosmetics. Recently, an outbreak of patients with leukoderma occurred in Japan with the use of cosmetics containing rhododendrol. Patients developed leukoderma mostly at the contact site, but some at nonexposed areas, too. The intensity of rhododendrol exposure did not correlate to the severity of depigmentation. In most cases, repigmentation is observed after treatment discontinuation.[9]

Cosmetic preparations containing mercury

Preparations containing mercury are still available in many developing countries, and their contents are poorly controlled (Figure 24.1). Peregrino et al. analyzed whitening creams in Mexico and found that mercury content varied between 878 and 36,000 ppm, despite the fact that the FDA has determined that the limit for mercury in creams should be less than 1 ppm.[10]

Plant extracts

Plant extracts and newer TYR inhibitors such as kojic acid derivatives are popular ingredients in skin lightening products. The majority of active compounds isolated from plants inhibit melanogenesis without melanocytotoxicity;[11] thus, hypopigmentation is rarely observed after use of kojic dipalmitate, liquorice extract, *Mitracarpus scaber* extract, and lemon toner.[11–13]

Oral submucous fibrosis (OSF) is a chronic disorder, predominantly encountered in South Asian and Southeast Asian countries. It has been established that OSF is etiologically linked to the consumption of the *Areca* nut in flavored formulations or as an ingredient in the betel quid. Depigmentation of the lips may be the earliest feature to develop in the natural history of OSF (Figure 24.2).[14]

Clinical features

The hypopigmentation may develop not only at the site of chemical contact (Figures 24.3 and 24.4), but also remotely (Figure 24.5). The mechanism responsible for this distant spread is unclear. Depigmented areas may continue to appear even after discontinuation of contact with the suspected chemicals. Repigmentation may or may not occur despite discontinuation of the offending agents. The presence of confetti or pea-sized macules (Figure 24.5) is characteristic of chemical leukoderma, albeit not diagnostic.[4]

Diagnosis

Relevant diagnostic elements are the history of exposure to a depigmenting agent and distribution corresponding to sites of chemical exposure. Despite its limitations, patch testing is important in patients with suspected chemical leukoderma. However, no guidelines exist for standardized

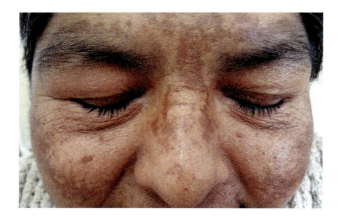

Figure 24.1 Irregular hypopigmented areas following exposure to mercury-containing lightening product for melasma.

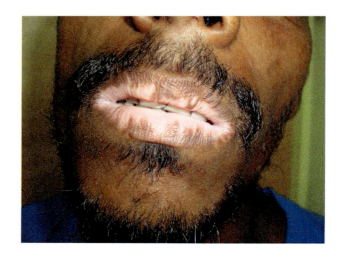

Figure 24.2 Depigmentation of the lips as the manifestation of oral submucous fibrosis.

Hypopigmentation from physical agents 161

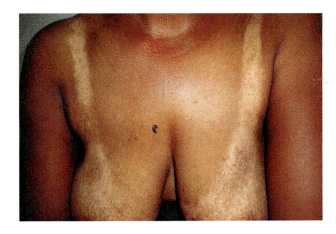

Figure 24.3 Chemical leukoderma. Depigmentation at the site of contact with black underwear.

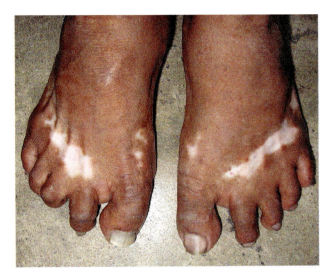

Figure 24.4 Chemical leukoderma from rubber sandals.

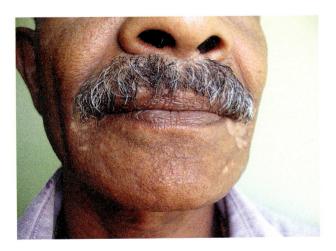

Figure 24.5 Chemical leukoderma due to hair dye applied on moustache. A few depigmented satellite macules can also be observed.

performance of the patch testing in chemical leukoderma, and the diagnostic value of this procedure depends on the choice of vehicle (petrolatum, dimethyl sulfoxide, and propylene glycol are recommended), substance concentration (elevated, between 2% and 10%, if possible), and results interpretation (not only after 48–96 hours, but after 1 or more months as well).[4] The open application test is not useful in chemical leukoderma. Chemical leukoderma should be differentiated from post-inflammatory leukoderma and Koebner phenomenon in vitiligo.[4,5]

Treatment

Depigmentation often resolves spontaneously after discontinuation of the offending agent. Treatment options for persistent hypopigmentation include topical steroids, tacrolimus, oral steroid pulse, phototherapy, and techniques of surgical repigmentation.[4]

HYPOPIGMENTATION FROM PHYSICAL AGENTS

Destruction or inhibition of melanocytes can result from exposure to a numerous physical agents, including mechanical and thermal injuries, ionizing and nonionizing radiation, and various types of burns. Some physical agents can induce a biological stress response in melanocytes that are not directly exposed, a phenomenon known as cellular bystander effect.[15]

Hypopigmentation from physical agents manifests as macules distributed on the site of skin injury. The macules may have an indistinct outline, in contrast to the discrete border seen in vitiligo.[16]

Repigmentation depends on the depth and width of the injury. In deep injuries in which all adnexal elements have been destroyed, the only available source for melanocytes will be the wound edges. These wounds will take longer to heal and will heal with a hypopigmented center in contrast to the surrounding unwounded skin.[17]

The hypopigmentation is usually transient and resolves over time. There are various methods to treat permanently hypopigmented skin, such as split skin grafting, lasers, cultured skin cell transplantation, medical needling, and noncultured skin cell suspension.[3,17]

Mechanical injuries

Hypopigmentation or hypopigmented scars can occur after various mechanical injuries, including surgical (Figure 24.6) and accidental injury, pressure sores, frictional forces, acne excoriée, and factitious disorder (Figure 24.7).[16,17] Skin signs of torture as well as child abuse can also result in residual hypopigmentation; lack of symmetry and linear lesions in irregular or criss-cross arrangements are supportive of external infliction.[18]

Cold injuries

Melanocytes are delicate and only require a temperature of −5°C for destruction, resulting in hypopigmentation in darker-skinned individuals.[19–21] Frostbite or congelation is tissue injury resulting from exposure to temperatures below 0°C. Cells are damaged by ice formation in their

162 Hypopigmentation from chemical and physical agents

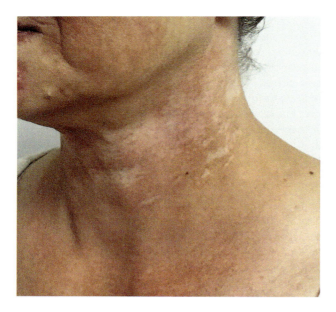

Figure 24.6 Depigmentation after microdermabrasion.

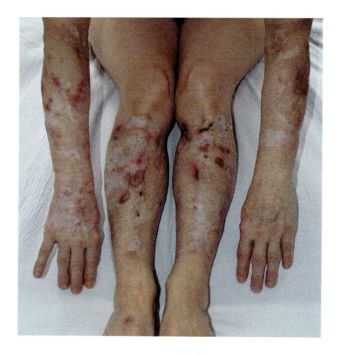

Figure 24.7 Hypopigmentation in dermatitis artefacta. Self-induced skin lesions caused by scratching, picking, and pouring chemicals on the skin.

structures and denaturation of lipid–protein complexes as well as by vascular supply disruption.[20]

Burns

In burn injuries, skin and appendageal structures are damaged by mechanical friction, heat, electrical discharge, chemicals, and radiation. Pigment changes persist for months (Figure 24.8). The repigmentation

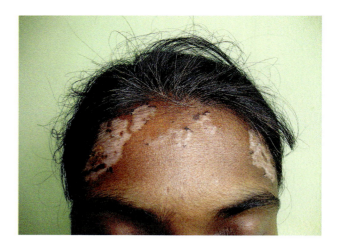

Figure 24.8 Hypopigmentation following topical application of crushed garlic for headache.

process often takes over a year to be completed. Permanent depigmentation occasionally develops after deep partial-thickness and full-thickness burn injuries.[22]

Laser and intense pulsed light (IPL) used for medical and cosmetic purposes can cause pigmentary side effects such as PIH, mottling, and "confetti-like" or "guttate" hypomelanosis.[23]

REFERENCES

1. Ruiz-Maldonado R, Orozco-Covarrubias ML. Postinflammatory hypopigmentation and hyperpigmentation. *Semin Cutan Med Surg*. 1997;16:36–43.
2. Dubey SK, Misra K, Tiwari A, Bajaj AK. Chemically induced pigmentary changes of human skin, interaction of some azo dyes with human DNA. *J Pharmacol Toxicol*. 2006;1:234–247.
3. Ortonne JP, Bahadoran P, Fitzpatrick TB et al. Hypomelanoses and hypermelanoses. In: Freedberg IM, Eisen AZ, Wolff K, Austen KF, Goldsmith LA, Katz SI, eds. *Fitzpatrick's Dermatology in General Medicine*. New York: McGraw-Hill, 2003:836–881.
4. Bonamonte D, Vestita M, Romita P et al. Chemical leukoderma. *Dermatitis*. 2016;27(3):90–99.
5. Ghosh SK, Bandyopadhyay D. Chemical leukoderma induced by colored strings. *J Am Acad Dermatol*. 2009;61(5):909–910.
6. Benn EKT, Alexis A, Mohamed N et al. Skin bleaching and dermatologic health of African and Afro-Caribbean populations in the US: New directions for methodologically rigorous, multidisciplinary, and culturally sensitive research. *Dermatology and Therapy*. 2016;6(4):453–459.
7. Nordlund JJ, Grimes PE, Ortonne JP. The safety of hydroquinone. *J Eur Acad Dermatol Venereol*. 2006;20:781–787.
8. Mohamed M, Toumi A, Soua Y et al. Confetti leukoderma following application of mequinol: A case report. *J Clin Dermatol Ther*. 2018;4:028.

9. Yoshikawa M, Sumikawa Y, Hida T et al. Clinical and epidemiological analysis in 149 cases of rhododendrol-induced leukoderma. *J Dermatol.* 2017;44(5):582–587.

10. Peregrino CP, Moreno MV, Miranda SV et al. Mercury levels in locally manufactured Mexican skin-lightening creams. *Int J Environ Res Public Health.* 2011;8(6):2516–2523.

11. Zhu W, Gao J. The use of botanical extracts as topical skin-lightening agents for the improvement of skin pigmentation disorders. *J Investig Dermatol Symp Proc.* 2008;13(1):20–24.

12. Madhogaria S, Ahmed I. Leucoderma after use of a skin-lightening cream containing kojic dipalmitate, liquorice root extract and *Mitracarpus scaber* extract. *Clin Exp Dermatol.* 2010;35(4):e103–e105.

13. Gye J, Nam CH, Kim JS et al. Chemical leucoderma induced by homemade lemon toner. *Australas J Dermatol.* 2014;55(1):90–92.

14. Sitheeque M, Ariyawardana A, Jayasinghe R, Tilakaratne W. Depigmentation of oral mucosa as the earliest possible manifestation of oral submucous fibrosis in Sri Lankan preschool children. *J Investig Clin Dent.* November 2010;1(2):156–159.

15. Redmond RW, Rajadurai A, Udayakumar D et al. Melanocytes are selectively vulnerable to UVA-mediated bystander oxidative signaling. *J Invest Dermatol.* 2013;134(4):1083–1090.

16. Vachiramon V, Thadanipon K. Postinflammatory hypopigmentation. *Clin Exp Dermatol.* 2011;36(7):708–714.

17. Chadwick S, Heath R, Shah M. Abnormal pigmentation within cutaneous scars: A complication of wound healing. *Indian J Plast Surg.* 2012;45(2):403–411.

18. Danielsen L, Rasmussen OV. Dermatological findings after alleged torture. *Torture.* 2006;16(2):108–127.

19. Eryilmaz T, Tuncer S, Uygur S, Ayhan S. Finger tip defect after cryotherapy. *Dermatol Surg* 2009;35:550–551.

20. Sachs C, Lehnhardt M, Daigeler A, Goertz O. The triaging and treatment of cold-induced injuries. *Dtsch Arztebl Int.* 2015;112(44):741–747.

21. Damevska K, Duma S, Pollozhani N. Median canaliform dystrophy of Heller after cryotherapy. *Pediatr Dermatol.* 2017;34(6):726–727.

22. Greenhalgh DG. A primer on pigmentation. *J Burn Care Res.* 2015;36(2):247–257.

23. Cil Y. Second-degree skin burn after intense pulsed light therapy with EMLA cream for hair removal. *Int J Dermatol.* 2009;48(2):206–207.

Guttate hypomelanosis and progressive hypomelanosis of the trunk (progressive macular hypomelanosis)

25

ALEXANDER KATOULIS and EFTHYMIA SOURA

CONTENTS

Guttate hypomelanosis	165	References	173
Progressive hypomelanosis of the trunk (progressive macular hypomelanosis)	170		

GUTTATE HYPOMELANOSIS

Introduction

Idiopathic guttate hypomelanosis (IGH) is a very common skin disorder that mainly affects the older population. IGH was first described by Costa in 1951 as "symmetric progressive leukopathy of the extremities." Soon after, Cummings and Cottel described the same condition in a group of patients, naming the disorder "idiopathic guttate hypomelanosis," a term that is still used today.[1] The pathogenesis of this condition has not been clearly elucidated, but aging, sun exposure, and genetic predisposition have been described as possible etiopathologic factors. In general, IGH is characterized by a benign course, although it may be a cause for concern for patients who frequently seek medical care for cosmetic reasons.[2,3]

Clinical presentation

IGH presents as small (0.5–6 mm), asymptomatic, sharply circumscribed, round, porcelain-white macules.[2] Although IGH lesions do not tend to increase in size or coalesce to form plaques, lesions up to 2.5 cm in diameter have been reported in the literature.[2,4] However, in a study performed by Shin et al., 16% of patients reported a progressive increase in lesion size.[4] It cannot be stated whether this was a true or subjective observation of patients as a result of cosmetic concerns.

IGH is usually located on sun-exposed areas of the skin and more commonly on the dorsal areas of arms and legs (distal sites more common than proximal sites) and very rarely on the face or trunk.[2,4] In some patients, lesions may be present on non-sun-exposed areas as well.[4] Hairs on the affected areas retain their pigment, and adnexal structures are normal. Three types of morphological distributions have been described for this disorder: hypopigmented macules on chronically sun-damaged skin (Figures 25.1 and 25.2); single porcelain-white, well-circumscribed, small whitish macules (can be sclerotic) observed in both sun-exposed and non-sun-exposed areas; and small, well-circumscribed hypopigmented macules presenting with hyperkeratosis and a scalloped border.[5] It is unclear whether these variants share the same etiopathogenesis.

Epidemiology

The exact prevalence of IGH is largely unknown, but it is believed that the disorder tends to be underdiagnosed in many populations. In previous studies, it has been shown that the probability of acquiring IGH tends to increase with age and may range from 80% to 97% in patients who are older than 40 years.[2,4] More specifically, Shin et al. reported that in a study that included 646 patients with IGH, the disorder was present in 47% of patients aged 31–40 years, in 80% of patients aged 41–50 years, and in 97% of patients aged 81–90 years.[4] However, it must be mentioned that in rare cases, IGH may be present in younger patients as well.[6] The condition can appear in any skin phototype but tends to be more visible in patients of darker skin phototypes (Figure 25.3). The incidence of IGH seems to be similar in males and females.[4]

Pathogenesis

The exact etiopathogenesis of IGH remains unclear. Until now, various hypotheses have been stated regarding the eliciting factors and pathogenesis of IGH, including chronic UV exposure, local melanogenesis abnormalities, cell senescence, possible genetic factors, trauma, and autoimmunity.[2] Overall, it is believed that the pathogenesis of IGH is multifactorial, with more than one factor being implicated in the appearance of the disorder at different ages (older versus younger) and at different localizations (sun exposed versus non-sun exposed).

The most prevalent of hypotheses is linked to chronic UV radiation exposure. This theory can be supported by the fact that IGH lesions tend to appear mainly on sun-exposed areas, and by small case series reporting the appearance of IGH lesions in patients receiving psoralen ultraviolet A (PUVA) radiation therapy or narrowband-ultraviolet B (nb-UVB) radiation for the treatment of mycosis fungoides.[7,8] In addition, the skin of patients with IGH lesions commonly exhibits histopathologic

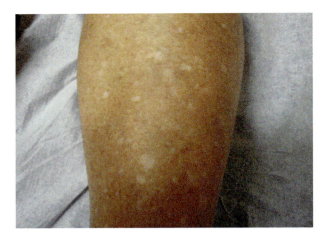

Figure 25.1 Presence of hypopigmented macules on chronically sun-damaged skin on the anterior surface of a female patient's tibia.

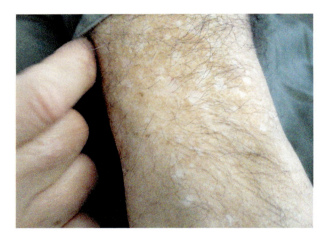

Figure 25.2 Idiopathic guttate hypomelanosis on the dorsal area of a male patient's wrist.

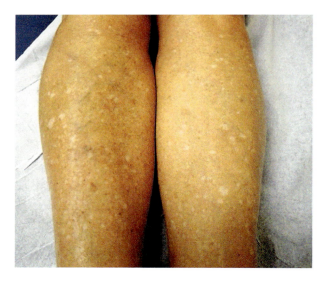

Figure 25.3 Idiopathic guttate hypomelanosis can be more evident in patients with darker skin color.

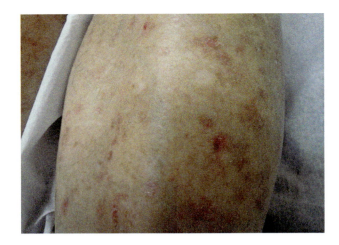

Figure 25.4 Idiopathic guttate hypomelanosis on the skin of a patient with solar elastosis. Adjacent to the IGH lesions, several actinic keratoses and lentigos can be seen.

and ultrastructural signs of solar elastosis[4,9] (Figure 25.4). However, it should be mentioned that IGH is not limited to sun-exposed areas, while heavily sun exposed areas (such as the face) are only rarely affected by the disorder.[6]

It is uncertain whether genetic factors play a role in the pathogenesis of IGH, although a correlation with specific HLAs (human leukocytic antigens) has been established.[10,11] One the other hand, continuous microtrauma may play an important role in the appearance of IGH.[4] Defective local melaninogenesis has also been included in the possible causes of IGH.[12–15]

Diagnostic modalities

Histopathology

The main histopathological findings commonly associated with IGH lesions are basket-weave hyperkeratosis (stratum corneum), acanthosis, and a decreased number of melanocytes.[4] Decreased melanin pigmentation is observed in the epidermis, and melanocytes may exhibit a decreased number of melanosomes, swelled mitochondria, and attenuated dendrites.[4,6] In some instances, the epidermis can be atrophic and the rete ridges flattened.[4,6,10] No dermal changes associated with IGH are usually seen; however, solar elastosis (and other histopathologic features of sun exposure) may be present.[9] A thicker Grenz zone and increased glycosaminoglycan presence may be demonstrated if Hale staining is used.[16]

Electron microscopy

Very few data are available regarding the ultrastructural characteristics of IGH. Kim et al. and Ortonne et al. reported characteristics such as melanocyte degeneration, decreased numbers of melanosomes, attenuation or absence of melanocyte dendrites, dilatation of the endoplasmic reticulum, and swelling of the mitochondria.[6,15] In addition, Wilson et al. and Ploysangam et al. have observed a decreased content of melanosomes in the keratinocytes neighboring melanocytes.[14,17] Other authors did not observe a decreased number or melanosomes in the melanocytes, but rather a decreased number of melanosomes in keratinocytes, suggesting an error in melanosome uptake from keratinocytes as opposed to decreased melanosome production.[9]

Dermoscopy

The dermoscopic findings in IGH are usually nonspecific. Recently, Ankad et al. reported the dermoscopic features of IGH lesions in 31 patients. Patterns that were described by the authors as "amoeboid," "feathery," "petaloid," and "nebuloid," as well as combinations of these patterns, were the most frequently observed.[18] Interestingly, the authors observed that the "feathery" pattern was more common in older lesions, while the "nebuloid" pattern was more common in newer lesions and in older patients[18] (Figure 25.5).

Differential diagnosis

The differential diagnosis of IGH includes all conditions that are characterized by macular hypopigmentation. These include vitiligo (early stages), pityriasis versicolor, pityriasis alba, hypopigmented flat warts, and post-inflammation hypomelanosis.[2,4,7] In addition, in the rare instances where IGH presents with characteristics of skin sclerosis, tuberous sclerosis, lichen sclerosus and atrophicus, and guttate morphea might also be considered.[2,4,7] Progressive macular hypomelanosis may also resemble IGH; however, the two disorders can be distinguished through various clinical features (summarized in Table 25.1). Differentiating IGH from early-stage vitiligo may also pose a problem and is a source of concern for most patients.[19] In general, vitiligo presents at younger ages compared to IGH, exhibits a different pattern of distribution, and is characterized by larger and irregularly circumscribed lesions.[2,4]

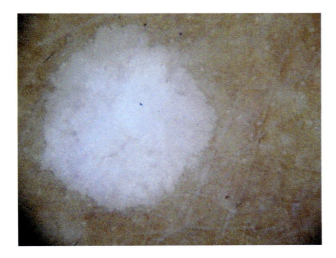

Figure 25.5 Dermoscopic image of a patient with IGH. No specific dermoscopic features can be identified besides a "nebuloid/cloudy"-type appearance.

Treatment

Until this point, no specific regimen has been considered the gold standard for the treatment of IGH. However, various modalities have been investigated, including topical retinoids and calcineurin inhibitors, tattooing with 5-fluorouracil (5-FU), lasers, dermabrasion, chemical peels, skin grafting, and cryotherapy.

The efficacy of topical tretinoin in the treatment of IGH has been investigated in a small clinical trial. Pagnogni et al. administered tretinoin cream to four female patients with photoaged skin and IGH. The patients received tretinoin cream on one arm and placebo cream on the other.[16] After 4 months of treatment, repigmentation of IGH lesions was observed, a result that was found statistically significant when the results from both arms were compared.[16] The authors suggested that increased melanin pigmentation after topical tretinoin use could be a result of melanin transfer improvement to keratinocytes or stimulation of melanin synthesis.[16]

Topical calcineurin inhibitors have also been investigated in the treatment of IGH. In a study by Asawanonda et al., four patients with IGH received treatment with 1% pimecrolimus cream for 8 weeks. The results were acceptable, as three out of four patients reported some improvement in their lesions (25%–75%).[20] Similar results were reported in a double-blinded placebo-controlled study by Rerknimitr et al., which involved 26 patients with IGH.[21] More specifically, patients received 0.1% topical tacrolimus ointment two times per day for 6 months on one side of the body and placebo cream on the other. Patients reported a better outcome and higher repigmentation on the tacrolimus-treated side compared to the placebo treated side after 6 months of treatment.[21] In addition, physician's improvement grading score showed that 11% of the patients demonstrated improvement of their skin lesions on the treated side after 6 months of treatment. Adverse events included mild burning sensation in about 20% of patients.[21] Topical calcineurin inhibitors may be considered an option for the treatment of IGH; however, when used, long-term therapeutic regimens are probably required.

In recent years, topical injections with 5-FU have been used as a possible treatment for IGH. Arbache et al. recently published the preliminary results of a small study that included eight patients with IGH.[22] A specific microneedling device was used (tattooing) to inject lesions with either 5-FU or placebo. According to the authors, 73.5% of lesions receiving 5-FU exhibited repigmentation compared to only 33.8% of lesions receiving placebo.[22] Wambier et al. used a similar technique to inject 5-FU 50 mg/mL solution to IGH lesions.[23] Results were noticeable within the first month and were persistent. Possible adverse events included irritation and transient post-inflammatory hyperpigmentation.[23]

Chemical peels have been also been used in the treatment of IGH, with acceptable results. In a study by Ravikiran et al., 88% phenol solution was topically applied in 20 patients with a total of 149 IGH lesions.[24] The authors reported that

Table 25.1 Differential diagnosis of progressive macular hypopigmentation

Disorder	Clinical presentation	Histologic findings	Dermoscopic findings	Laboratory tests
Progressive macular hypopigmentation	Hypopigmented, ill-defined, nummular, macules (trunk, abdomen), no scales or pruritus	Unremarkable, decreased melanin in epidermis, perifollicular Gram+ staining	Ill-defined whitish area without scaling	• Red follicular fluorescence on lesional skin (Wood's light) • Negative KOH preparations • Presence of follicular *P. acnes*
Pityriasis alba	Oval macules commonly located on the face, neck, and arms covered by thin scales	Hypopigmentation of epidermis, eczematous changes in the epidermis and dermis	N/A	• Negative KOH preparations • Positive history of atopic dermatitis
Idiopathic guttate hypomelanosis	Hypopigmented, well-circumscribed circular/oval macules on sun-damaged skin in middle-aged and older patients	Decreased melanocyte and melanin content, epidermal atrophy	"Cloudy sky-like" or "cloudy" patterns	Unremarkable, clinical diagnosis
Post-inflammatory hypopigmentation	Positive history of previous skin disorder, restricted to sites of initial lesions	Decreased melanin in basal layer, pigment-containing melanophages in upper dermis, characteristics of previous disorder	Dermoscopic findings associated with initial lesions	N/A, clinical diagnosis based on patient history
Guttate vitiligo	Hypopigmented/depigmented, well-circumscribed macules with variable distribution (can be symmetric), no scales	Complete loss of melanocytes	Well-circumscribed, dense/glowing, whitish areas, perifollicular hyperpigmentation	N/A, clinical diagnosis based on patient history
Achromic tinea (pityriasis) versicolor	Hypopigmented irregular asymmetric circular/oval, well-circumscribed macules, commonly on trunk, thin scales	Hypopigmentation of epidermis, yeast and hyphae present in stratum corneum, dermal inflammation	Well-circumscribed whitish area with thin scales present in the skin furrows	• Positive KOH preparation • Blue-green fluorescence of scales under Wood's lamp • *Pityrosporum ovale* in culture

(Continued)

Disorder	Clinical presentation	Histologic findings	Dermoscopic findings	Laboratory tests
Mycosis fungoides (hypopigmented)	Hypopigmented oval macules located on trunk and extremities, can be symmetric, often pruritic	Decreased epidermal melanin, no epidermal atrophy, epidermotropism of lymphocytes, minimal dermal involvement, presence of Paultrier microabscesses	Polygonal structures consisting of lobule of white storiform streaks with septa of pigmented dots, fine red dots or hairpin vessels present	• Histopathology • Immunohistochemistry findings (clonal T-cell proliferation)
Tuberculoid and borderline tuberculoid leprosy	Well-circumscribed hypopigmented macules, induration may be present, asymmetric	Loss of epidermal pigment, granulomatous inflammation	White areas, decreased density of hairs, presence of yellow globules, branching vessels	• Lepromin test • Clinical history • Should be suspected only in endemic areas
Pinta	Hypo- or hyperpigmented lesions of variable distribution	Decreased epidermal melanin content, dermal lymphoplasmacytic infiltrate, treponemes may be present in early lesions (silver stain)	N/A	• Positive syphilis serology • Dark-field microscopy (*Tr. carateum*) • Should be suspected only in endemic areas
Dermal leishmaniasis (post-kala-azar)	Hypopigmented macules with variable distribution	Hypopigmentation of basal cell layer, dermal infiltration by lymphocytes and macrophages, parasites may be present	Erythema, various configurations of vascular structures, white starburst-like patterns, central ulcers, "yellow tears," hyperkeratosis	• Positive history of visceral leishmaniasis • Should be suspected only in endemic areas

64% of the lesions exhibited acceptable repigmentation.[24] Adverse events included persistent crusting (17.2% of lesions), post-inflammatory hyperpigmentation (11.5%), ulceration (7.9%), secondary infection (8.6%), and scarring (5.6%).[24] Therapeutic wounding with 88% phenol solution was also investigated in a more recent study by Gupta et al., with acceptable results.[25]

Various lasers have been used in the treatment of IGH. These include fractional carbon dioxide (CO_2FL), ytterbium/erbium fiber, and excimer lasers. In a recent pilot study by Gordon et al., six patients received treatment with an excimer laser (wavelength of 308 nm) twice weekly for 12 weeks.[26] Improvement was observed in all patients, while at the end of the study, 50% of patients reported full repigmentation of lesions.[26] No adverse events were reported besides mild transient erythema after the application of the laser treatment.[26]

Fractional carbon dioxide lasers have also shown acceptable efficacy in the treatment of IGH. In a pilot study by Shin et al., 40 patients received treatment with CO_2FL once, and repigmentation was assessed 2 months following treatment.[27] According to the authors, at least 50% improvement of lesions was observed in 90% (36) of patients.[27] In addition, patient satisfaction was high, as 82.5% (33) of patients reported being very satisfied or satisfied with just this one session of CO_2FL treatment, while the results remained stable at 1 year follow-up.[27] Adverse events included pain, burning sensation, and appearance of erythema during the procedure. Post-inflammatory hyperpigmentation was also observed in four patients. In a similar study by Goldust et al., 240 patients received treatment with a 10,600-nm CO_2FL.[28] A single treatment session was performed and the patients were assessed 2 months later. According to the authors, 47.9% (115) and 41.6% (100) of patients had achieved >75% and 51%–75% clinical improvement, respectively.[28] No recurrences were observed at 1 year follow-up. Patient satisfaction was high in this study as well, with 39.6% (95) and 42.5% (102) of patients reporting being "very satisfied" and "satisfied" with the results, respectively.[28]

Fractional 1550-nm ytterbium/erbium fiber laser was used by Rerknimitr et al. in a study that included 30 patients with a total of 120 IGH lesions.[29] Patients received four treatments at 4-week intervals. Assessment was performed with colorimetry, digital photography, and digital dermoscopy at weeks 0, 4, 8, 12, and 16.[29] According to the authors, 83.34% of the lesions that received treatment exhibited some type of improvement compared to only 18.34% of the control group lesions.[29] Adverse events included transient mild erythema and edema.[29] No post-inflammatory pigmentation was observed, possibly making this laser a more suitable option for patients with darker skin phototypes. In a more recent study by Chitvanich et al., 30 patients received treatment with fractional 1550-nm ytterbium/erbium fiber laser every 4 weeks combined with twice daily topical application of 0.1% tacrolimus ointment on lesions on one side and placebo on lesions of the other side of their body.[30] Photographic evaluations demonstrated that 91.67% of lesions in the treatment group exhibited some improvement compared to 18.34% in the control group.[30] Similarly, the relative lightness index of IGH reached statistical significance at week 12, after three sessions of laser treatment (p = 0.026).[30] The authors suggest that the use of erbium laser may improve the absorption of tacrolimus in the skin, further potentiating its efficacy.[30] Adverse events included transient erythema and edema.[30]

Cryotherapy and dermabrasion are two more modalities that have been investigated for the treatment of IGH. In a recent study by Laosakul et al., tip cryotherapy was applied for 5 seconds in a single treatment session.[31] A total of 29 patients were included in the study and lesions on both sides of the body were randomized to either receive treatment or be used as controls.[31] The authors of this study reported that 94.9% of treated lesions exhibited improvement after 4 weeks, while at week 16, 82.3% of the treated sites exhibited more than 75% improvement compared to just 2.0% of sites in the control group (p < 0.001).[31] Adverse events included mild burning sensation, post-inflammatory hyperpigmentation, erythema, and blister formation.[31]

The efficacy of classic cryotherapy was investigated in previous clinical trials, with acceptable results.[5,17] In general, no more than 3–5 seconds of liquid nitrogen application was required. However, it is strongly recommended that a well-trained health care professional perform the treatment, as there is always the possibility of scarring if lesions are overtreated.[2,5]

Dermabrasion may also be considered an option in specific cases. A disadvantage of this method is that it is applied in larger areas (whereas IGH is composed of small lesions) and requires expert supervision when performed. In a study by Hexsel et al., 20 patients with IGH lesions smaller than 5 cm were treated with a standard dermabrader, with acceptable results.[32] According to the authors of this study, 80% of patients exhibited satisfactory repigmentation after treatment.[32] However, crust formation and persistent erythema (6 months) were reported as treatment-associated adverse effects.[32]

PROGRESSIVE HYPOMELANOSIS OF THE TRUNK (PROGRESSIVE MACULAR HYPOMELANOSIS)

Introduction

Progressive hypomelanosis of the trunk (progressive macular hypomelanosis; PMH) is a skin condition that is poorly understood and often misdiagnosed. It was first described by Guillet et al.[33] in French people of mixed racial ancestry (Caucasian and African). The condition was later described by other investigators as well, and they assigned several terminologies to it, including "cutis trunci variata," "Creole dyschromia," and "idiopathic multiple large macule hypomelanosis."[34–36]

Clinical presentation

This dermatologic entity is characterized by the appearance of asymptomatic, poorly defined nummular, symmetric,

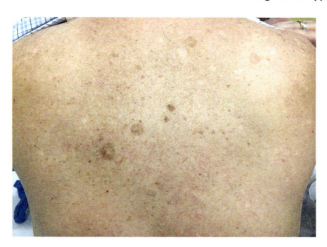

Figure 25.6 Typical clinical picture of PMH on the trunk of a male patient. Presence of nonscaly symmetric, hypopigmented macules.

hypopigmented macules that coalesce into patches and are usually nonscaly.[34–36] In general, the lesions are distributed in the trunk (back, lumbar, and abdominal areas), but can also extend to the neck and proximal extremities[34] (Figure 25.6). The hands of the patients are never affected by the condition, while lesions on the face are considered extremely uncommon.[35,36]

Epidemiology

The exact prevalence of PMH is currently unknown and may be difficult to determine, as it could vary widely from country to country based on the type of population.[33–37] PMH usually appears during adolescence or early adulthood, with reported patient ages ranging from 13 to 45 years.[34–36] In general, it is considered more common in female patients, with the Netherlands Institute for Pigment Disorders reporting a 7:1 female-to-male ratio.[34–36]

Pathogenesis

A theory has suggested that the lesions of PMH tend to appear in areas of the body with a high concentration of sebaceous glands.[34–36] More specifically, the microbial flora of sebaceous glands may play an important role in disease pathogenesis.[38] A specific strain of *P. acnes,* different from that isolated in acne patients, has been identified in several patients with PMH.[39–41] To further support the theory of the implication of *P. acnes* in the pathogenesis of PMH, various case series have shown that antimicrobial treatment may improve pigmentation of the affected areas in some patients.[42,43] Another theory has suggested that PMH is a type of post-inflammatory hypopigmentation that persists after a fungal infection has resolved, but very few data support this hypothesis.[35] Other authors have suggested that PMH could be a type of genodermatosis. This theory was considered because the condition is commonly seen in members of the same family; however, there are very few scientific data to support it.[37] Finally, hormonal reasons may also play a role in the pathogenesis of PMH. Although the role of hormones remains obscure, it could be supported by the high female-to-male ratio observed in this disorder.

Diagnostic modalities

Histopathology

Very subtle histopathologic differences are observed between lesional and nonlesional skin in patients with PMH. Overall, the dermis appears normal, while a decrease in melanin content in the epidermis, compared with that in normal adjacent skin, may be present.[35,36] There are no signs of spongiosis or other histopathological features of inflammation present,[38] although Gram+ material may be observed in areas adjacent to the pilosebaceous units of the skin. This material is probably associated with the presence of *P. acnes*.[35,36]

Electron microscopy

It is believed by many authors that the hypopigmentation observed in patients with PMH should be attributed to alterations in the melanogenesis pathway rather than changes in the melanosome transfer or degradation processes. This belief is based on electron microscope findings that indicate a decreased production of melanosomes and the transfer of less melanized melanosomes and aggregated melanosomes in the lesional skin of PMH patients with Fitzpatrick skin types V and VI.[35,36,44] More specifically, Kumarasinghe et al. observed a statistically significant ($p = 0.047$) higher ratio of stage IV and late stage III (dark) melanosomes in normal versus lesional skin in eight Chinese patients with PMH.[45] Similar findings were also reported in previous studies.[33,44] No other significant ultrastructural differences between lesional and nonlesional skin of patients with PMH have been reported.

Dermoscopy

Similar to histopathology, the dermoscopic picture of PMH is unremarkable, with lesions presenting as an ill-defined whitish area without scaling[46] (Figure 25.7). A distinction can be made from other hypopigmented macular diseases of the skin based on very subtle differences. For instance, achromic pityriasis versicolor presents as a well-demarcated whitish area with fine scaling in the skin furrows, guttate vitiligo as a dense and well-demarcated white area with perifollicular hyperpigmentation, and idiopathic guttate hypomelanosis as a "cloudy sky-like" or "cloudy" pattern[46,47] (Figure 25.5).

Wood's lamp

The use of a Wood's lamp may assist greatly in the diagnosis of PMH. The hypopigmented macules are more clearly visible under a Wood's lamp, and a typical coral-red follicular/ perifollicular fluorescence, observed only in lesional skin and not in adjacent nonlesional skin, can be seen when lesions are inspected under a powerful Wood's lamp in a pitch-black room.[38] This type of fluorescence is most probably caused by an agent produced by the *P. acnes*

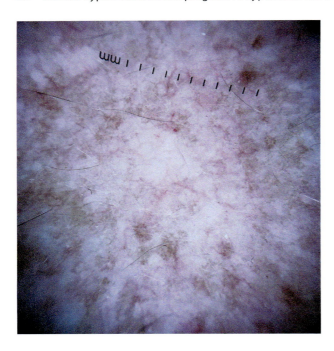

Figure 25.7 Dermoscopic image of PMH. There are no specific dermoscopic characteristics, and lesions present as asymmetrical, ill-defined whitish macules.

strain that is associated with the appearance of PMH[48] and has been shown to be almost universally present in patients with the disorder.[48,49]

Differential diagnosis

PMH should mainly be distinguished from other acquired disorders characterized by macular hypopigmentation localized in the area of the trunk. These disorders can be caused by nonmicrobial skin inflammation (i.e., pityriasis alba, post-inflammatory hypopigmentation, idiopathic guttate hypopigmentation), by infection-associated skin inflammation, by fungi (i.e., pityriasis versicolor) or bacteria/other infectious agents (i.e., tuberculoid or borderline tuberculoid leprosy, pinta, etc.), or by proliferative neoplastic disorders (e.g., mycosis fungoides). Progressive macular hypopigmentation can be differentiated from several of these conditions due to the lack of pruritus and desquamation. In addition, in cases of post-inflammatory hypopigmentation, a positive history for an inflammatory dermatosis precedes the appearance of lesions. A summary of conditions that are included in the differential diagnosis of PMH and their differences can be seen in Table 25.1.[34–36,50–52]

Treatment

There is no specific treatment algorithm for PMH. In the past, various topical and systemic corticosteroids and antifungal agents have been used in the treatment of PMH, with limited effectiveness.[35,36] Due to the recent data that indicate that the presence of *P. acnes* plays a major pathogenetic role in the appearance of the disease, various authors have attempted the use of topical antimicrobial agents in the treatment of this disorder. More specifically, Relyveld et al. investigated the effectiveness of combination therapy with benzoyl peroxide 5% hydrogel, clindamycin 1% lotion, and UVA irradiation compared to the combination of fluticasone 0.05% cream and UVA irradiation in patients with PMH.[42] A total of 45 patients were enrolled in the study, and each regimen was administered in a preselected side of every patient's face (left and right). Patients received the treatments for 14 weeks, followed by a 12-week follow-up period to evaluate repigmentation rates. The antimicrobial combination regimen showed strong superiority to the anti-inflammatory combination regimen (photometric measurements $p = 0.007$, patient assessment $p < 0.0001$, and dermatologist assessment $p < 0.0001$).[42] In addition, repigmentation rates were reported to be slower on the side of the face that had received the antimicrobial combination regimen treatment.[42] Similar results were reported by Santos et al. in a double-blinded, placebo-controlled study that included 23 patients with PMH.[53] In this study, 10 patients received treatment with placebo and 13 a combination of topical benzoyl peroxide 5% and clindamycin 1%, for a total duration of 12 months.[53] A statistically significant improvement was observed for the patients receiving the antimicrobial regimen after this period. There were no follow-up results reported.[53] Although both of these studies have many limitations (e.g., subjective methods of result evaluation and low patient numbers), they both report encouraging results for the use of antimicrobial agents, suggesting that this could be considered a treatment of choice for patients with PMH.

Phototherapy has also been evaluated in the treatment of PMH. Previous studies have reported acceptable efficacy for the use of PUVA or narrowband UVB in patients with the disorder. In a study by Duarte et al., 85 patients received treatment with either PUVA or nb-UVB, with the majority of patients reporting at least 50% repigmentation after 16 phototherapy sessions.[54] Although 65% of patients were reported as "cured or much improved," 72% relapsed soon after treatment cessation.[54] There were no statistically significant differences between the efficacy of PUVA and nb-UVB reported in this study.[54] Similar results were reported in a small, uncontrolled study by Kim et al. that included 17 patients with PMH.[55] More specifically, nb-UVB therapy was successfully used in 56.2% of patients, who demonstrated more than 90% repigmentation.[55] Interestingly, the beneficial results of the treatment seemed to have an acceptable duration, as 68.7% of the responders did not show signs of relapse after 13.2 ± 8.2 (mean, SD) months of follow-up.[55] In general, case reports and a short case series corroborate these results, although the duration of response is still debated.[56,57]

Finally, oral isotretinoin has also been used in the treatment of PMH, with mixed results. In a previous case report, 10 mg of oral isotretinoin were administered in a patient with PMH and rosacea, with complete response of PMH lesions reported after 1 month of treatment.[58] The authors reported that no relapse was observed after

10 months of follow-up.[58] However, in a recent case report, oral isotretinoin proved ineffective in the treatment of a 22-year-old male with long-standing lesions of PMH (5 years).[59] Although the use of isotretinoin could be considered logical due to the implication of *P. acnes* in the pathogenesis of PMH, more data are required in order to evaluate the effectiveness of this treatment.

Prognosis

The prognosis of the condition remains uncertain, with various authors reporting mixed data. More specifically, Guillet et al. have reported that PMH resolves spontaneously after 3–5 years,[33] while others report a more long-standing, or even persistent, course for the disease.[35,57,59] In general, more epidemiological data are required to establish the prognosis of the disease, as the fact that PMH is never observed in older ages may indicate a spontaneous disappearance after adolescence or early adulthood.[35]

REFERENCES

1. Cummings KI, Cottel WI. Idiopathic guttate hypomelanosis. *Arch Dermatol.* 1966;93(2):184–186.
2. Juntongjin P, Laosakul K. Idiopathic guttate hypomelanosis: A review of its etiology, pathogenesis, findings, and treatments. *Am J Clin Dermatol.* 2016;17(4):403–411.
3. Brown F, Crane JS. *Idiopathic Guttate Hypomelanosis.* Stat Pearls. Treasure Island, FL: StatPearls Publishing, 2018.
4. Shin MK, Jeong KH, Oh IH et al. Clinical features of idiopathic guttate hypomelanosis in 646 subjects and association with other aspects of photoaging. *Int J Dermatol.* 2011;50(7):798–805.
5. Kumarasinghe SP. 3-5 second cryotherapy is effective in idiopathic guttate hypomelanosis. *J Dermatol.* 2004;31(5):437–439.
6. Kim SK, Kim EH, Kang HY et al. Comprehensive understanding of idiopathic guttate hypomelanosis: Clinical and histopathological correlation. *Int J Dermatol.* 2010;49(2):162–166.
7. Kaya TI, Yazici AC, Tursen U et al. Idiopathic guttate hypomelanosis: Idiopathic or ultraviolet induced? *Photodermatol Photoimmunol Photomed.* 2005;21(5):270–271.
8. Friedland R, David M, Feinmesser M et al. Idiopathic guttate hypomelanosis-like lesions in patients with mycosis fungoides: A new adverse effect of phototherapy. *J Eur Acad Dermatol Venereol.* 2010;24(9):1026–1030.
9. Kakepis M, Havaki S, Katoulis A et al. Idiopathic guttate hypomelanosis: An electron microscopy study. *J Eur Acad Dermatol Venereol.* 2015;29(7):1435–1438.
10. Falabella R, Escobar C, Giraldo N et al. On the pathogenesis of idiopathic guttate hypomelanosis. *J Am Acad Dermatol.* 1987;16(1 Pt 1):35–44.
11. Arrunategui A, Trujillo RA, Marulanda MP et al. HLA-DQ3 is associated with idiopathic guttate hypomelanosis, whereas HLA-DR8 is not, in a group of renal transplant patients. *Int J Dermatol.* 2002;41(11):744–747.
12. Gilhar A, Pillar T, Eidelman S et al. Vitiligo and idiopathic guttate hypomelanosis. Repigmentation of skin following engraftment onto nude mice. *Arch Dermatol.* 1989;125(10):1363–1366.
13. Rani S, Kumar R, Kumarasinghe P et al. Melanocyte abnormalities and senescence in the pathogenesis of idiopathic guttate hypomelanosis. *Int J Dermatol.* 2018;57(5):559–565.
14. Wilson PD, Lavker RM, Kligman AM. On the nature of idiopathic guttate hypomelanosis. *Acta Derm Venereol.* 1982;62(4):301–306.
15. Ortonne JP, Perrot H. Idiopathic guttate hypomelanosis. Ultrastructural study. *Arch Dermatol.* 1980;116(6):664–668.
16. Pagnoni A, Kligman AM, Sadiq I et al. Hypopigmented macules of photodamaged skin and their treatment with topical tretinoin. *Acta Derm Venereol.* 1999;79(4):305–310.
17. Ploysangam T, Dee-Ananlap S, Suvanprakorn P. Treatment of idiopathic guttate hypomelanosis with liquid nitrogen: Light and electron microscopic studies. *J Am Acad Dermatol.* 1990;23(4 Pt 1):681–684.
18. Ankad BS, Beergouder SL. Dermoscopic evaluation of idiopathic guttate hypomelanosis: A preliminary observation. *Indian Dermatol Online J.* 2015;6(3):164–167.
19. Morrison B, Burden-Teh E, Batchelor JM et al. Quality of life in people with vitiligo: A systematic review and meta-analysis. *Br J Dermatol.* 2017;177(6):e338–e39.
20. Asawanonda P, Sutthipong T, Prejawai N. Pimecrolimus for idiopathic guttate hypomelanosis. *J Drugs Dermatol.* 2010;9(3):238–239.
21. Rerknimitr P, Disphanurat W, Achariyakul M. Topical tacrolimus significantly promotes repigmentation in idiopathic guttate hypomelanosis: A double-blind, randomized, placebo-controlled study. *J Eur Acad Dermatol Venereol.* 2013;27(4):460–464.
22. Arbache S, Roth D, Steiner D et al. Activation of melanocytes in idiopathic guttate hypomelanosis after 5-fluorouracil infusion using a tattoo machine: Preliminary analysis of a randomized, split-body, single blinded, placebo controlled clinical trial. *J Am Acad Dermatol.* 2018;78(1):212–215.
23. Wambier CG, Perillo de Farias Wambier S, Pereira Soares MT et al. 5-fluorouracil tattooing for idiopathic guttate hypomelanosis. *J Am Acad Dermatol.* 2018;78(4):e81–e82.
24. Ravikiran SP, Sacchidanand S, Leelavathy B. Therapeutic wounding—88% phenol in idiopathic guttate hypomelanosis. *Indian Dermatol Online J.* 2014;5(1):14–18.
25. Gupta K, Tripathi S, Kaur M. Evaluation of placental extracts as an adjuvant therapy to phenol in treatment of idiopathic guttate hypomelanolsis. *J Clinical Diagn Res.* 2016;10(8):Wc01–Wc03.

26. Gordon JR, Reed KE, Sebastian KR et al. Excimer light treatment for idiopathic guttate hypomelanosis: A pilot study. *Dermatol Surg.* 2017;43(4):553–557.

27. Shin J, Kim M, Park SH et al. The effect of fractional carbon dioxide lasers on idiopathic guttate hypomelanosis: A preliminary study. *J Eur Acad Dermatol Venereol.* 2013;27(2):e243–e246.

28. Goldust M, Mohebbipour A, Mirmohammadi R. Treatment of idiopathic guttate hypomelanosis with fractional carbon dioxide lasers. *J Cosmet Laser Ther.* 2013.

29. Rerknimitr P, Chitvanich S, Pongprutthipan M et al. Non-ablative fractional photothermolysis in treatment of idiopathic guttate hypomelanosis. *J Eur Acad Dermatol Venereol.* 2015;29(11):2238–2242.

30. Chitvanich S, Rerknimitr P, Panchaprateep R et al. Combination of non-ablative fractional photothermolysis and 0.1% tacrolimus ointment is efficacious for treating idiopathic guttate hypomelanosis. *J Dermatolog Treat.* 2016;27(5):456–460.

31. Laosakul K, Juntongjin P. Efficacy of tip cryotherapy in the treatment of idiopathic guttate hypomelanosis (IGH): A randomized, controlled, evaluator-blinded study. *J Dermatolog Treat.* 2017;28(3):271–275.

32. Hexsel DM. Treatment of idiopathic guttate hypomelanosis by localized superficial dermabrasion. *Dermatol Surg.* 1999;25(11):917–918.

33. Guillet G, Helenon R, Gauthier Y et al. Progressive macular hypomelanosis of the trunk: Primary acquired hypopigmentation. *J Cutan Pathol.* 1988;15(5):286–289.

34. Elmariah SB, Kundu RV. Progressive macular hypomelanosis. *J Drugs Dermatol.* 2011;10(5):502–506.

35. Relyveld GN, Menke HE, Westerhof W. Progressive macular hypomelanosis: An overview. *Am J Clin Dermatol.* 2007;8(1):13–19.

36. Desai S, Owen J. Progressive macular hypomelanosis: An update. *Pigment Int.* 2014;1(2):52–55.

37. Borelli D. [Cutis "trunci variata." A new genetic dermatosis]. *Medicina Cutanea Ibero-Latino-Americana.* 1987;15(4):317–319.

38. Westerhof W, Relyveld GN, Kingswijk MM et al. *Propionibacterium acnes* and the pathogenesis of progressive macular hypomelanosis. *Arch Dermatol.* 2004;140(2):210–214.

39. Relyveld GN, Westerhof W, Woudenberg J et al. Progressive macular hypomelanosis is associated with a putative *Propionibacterium* species. *J Invest Dermatol.* 2010;130(4):1182–1184.

40. Barnard E, Liu J, Yankova E et al. Strains of the *Propionibacterium acnes* type III lineage are associated with the skin condition progressive macular hypomelanosis. *Sci Rep.* 2016;6:31968.

41. Cavalcanti SM, de Franca ER, Lins AK et al. Investigation of *Propionibacterium acnes* in progressive macular hypomelanosis using real-time PCR and culture. *Int J Dermatol.* 2011;50(11):1347–1352.

42. Relyveld GN, Kingswijk MM, Reitsma JB et al. Benzoyl peroxide/clindamycin/UVA is more effective than fluticasone/UVA in progressive macular hypomelanosis: A randomized study. *J Am Acad Dermatol.* 2006;55(5):836–843.

43. Cavalcanti SM, Querino MC, Magalhaes V et al. The use of lymecycline and benzoyl peroxide for the treatment of progressive macular hypomelanosis: A prospective study. *Anais Brasileiros de Dermatol.* 2011;86(4):813–814.

44. Relyveld GN, Dingemans KP, Menke HE et al. Ultrastructural findings in progressive macular hypomelanosis indicate decreased melanin production. *J Eur Acad Dermatol Venereol.* 2008;22(5):568–574.

45. Kumarasinghe SP, Tan SH, Thng S et al. Progressive macular hypomelanosis in Singapore: A clinico-pathological study. *Int J Dermatol.* 2006;45(6):737–742.

46. Errichetti E, Stinco G. Dermoscopy in general dermatology: A practical overview. *Dermatol Ther.* 2016;6(4):471–507.

47. Errichetti E, Stinco G. Dermoscopy of idiopathic guttate hypomelanosis. *J Dermatol.* 2015;42(11):1118–1119.

48. Pflederer RT, Wuennenberg JP, Foote C et al. Use of Wood's lamp to diagnose progressive macular hypomelanosis. *J Am Acad Dermatol.* 2017;77(4):e99–e100.

49. Wu XG, Xu AE, Song XZ et al. Clinical, pathologic, and ultrastructural studies of progressive macular hypomelanosis. *Int J Dermatol.* 2010;49(10):1127–1132.

50. Xu P, Tan C. Dermoscopy of poikilodermatous mycosis fungoides (MF). *J Am Acad Dermatol.* 2016;74(3):e45–e47.

51. Ankad BS, Sakhare PS. Dermoscopy of borderline tuberculoid leprosy. *Int J Dermatol.* 2018;57(1):74–76.

52. Jha A, Sonthalia S, Lallas A. Dermoscopy of post kala-azar dermal leishmaniasis. *Indian Dermatol Online J.* 2018;9(1):78–79.

53. Santos JB, Almeida OLS, Silva LMD et al. Eficácia da combinação tópica de peróxido de benzoíla 5% e clindamicina 1% para o tratamento da hipomelanose macular progressiva: um estudo randomizado, duplo-cego, placebo-controlado. *Anais Brasileiros de Dermatol.* 2011;86:50–54.

54. Duarte I, Nina BI, Gordiano MC et al. Progressive macular hypomelanosis: An epidemiological study and therapeutic response to phototherapy. *Anais Brasileiros de Dermatol.* 2010;85(5):621–624.

55. Kim MB, Kim GW, Cho HH et al. Narrowband UVB treatment of progressive macular hypomelanosis. *J Am Acad Dermatol.* 2012;66(4):598–605.

56. Chung YL, Goo B, Chung WS et al. A case of progressive macular hypomelanosis treated with narrow-band UVB. *J Eur Acad Dermatol Venereol.* 2007;21(7):1007–1009.

57. Menke H, Relyveld G, Westerhof W. Comment on the letter by Chung et al. about progressive macular hypomelanosis. *J Eur Acad Dermatol Venereol.* 2008;22(8):1029–1030.
58. Kim YJ, Lee DY, Lee JY et al. Progressive macular hypomelanosis showing excellent response to oral isotretinoin. *J Dermatol.* 2012;39(11):937–938.
59. Damevska K, Pollozhani N, Neloska L et al. Unsuccessful treatment of progressive macular hypomelanosis with oral isotretinoin. *Dermatol Ther.* 2017;30(5).

Index

A

Acid-fast bacillus (AFB), 135
Afamelanotide, 86
Albinism, 93; *see also* Oculocutaneous albinism
    red, 94
Albinoid disorders, 93
Alezzandrini syndrome, 113
    clinical presentation, 114–115
    differential diagnosis, 115
    epidemiology, 113
    pathophysiology, 113–114
    treatment, 115
Alopecia areata (AA), 103
Angiofibromas, 91; *see also* Tuberous sclerosis
    complex
Antibody-dependent cellular cytotoxicity
    (ADCC), 36
Antimalarial drugs, 154; *see also* Systemic
    drugs
Atopic dermatitis (AD), 128

B

Birt-Hogg-Dubé syndrome (BHD syndrome), 91
Blaschko lines, 118, 119; *see also* Mosaic
    hypopigmentation
    hypomelanosis following, 118–120
Bleeding diathesis, 97
Borderline lepromatous (BL), 135; *see also*
    Leprosy
Borderline tuberculoid (BT), 135; *see also*
    Leprosy
Burns, 162; *see also* Hypopigmentation

C

Café au lait macules (CALMs), 101, 103
Calcineurin inhibitors, 49, 53–54; *see also*
    Vitiligo treatments
CALMs, *see* Café au lait macules
Catalase/dismutase superoxide (C/DSO), 52
Cell–cell crosstalk, 7; *see also* Melanocyte
    melanocyte-endothelial cell interactions, 9
    melanocyte-fibroblast interactions, 8–9
    melanocyte-keratinocyte interactions, 7–8
    stimulating and inhibiting bioactive
        mediators, 8
Cellular transplantation, 73–76; *see also*
    Vitiligo surgical treatment
Chediak-Higashi syndrome (CHS), 15, 17, 98,
    113; *see also* Hypopigmentation
    clinical presentation, 114–115
    diagnosis, 98–99
    differential diagnosis, 115
    epidemiology, 113
    management, 99
    pathophysiology, 113–114
    prevalence and prognosis, 98
    treatment, 115
Childhood vitiligo (CV), 43; *see also*
    Post-childhood vitiligo
    clinical presentation, 43–44
    comorbidities, 44
    differential diagnosis, 45
    epidemiology, 43
    halo nevi, 44–45
    leukotrichia, 43
    nonsegmental, 44
    phototherapy, 46
    psychological burden of vitiligo, 45
    segmental, 44
    surgical treatment, 46–47
    308-nm excimer laser, 46
    topical treatment, 45–46
    treatment, 45–47

Cold injuries, 161–162; *see also*
    Hypopigmentation
Confetti-like hypopigmentation, 91; *see also*
    Tuberous sclerosis complex
Conradi-Hünermann-Happle syndrome, 123;
    see also Mosaic hypopigmentation
Contact leukoderma, *see* Leukoderma, chemical
Corticotropin-releasing hormone (CRH), 36
Cosmetic preparations containing mercury,
    160; *see also* Skin-lightening agents
Cross syndrome, 113
    clinical presentation, 114–115
    differential diagnosis, 115
    epidemiology, 113
    pathophysiology, 113–114
    treatment, 115
Cytotoxic T-lymphocyte-associated antigen 4
    (CTLA-4), 145

    agonists, 87

D

Dasatinib, 153; *see also* Tyrosine kinase
    inhibitors
Dermatitis/eczema, 129–130; *see also* Post-
    inflammatory hypopigmentation
Discoid lupus erythematosus (DLE), 128
Drug-induced hypopigmentation, 153
    systemic drugs, 153–155
    topical drugs, 155–156
Durvalumab, 154; *see also* Immune checkpoint
    inhibitors

E

Endemic treponematoses, 140; *see also*
    Treponematoses
Endothelin-1 (ET-1), 7
Endothelin receptor (EDNR), 108; *see also*
    Waardenburg syndrome
Endothelin receptor type B (EDNRB), 7
Endothelins (EDNs), 108; *see also* Waardenburg
    syndrome
ENL, *see* Erythema nodosum leprosum
Epidermal nevus, 120, 122; *see also* Mosaic
    hypopigmentation
Erythema nodosum leprosum (ENL), 135;
    see also Leprosy
Extracellular matrix (ECM), 9; *see also*
    Melanocyte

F

Fibrous cephalic plaques, 91; *see also* Tuberous
    sclerosis complex
Fine-needle aspiration cytology (FNAC), 138
Focal dermal hypoplasia, *see* Goltz syndrome

G

Genetic mosaicism, 124; *see also* Mosaic
    hypopigmentation
Goltz syndrome, 123–124; *see also* Mosaic
    hypopigmentation
Granulocyte-macrophage colony-stimulating
    factor (GM-CSF), 7
Griscelli syndrome (GS), 17, 99, 113; *see also*
    Hypopigmentation
    clinical presentation, 114–115
    differential diagnosis, 115
    epidemiology, 113
    pathophysiology, 113–114
    subtypes, 114
    treatment, 115
Griscelli syndrome type 1–3 (GS1–3), 15
Guttate hypomelanosis, *see* Idiopathic guttate
    hypomelanosis

H

Hair depigmentation, 109; *see also*
    Waardenburg syndrome
Hair hypopigmentation, 109
Halo nevus (HN), 44–45, 149
    clinical course, 149–150
    dermoscopy, 149
    differential diagnosis, 150
    epidemiology, 149
    features, 149
    histologic features, 149
    management, 151
    medium-sized congenital, 150
    multiple, 150
    pathogenesis, 150–151
    and vitiligo, 151
Halo phenomenon, 146; *see also* Melanoma
    leukoderma
Hansen disease, *see* Leprosy
Hematopoietic stem cell transplantation
    (HSCT), 99, 115, 154–155; *see also*
    Systemic drugs
Hemophagocytic lymphohistiocytosis
    (HLH), 113
Hepatocyte growth factor (HGF), 7
Hermansky-Pudlak syndrome (HPS), 17, 97,
    113; *see also* Hypopigmentation
    clinical features, 97, 114–115
    diagnosis, 97–98
    differential diagnosis, 115
    disorder types, 114
    epidemiology, 113
    management, 98
    pathophysiology, 113–114
    prevalence and prognosis, 97
    treatment, 115
Hermansky-Pudlak syndrome type 1–7
    (HPS1–7), 15
Heterochromia, partial, 109; *see also*
    Waardenburg syndrome
High-resolution computed tomography of the
    chest (HRCT), 97
Histamine, 55; *see also* Topical agents
Human pigmentation; *see also* Melanocyte
    adaptation of, 1–2
    in dark and light skin, 4
Hydroquinone (HQ), 159, 160; *see also* Skin-
    lightening agents
Hypomelanosis, 118–120, 128; *see also* Mosaic
    hypopigmentation
    in checkerboard pattern, 120, 122
    linear, 118, 122
Hypopigmentation, 13, 127, *see*
    Leukoderma, chemical; Mosaic
    hypopigmentation; Post-
    inflammatory hypopigmentation;
    Tuberous sclerosis complex;
    Waardenburg syndrome
    acquired disorders of, 17
    burns, 162
    from chemical and physical agents, 159
    classification of, 14
    cold injuries, 161–162
    congenital, 14–15
    considerations, 14
    depigmentation of lips, 160
    in dermatitis artefacta, 162
    diagnostic approach to, 13–14
    differential diagnosis, 16, 18
    disorders involving, 13, 129
    distribution of, 14
    drug-induced, *see* Drug-induced
        hypopigmentation

178 Index

Hypopigmentation (*Continued*)
    epidermal nevus, 122
    due to gene defects, 15, 17
    infectious and parasitic causes of, 133
    leprosy, 135–139
    macules, 90–91
    mechanical injuries, 161
    melanocyte and genes controlling
            pathway, 15
    due to mercury-based lightening
            product, 160
    after microdermabrasion, 162
    noncongenital, 17
    onchocerciasis, 139
    from physical agents, 161
    pityriasis versicolor, 133–135
    of skin, 109
    due to topical application of garlic, 162
    due to topical steroid abuse, 155
    treponematoses, 139–141
    tuberous sclerosis complex, 17
Hypopigmented MF (HMF), 131; *see also* Post-
        inflammatory hypopigmentation

I
Idiopathic guttate hypomelanosis (IGH),
        165; *see also* Progressive macular
        hypomelanosis
    clinical presentation, 165
    dermoscopy, 167
    diagnostic modalities, 166
    differential diagnosis, 167
    electron microscopy, 166–167
    epidemiology, 165
    histopathology, 166
    pathogenesis, 165–166
    treatment, 167, 170
Imatinib, 153; *see also* Tyrosine kinase
        inhibitors
Imiquimod-induced hypopigmentation, 155
Immune checkpoint inhibitors (ICIs), 154; *see
        also* Systemic drugs
Immune regulatory cells, 76
Immune-related adverse events (irAEs), 154
Incontinentia pigmenti (IP), 17, 122–123; *see
        also* Hypopigmentation; Mosaic
        hypopigmentation
Indeterminate leprosy (IL), 135; *see also*
        Leprosy
Inflammatory dermatoses, 127
Intense pulsed light (IPL), 162
Interferon gamma (IFN-γ), 8, 36

J
Janus kinases (JAKs), 36, 55, 87
Juvenile localized scleroderma (JLS), 131

K
Keratinocyte growth factor (KGF), 8
Keratinocytes, 7
Koenen tumors, 91; *see also* Tuberous sclerosis
        complex

L
L-3,4-dihydroxyphenylalanine (L-DOPA), 4
Lasers, 79; *see also* Phototherapy
Lepromatous leprosy (LL), 135; *see also* Leprosy
Leprosy, 135; *see also* Hypopigmentation
    borderline lepromatous, 135, 136
    borderline tuberculoid, 135, 136
    classification, 136
    diagnosis, 137
    differential diagnosis, 139
    epidemiology, 136
    erythema nodosum leprosum, 135, 137
    Fite stain, 138
    granuloma, 138
    lepromatous leprosy, 135, 137
    treatment and prognosis, 139
    tuberculoid leprosy, 135, 136
    well-formed granuloma, 138

Leucoderma in chronic GvHD, 155
Leukoderma, chemical, 159
    clinical features, 160
    cosmetics with mercury, 160
    depigmentation at site of contact, 161
    diagnosis, 160–161
    due to hair dye, 161
    hydroquinone, 160
    mequinol, 160
    plant extracts, 160
    rhododendrol, 160
    from rubber sandals, 161
    skin-lightening agents, 159
    treatment, 161
Leukoderma in DLE lesions, 130; *see also* Post-
        inflammatory hypopigmentation
Leukotrichia, 43
Lichen sclerosus (LS), 128, 130–131;
            see also Post-inflammatory
            hypopigmentation
Linear hypomelanosis, 118, 122; *see also* Mosaic
        hypopigmentation
LS-associated leukoderma, 130; *see also* Post-
        inflammatory hypopigmentation
Lucio phenomenon (LP), 135; *see also* Leprosy
Lupus erythematosus, 130; *see also* Post-
        inflammatory hypopigmentation
Lymphangioleiomyomatosis (LAM), 89
Lysosome-related organelles (LROs), 114

M
Margolis syndrome, *see* Ziprkowski-Margolis
        syndrome
Marinesco-Sjögren syndrome (MSS), 115
Mechanical injuries, 161; *see also*
        Hypopigmentation
Melagenina, 55; *see also* Topical agents
Melanin
    biosynthetic pathway, 5
    synthesis, 3–4
Melanocortin 1 receptor (MC1R), 7, 36
Melanocyte, 1, 9
    cell–cell crosstalk, 7–9
    DOPA staining, 2
    double immunofluorescence staining, 6
    epidermal-melanin unit, 3
    extracellular microenvironment, 9
    homeostasis, 9
    keratinocytes, 4–6
    markers, 3
    and melanin synthesis, 2, 3–4, 5
    melanosome, 2
    melanosome maturation within, 5
    melanosome transport, 1–6
    microscopic analysis, 2
    MITF expression analysis, 7
    pigmentation adaptation, 1–2
Melanogenesis, 128; *see also* Post-inflammatory
        hypopigmentation
Melanoma antigen recognized by T cells 1
        (MART1), 3, 146
Melanoma-associated depigmentation
        (MAD), 145
Melanoma-associated hypopigmentation
        (MAH), 145
Melanoma-associated leukoderma (MAL), 145
Melanoma-associated vitiligo (MAV), 145
Melanoma leukoderma, 145
    halo phenomenon, 146
    melanoma regression, 146
    pathogenesis, 145
    prognosis, 147
    vitiligo-like depigmentation, 146
    vitiligo-like lesions, 146
Melanophilin (MLPH), 99
Melanosome, 2
    maturation, 5
    transfer to keratinocytes, 4–6
Membrane-associated transport protein
        (MATP), 93
MEN1, *see* Multiple endocrine neoplasia type 1

Mequinol, 160; *see also* Skin-lightening agents
Metastatic melanoma (MM), 154
Methionine sulfoxide reductase (MSR), 86
5-methoxypsoralen (5-MOP), 24
8-methoxypsoralen (8-MOP), 24
Methylprednisolone (MPD), 60
Microphthalmia-associated transcription
        factor (MITF), 3, 7, 107–108; *see also*
        Waardenburg syndrome
Million units (MU), 140
Minimal erythema dose (MED), 80
Mini-punch grafting, 73; *see also* Vitiligo
        surgical treatment
    vs. noncultured epidermal cell
            suspension, 75
Mixed vitiligo (MV), 39
Monoamine oxidase (MAO), 36
Monochromatic excimer light (MEL) 81, 85; *see
        also* Phototherapy
Mosaic, 117
Mosaic hypopigmentation, 117, *see*
            Hypopigmentation
    Blaschko lines, 118, 119, 120
    clinical manifestations, 118–124
    comparison of principal diseases of, 121
    Conradi-Hünermann-Happle
            syndrome, 123
    cutaneous mosaicism pattern, 113
    diagnosis, 124
    epidermal nevus, 120, 122
    follow-up and treatment, 124
    genetic mosaicism, 124
    genomic and epigenetic mosaicism, 117
    Goltz syndrome, 123–124
    hypomelanosis, 118–120, 122
    incontinentia pigmenti, 122–123
    mosaicism, 117–118, 120
    nevus achromicus, 122
    Pallister-Killian syndrome, 123
    phylloid hypomelanosis, 123
    postzygotic mutation, 117
    segmental expression of nonlethal
            disorders, 118
Mosaicism, 117; *see also* Mosaic
        hypopigmentation
    cutaneous, 118
    genetic, 124
    genomic and epigenetic, 117
    mechanisms of, 117–118
    patterns of, 120
Multibacillary (MB), 135
Multiple drug therapy (MDT), 135
Multiple endocrine neoplasia type 1
        (MEN1), 91
Mycophenolate mofetil, 55; *see also* Topical
        agents
Mycosis fungoides (MF), 128, 131–132;
            see also Post-inflammatory
            hypopigmentation

N
Narrowband ultraviolet B (NB-UVB), 46, 52,
        79, 81, 85
Nerve growth factor (NGF), 7
Neurochemical mediators, 36
Neurofibromatosis 1 (NF1), 101
Nevus achromicus, 122; *see also* Mosaic
        hypopigmentation
Nivolumab, 154; *see also* Immune checkpoint
        inhibitors
Noncultured epidermal cell suspension
        (NCES), 74; *see also* Vitiligo surgical
        treatment
    mini-punch graft vs., 75
    modifications of transplantation, 75
    preparation method, 74
Noncultured, extracted follicular outer root
        sheath suspension (NC-EHF-
        ORS-CS), 87
Nonsegmental vitiligo (NSV), 17, 29, 43;
            see also Hypopigmentation

O

Occupational leukoderma, *see* Leukoderma, chemical
Oculocerebral hypopigmentation syndrome (OCHS), 114, *see* Cross syndrome
Oculocutaneous albinism (OCA), 17, 93; *see also* Hypopigmentation
  clinical manifestations, 93–94
  diagnosis, 94–95
  epidemiology, 93
  etiology, 93
  histology, 94
  pathogenesis, 93
  prevalence and genetics of, 94
  prognosis, 95
  red albinism, 94
  treatment, 95
Onchocerciasis, 139; *see also* Hypopigmentation
Oral corticosteroids, 60, 81
Oral submucous fibrosis (OSF), 160

P

Pallister-Killian syndrome (PKS), 123; *see also* Mosaic hypopigmentation
Partial heterochromia, 109; *see also* Waardenburg syndrome
Paucibacillary (PB), 135
PAX3, 107; *see also* Waardenburg syndrome
Pazopanib, 153; *see also* Tyrosine kinase inhibitors
Pembrolizumab, 154; *see also* Immune checkpoint inhibitors
Peroxisome proliferator-activated receptor-γ (PPAR-γ), 7
Phenylalanine hydroxylase (PAH), 35
Pheomelanin, 4
Phosphate buffer saline (PBS), 74
Phosphatidylinositol (PI), 7
Photo(chemo) therapy, 24; *see also* Vitiligo
Phototherapy, 46, 79, 80
  and carcinogenicity, 80
  combination treatments with, 81
  hospital and home, 79–80
  mechanism of action of, 79
  monochromatic excimer light, 81
  oral corticosteroids and, 81
  side effects and contraindications, 80
  targeted phototherapy devices, 80–81
  topical cancineurin inhibitors and, 81
  topical steroids and, 81
  using NB-UVB B, 80
  vitamin D analogues and, 81
Phylloid hypomelanosis, 123; *see also* Mosaic hypopigmentation
Piebaldism, 15, 101; *see also* Hypopigmentation
  amelanotic macules, 102
  Café au lait macule, 101, 103
  clinical presentation, 101
  differential diagnosis, 103
  different phenotypes, 102
  epidemiology, 101
  etiopathogenesis, 101
  histopathology, 103
  leukodermatous patches, 103
  sparring of dorsal midline, 102
  treatment, 103–104
  white forelock and triangularly shaped leukoderma, 102
Pityriasis alba (PA), 129; *see also* Post-inflammatory hypopigmentation
Pityriasis versicolor (PV), 133; *see also* Hypopigmentation
  clinical features, 133
  diagnostic methods of, 135
  differential diagnoses of, 135
  epidemiology, 133
  etiopathogenesis, 133
  follicular variant of, 134
  histopathology, 134

hyperpigmented variant of, 134
  with hypopigmented patches with fine scaling, 134
  with pink scaly patches, 134
  prognosis, 135
  RDPV, 133
  treatment, 135
  yeast within stratum corneum, 134
Plant extracts, 160; *see also* Skin-lightening agents
Platelet-derived growth factor receptor (PDGFR), 153
Platelet transmission electron microscopy (PTEM), 98
Point-of-care (PoC), 140
Polypodium leucotomos (PL), 64, 86
Post-childhood vitiligo (PCV), 43; *see also* Childhood vitiligo
  clinical presentation, 43–44
  comorbidities, 44
  differential diagnosis, 45
  epidemiology, 43
  halo nevi, 44–45
  phototherapy, 46
  psychological burden of vitiligo, 45
  surgical treatment, 46–47
  308-nm excimer laser, 46
  topical treatment, 45–46
  treatment, 45–47
Post-inflammatory hyperpigmentation (PIH), 160, 167, 170
Post-inflammatory hypopigmentation (PIH), 127, 132
  clinical features, 128
  course and prognosis, 129
  dermatitis/eczema, 129–130
  diagnosis, 128
  disorders with hypopigmentation, 129
  etiology, 127
  with fine scaling due to psoriasis, 127
  following resolution of AD eruption, 129–130
  histological features, 128
  hypopigmented MF, 131
  leukoderma in DLE lesions, 130
  lichen sclerosus, 130–131
  LS-associated leukoderma, 130
  lupus erythematosus, 130
  management, 128–129
  melanogenesis, 128
  mycosis fungoides, 131–132
  pathogenesis, 127–128
  pityriasis alba, 129
  sarcoidosis, 131
  scleroderma, 131
  skin disorders causing, 127, 132
Postzygotic mutation, 117
Programmed cell death protein 1 (PD-1), 145, 154
  PD-1 ligand, 87
Progressive hypomelanosis of trunk, *see* Progressive macular hypomelanosis
Progressive macular hypomelanosis (PMH), 170; *see also* Idiopathic guttate hypomelanosis
  clinical presentation, 170–171
  dermoscopy, 171, 172
  diagnostic modalities, 171
  differential diagnosis, 168–169, 172
  electron microscopy, 171
  epidemiology, 171
  histopathology, 171
  pathogenesis, 171
  prognosis, 173
  treatment, 172–173
  wood's lamp, 171–172
Pro-opiomelanocortin (POMC), 7, 36
Prostaglandins (PGs), 55, 59; *see also* Topical agents
Pseudocatalase, 52, 55, 58; *see also* Topical agents

Psoralen plus ultraviolet A (PUVA), 24, 46, 52, 69, 80, 115, 155; *see also* Phototherapy
Pterin-4a-carbinol-amine dehydratase (PCD), 151
Pure neuritic leprosy (PNL), 135; *see also* Leprosy
PUVA, *see* Psoralen plus ultraviolet A

R

Rapid plasma regain (RPR), 140
Reactive oxygen species (ROS), 1, 86
Recurrent and disseminated pityriasis versicolor (RDPV), 133; *see also* Pityriasis versicolor
Red albinism, 94; *see also* Oculocutaneous albinism
Reflectance confocal microscopy (RCM), 149
Restriction fragment length polymorphism (RFLP), 135
RFLP, *see* Restriction fragment length polymorphism
Rhododendrol, 160; *see also* Skin-lightening agents
River blindness, *see* Onchocerciasis

S

Sarcoidosis, 131; *see also* Post-inflammatory hypopigmentation
SCC, *see* Squamous cell carcinoma
Scleroderma, 131; *see also* Post-inflammatory hypopigmentation
Secreted frizzled-related protein 2 (sFRP2), 9
Segmental heterochromia, 109; *see also* Waardenburg syndrome
Segmental hypomelanosis, 120
Segmental vitiligo (SV), 17, 29, 32, 39, 43; *see also* Hypopigmentation
  classification on face, 41
  clinical features, 40
  differential diagnosis, 41
  epidemiology, 39–40
  features different from nonsegmental vitiligo, 40
  mixed vitiligo, 41
  monosegmental vitiligo, 40
  pathogenesis, 39
  treatment, 41–42
sFRP2, *see* Secreted frizzled-related protein 2
Shagreen patches, 91; *see also* Tuberous sclerosis complex
Signal transduction and transcription (STAT), 87
Skin depigmentation, 109; *see also* Waardenburg syndrome
Skin harvesting method, 72; *see also* Vitiligo surgical treatment
Skin-lightening agents, 159
  cosmetic preparations containing mercury, 160
  hydroquinone, 160
  mequinol, 160
  plant extracts, 160
  rhododendrol, 160
Skin-slit smear assessment (SSS assessment), 135
SNAI2, 108; *see also* Waardenburg syndrome
Sorafenib, 154; *see also* Tyrosine kinase inhibitors
SOX10, 108; *see also* Waardenburg syndrome
SPRED1, 101
Squamous cell carcinoma (SCC), 131
Squaric acid dibutylester (SADBE), 156
Stem cell factor (SCF), 7, 35, 153
Suction blister epidermal grafting, 73; *see also* Vitiligo surgical treatment
Sunitinib, 154; *see also* Tyrosine kinase inhibitors
Synophrys, 109–110; *see also* Waardenburg syndrome
Syphilis, 140–141; *see also* Treponematoses

180   Index

Systemic drugs of vitiligo, 60, 153; *see also*
  Drug-induced hypopigmentation
  antimalarial drugs, 154
  antioxidants, 64
  biologics and small molecules, 64
  corticosteroids, 60, 62
  hematopoietic stem cell transplantation,
    154–155
  immune checkpoint inhibitors, 154
  immunosuppressive treatments, 60, 63
  targeted antineoplastic agents, 153
  tyrosine kinase inhibitors, 153–154
Systemic sclerosis (SS), 131

T

Targeted antineoplastic agents, 153; *see also*
  Systemic drugs
Targeted phototherapy devices, 80–81; *see also*
  Phototherapy
12-Tetradecanoylphorbol 13 acetate (TPA), 74
T helper 2 (Th2), 133
308-nm excimer laser, 46
Thymic stromal lymphopoietin (TSLP), 35
Tietz syndrome, 17; *see also* Hypopigmentation
Tissue grafts, 69, 72–73; *see also* Vitiligo
  surgical treatment
Topical agents, 52
  histamine, 55
  melagenina, 55
  mycophenolate mofetil, 55
  prostaglandins, 55, 59
  pseudocatalase, 52, 55, 58
Topical calcineurin inhibitors (TCIs), 45, 49
  and phototherapy, 81
Topical drugs, 155; *see also* Drug-induced
  hypopigmentation
  corticosteroids, 45, 49, 50–51, 155
  hypopigmentation due to abuse of, 155
  imiquimod, 155–156
  immunotherapy, 156
  steroids and phototherapy, 81
  transdermal patch, 156
  for vitiligo therapy, 49–52, 61
Transdermal patch, 156; *see also* Topical drugs
T-regs, *see* T-regulatory cells
T-regulatory cells (T-regs), 76
Treponema pallidum particle agglutination
  (TPPA), 140
Treponematoses, 139; *see also*
  Hypopigmentation
  endemic, 140
  syphilis, 140–141
Tuberculoid leprosy (TT), 135; *see also* Leprosy
Tuberous sclerosis complex (TSC), 17, 89; *see
  also* Hypopigmentation
  angiofibromas, 91
  ash leaf spot, 90
  clinical features, 89–90
  confetti-like hypopigmentation, 91
  cutaneous manifestations of, 90
  diagnosis, 89
  fibrous cephalic plaques, 91
  hypopigmented macules, 90–91
  large hypopigmented macules with serrated
    margins, 90
  shagreen patches, 91

treatment of cutaneous lesions, 92
  ungual fibromas, 91
Tumor necrosis factor (TNF), 36, 128
  TNF-α, 8
Tyrosinase gene (TYR), 93
Tyrosinase-related protein 1 (TYRP-1), 3
  gene, 93
Tyrosinase-related protein 2 (TYRP-2), 4
Tyrosine hydroxylase (TH), 35
Tyrosine kinase 2 (TYK2), 87
Tyrosine kinase inhibitors (TKIs), 153; *see also*
  Systemic drugs
  dasatinib, 153
  imatinib, 153
  pazopanib, 153
  sorafenib, 154
  sunitinib, 154

U

Ultraviolet (UV), 1, 24, 52, 128
Ultraviolet A (UVA), 24, 79
Ultraviolet B (UVB), 1
Ultraviolet radiation (UVR), 1, 85
Ungual fibromas, 91; *see also* Tuberous sclerosis
  complex
U.S. Food and Drug Administration (FDA), 85

V

Vasoactive endothelial growth factor receptor
  (VEGFR), 153
VDRL, *see* Venereal Disease Research
  Laboratory
Venereal Disease Research Laboratory
  (VDRL), 140
Vici syndrome, 113
  clinical presentation, 114–115
  differential diagnosis, 115
  epidemiology, 113
  pathophysiology, 113–114
  treatment, 115
Vitamin D analogues, 52, 56–57
  and phototherapy, 81
Vitiligo, 17; *see also* Hypopigmentation
  autoimmune diseases associated with, 29
  classification, 28, 30
  clinical features, 28
  dyschromy, 22
  epidemiology, 27–28
  etiopathophysiological theories for, 27
  etymology, 21
  genes implicated in vitiligo pathogenesis, 28
  genetic alterations with comorbidities, 28
  halo nevi and, 151
  with inflammatory raised border, 129
  lesions, 86
  nonsegmental vitiligo, 30, 31
  pathogenesis, 85
  perceptios, 21–22
  photo(chemo) therapy, 24
  prognosis, 24
  in religious books, 21
  segmental, 32
  social stigma, 22
  topical calcineurin inhibitors, 24
  topical corticosteroid, 24
  treatment list, 23

treatment of, 22–24
  trigger factors, 29
  variants of, 29
  white macules of, 29
Vitiligo pathophysiology, 35, 37
  autoimmunity, 36
  genetic predisposition, 35
  neuroendocrine phenomena, 36
  oxidative stress, 35–36
Vitiligo surgical treatment, 69, 76
  area preparation, 69
  cellular transplantation, 73–76
  mini-punch grafting, 73
  NCES preparation method, 74
  noncultured epidermal cell suspension
    transplantation, 75
  patient selection, 69
  skin harvesting method, 72
  suction blister epidermal grafting, 73
  techniques, 70–71
  tissue grafts, 69, 72–73
  types of vitiligo surgery, 69
Vitiligo treatments, 85, 87; *see also* Calcineurin
  inhibitors; Lasers; Phototherapy;
  Vitiligo lesions

W

Waardenburg syndrome (WS), 17, 103; *see also*
  Hypopigmentation
  clinical findings, 108–109
  cutaneous features, 109
  depigmentation, 109
  diagnosis, 110
  diagnostic criteria of, 110
  EDN3 and EDNRB, 108
  genetic background, 107
  microphthalmia-associated transcription
    factor, 107–108
  partial/segmental heterochromia, 109
  PAX3, 107
  SNAI2, 108
  SOX10, 108
  subtypes and mode of inheritance, 108
  synophrys, 109–110
  treatment, 110
  variation in clinical features, 109
World Health Organization (WHO), 135

X

Xenon chloride device (XeCl device), 81
X-linked albinism-deafness syndrome (ADFN),
  114, *see* Ziprkowski-Margolis
  syndrome
X-linked ocular albinism (XLOA), 115; *see also*
  Oculocutaneous albinism
XLOA, *see* X-linked ocular albinism

Z

Ziprkowski-Margolis syndrome, 113
  clinical presentation, 114–115
  differential diagnosis, 115
  epidemiology, 113
  pathophysiology, 113–114
  treatment, 115